"Answering 1,500 questions about Hormones, Metabolism and Nutrition"

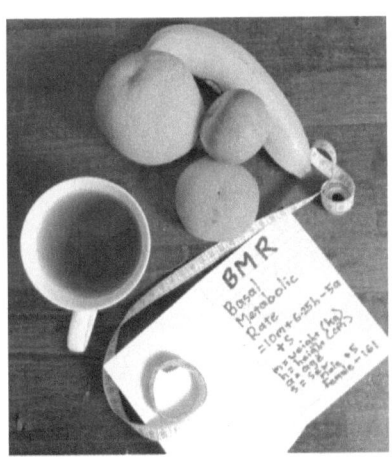

Dr. Mario Vega Carbó
Endocrinólogyst

First Edition, 2019

To my tutor, Dr. Silvia Marín, nutrition expert
To my parents, my wife and my children, who borrow me in time
To my cousin Miguel Carbó Riverón, may God have him in his glory
And every person who has in his health his most precious asset

Table of Contents

Introduction 11

The why of this book 12

The importance of Endocrinology..12

SECTION I. METABOLISM...15

Part I. DIETETICS 17

Chapter 1. Healthy Diet. Keys to healthy eating....................................18

Chapter 2. Mediterranean diet...22

Chapter 3. Vegetarian Diet...24

Chapter 4. Vegan Diet...28

Chapter 5. Hypercaloric Diet..31

Chapter 6. Low calorie diet..34

Chapter 7. Ketogenic Diet..37

Chapter 8. DASH diet to lower blood pressure......................................40

Chapter 10. Glycemic Index Diet...46

Chapter 11. Diet and dyslipidemia...49

Chapter 12. Diet for elevated uric acid..52

Chapter 13. Diet in case of renal lithiasis...56

Chapter 14. Diet for chronic kidney disease 59

Chapter 15. Diet for Gastritis and Gastroesophageal Reflux 62

Chapter 16. Diet for fatty liver and cirrhosis...65

Chapter 17. Diet for irritable bowel FODMAP.....................................68

Chapter 18. Biliary Protection Diet...71

Chapter 19. Diet for the control and prevention of thyroid diseases....74

Chapter 20. Diet for Polycystic Ovary Syndrome..............................77

Chapter 21. Gluten-free diet for celiac people 79

Chapter 22. Lactose free diet..82

Part II NUTRITION 85

3

Chapter 23. Endocrine disruptors. Invisible" contaminants that affect our health 86

Chapter 24. Extreme Thinness and its dangers 89

Chapter 25. Celiac Disease or Celiac Disease.................................91

Chapter 26. Anorexia nervosa 94

Chapter 27. Bulimiaa..97

Chapter 28. Hypercholesterolemia or high cholesterol 100

Chapter 29. Hypertriglyceridemia or high triglycerides 103

Chapter 30. Dyslipidemias 105

Chapter 31. Obesity, a serious chronic disease that grows year by year 107

Chapter 32. Morbid Obesity and its risks...110

Chapter 33. Obesity drugs: Orlistat and Phentermine 113

Chapter 34. Metabolic Syndrome and associated disorders...............116

Chapter 35. Non-Alcoholic Fatty Liver Disease 119

Chapter 36. Acanthosis Nigricans or Pigmented Acanthosis............121

Chapter 37. Acrocordones and skin lumps...123

Chapter 38. Hyperinsulinemia, Insulinoma and Diabetes.................125

Chapter 39. Insulinoma and Hypoglycemia 128

Chapter 40. Gout: what it is and how it is treated 130

Chapter 41. Hemochromatosis and excess iron in the body..............133

PART III DIABETES...136

Chapter 42. Prediabetes and how to solve it in time 137

Chapter 43. Type 2 Diabetes Mellitus..139

Chapter 44. MODY Diabetes 143

Chapter 45. LADA Diabetes 145

Chapter 46. Other specific types of Diabetes 147

Chapter 47. Acute Complication of Diabetes.....................................149

Chapter 48. Diabetic Hypoglycemia and its complications 152

Chapter 49. Hyperosmolar Hyperglycemic State..............................154

Chapter 50. Diabetic Ketoacidosis......................................156

Chapter 51. Diabetic Neuropathy and its complications...................158

Chapter 52. The Diabetic Foot and the possibilities of amputation ...160

Chapter 53. Diabetic Retinopathy and Eye Problems......................163

Chapter 54. The Heart and Diabetes.....................................166

Chapter 55. Diabetes and kidney disease................................169

Chapter 56. Surgery in the diabetic patient............................172

Chapter 57. Insulin Resistance: Metformin..............................175

Chapter 58. Hypoglycemic drugs...178

Chapter 59. Use of insulin for the control of Diabetes.................181

Chapter 60. Glucose monitoring and self-control........................185

SECTION II ENDOCRINOLOGY...189

Part IV Thyroid..192

Chapter 61. Ectopic Thyroid..193

Chapter 62. Goiter...195

Chapter 63. Ultrasound or ultrasound of the thyroid....................197

Chapter 64. Fine needle biopsy for the study of thyroid nodules.......199

Chapter 65. Thyroid Cancer...201

Chapter 66. Thyroid surgery and its complications......................204

Chapter 67. Hypothyroidism or Hypoactive Thyroid.......................207

Chapter 68. Medications for Hypothyroidism: Levothyroxine and
Lyothyronine...210

Chapter 69. Mixedematous Coma..213

Chapter 70. Chronic Hashimoto's Thyroiditis and Hypothyroidism..215

Chapter 71. Subacute thyroiditis and viral infections..................217

Chapter 72. Euthyroid Sick Syndrome....................................219

Chapter 73. Hyperthyroidism or overactive thyroid......................221

Chapter 74. Thyroid Orbitopathy..224

Chapter 75. Thyroid Storm or Thyrotoxic Crisis 226

Chapter 76. Treatments for hyperthyroidism: radioiodine and antithyroid 228

Chapter 77. Radioactive iodine post thyroiditis 231

Chapter 78. Nuclear Medicine for Thyroid 233

Part V. Calcium Metabolism 236

Chapter 79. Hypocalcaemia 237

Chapter 80. Hypocalcaemic Crisis 239

Chapter 81. Supplementation: calcium, vitamin D and magnesium ..241

Chapter 82. Rickets and lack of vitamin D 246

Chapter 83. Bone Densitometry and the diagnosis of Osteoporosis ..249

Chapter 84. Osteoporosis and bone weakness...................................252

Chapter 85. Hypoparathyroidism, calcium and vitamin D................255

Chapter 86. Hyperparathyroidism: causes, symptoms and consequences
....257

Chapter 87. Parathyroid Surgery 260

Chapter 88. Hypercalcemia and excess calcium 263

Chapter 89. Renal lithiasis: causes, consequences and treatment of the famous "stones" in the kidneys 266

Chapter 90. Bone Paget Disease...269

Chapter 91. Osteomalacia and bone softening 271

Part VI Kidney glands 273

Chapter 92. Lipotimias and Fainting..274

Chapter 93. Addison's disease and adrenal insufficiency..................277

Chapter 94. The Adrenal Crisis or Acute Adrenal Insufficiency 280

Chapter 95. Cortisol Replacement: Glucocorticoids.........................282

Chapter 96. Autoimmune Polyglandular Syndrome 286

Chapter 97. Vitiligo Loss of skin color 288

Chapter 98. Secondary Hypertension. Diseases that cause it............291

Chapter 99. Benign and Malignant Adrenal Incidentaloma.............294

Chapter 100. Hypercortisolism or Cushing's Syndrome...................297

Chapter 101. Pheochromocytoma and increased blood pressure.......300

Chapter 102. Primary Hyperaldosteronism and Blood Pressure........303

Chapter 103. Carcinoid Syndrome..306

Chapter 104. Multiple Endocrine Neoplasia....................................309

Chapter 105. Benign and Malignant Neuroendocrine Tumors 312

Part VII Hypothalamus and Pituitary...315

Chapter 106. Syndrome of Inappropriate Antidiuretic Hormone
Secretion...316

Chapter 107. Polyuria or excessive urination..................................318

Chapter 108. Care and treatment of diabetes insipidus...................321

Chapter 109. Hypopituitarism...324

Chapter 110. Sheehan syndrome and severe bleeding during childbirth
....327

Chapter 111. Empty Turkish Chair Syndrome.................................329

Chapter 112. Galactorrhea and abnormal breast secretion..............332

Chapter 113. Hyperprolactinemia and tumors in the pituitary gland .334

Chapter 114. Pituitary Tumors..336

Chapter 115. Acromegaly..339

Chapter 116. Craniopharyngioma..341

Chapter 117. Pineal Tumors and Early Puberty...............................344

Chapter 118. Pituitary Surgery...346

Chapter 119. Pituitary Stroke...349

SECTION III REPRODUCTION AND LIFE CYCLE 352

Part VIII Ovary..355

Capítulo 120. Disfunción Sexual Femenina.....................................356

Chapter 121. Hypoactive Sexual Desire Disorder............................359

Chapter 122. Hormone Therapy of Feminization 361

Chapter 123. Premenstrual Syndrome..364

Chapter 124. Endometriosis and severe pain during menstruation 367

Chapter 125. Treatment of abnormal uterine bleeding.....................370

Chapter 126. Amenorrhea or absence of menstruation 373

Chapter 127. Hormone Contraception and its different possibilities .376

Chapter 128. Female Infertility 380

Chapter 129. Fertility: ovulation inducers..383

Chapter 130. Female Androgenic Alopecia 387

Chapter 131. Hyperandrogenism, Hirsutism and Acne....................390

Chapter 132. Clitoromegaly or clitoral hypertrophy 394

Chapter 133. Symptoms and Treatment of Polycystic Ovary Syndrome
....397

Chapter 134. Antiandrogens: Finasteride, Spironolactone and
Flutamide..400

Chapter 135. Primary Ovarian Insufficiency 404

Chapter 136. Hormone replacement therapy during menopause 407

Chapter 137. Treatment with estrogen and progesterone..................410

Part IX Testicles 414

Chapter 138. Gender Identity Disorder 415

Chapter 139. Hormone therapy of masculinization..........................418

Chapter 140. The micropenis and its treatment................................421

Chapter 141. Gynecomastia and enlarged breasts in men.................423

Chapter 142. Klinefelter syndrome 426

Chapter 143. Kallmann syndrome and the sense of smell 429

Chapter 144. Causes and main symptoms of Noonan Syndrome 432

Chapter 145. Erectile Dysfunction 434

Chapter 146. Male Infertility...437

Chapter 147. Spermatogram...440

Chapter 148. Hypogonadism and the sex glands 443

Chapter 149. Andropause or "male menopause".................................446

Chapter 150. Testosterone Treatment 449

Chapter 151. Anabolic Steroids and their dangers 452

Chapter 152. Male Androgenic Alopecia..455

Part X. Endocrinology in Pediatrics 457

Capítulo 153. Endocrinología Pediátrica..458

Chapter 154. Diagnosis and care of Congenital Adrenal Hyperplasia
....461

Chapter 155. Ambiguous Genitals 464

Chapter 156. Cryptorchidism or undescended testicle.....................468

Chapter 157. Diagnosis and treatment of Congenital Hypothyroidism
....470

Chapter 158. Children with growth problems 473

Chapter 159. Precocious Puberty 477

Chapter 160. Delayed Puberty..479

Chapter 161. Turner Syndrome care and treatments 481

Chapter 162. Hyperhidrosis and excessive sweating 484

Chapter 163. Type 1 Diabetes or Juvenile Diabetes 487

Chapter 164. Obesity in childhood...490

Part XI Endocrinology in Obstetrics..493

Chapter 165. Nutrition and pregnancy 494

Chapter 166. Obesity and pregnancy 497

Chapter 167. Diabetes and pregnancy...500

Chapter 168. Recurring Abortions 503

Chapter 169. Hypothyroidism and pregnancy...................................506

Chapter 170. Hyperthyroidism and pregnancy..................................509

Chapter 171. Prolactinoma and pregnancy.......................................512

Chapter 172. Cushing Syndrome and Pregnancy 514

Part XII Endocrinology in Geriatrics..517

Chapter 173. Endocrinopathies in the elderly 518

Chapter 174. Nutrition in older adults....................................521

Chapter 175. Sarcopenia and muscle weakness 524

Chapter 176. Osteoporosis in the elderly 527

Chapter 177. Obesity in older adults 530

Chapter 178. Diabetes in older adults 532

Chapter 179. Peripheral Neuropathy and Numbness of Hands and Feet 535

Chapter 180. Reversible Dementias 538

Chapter 181. Hypothyroidism in older adults 541

Chapter 182. Hyperthyroidism in older adults 543

Chapter 183. Thyroid Cancer in Older Adults 545

Chapter 184. Multiple Myeloma and its disorders 547

Chapter 185. The practice of exercise in older adults 550

Epilogue...553

The interview..555

Interview conducted by: 556

Synopsis..557

Introduction

Medicine and the specific terms of the profession can sometimes be too confusing and difficult for the general public to understand.

Health professionals are accustomed to technicalities and, when making their diagnoses and advising treatments, they often forget that the patients in front of them or their relatives are not work colleagues who handle the same lexicon as them.

On many occasions people, who are already overwhelmed by a disease, need to understand clearly and concisely what happens to them, what are the causes of their ailments and how they should face them.

To help them with this task, Dr. Mario Vega Carbó presents "I answer 1,500 questions about Hormones, Metabolism and Nutrition", an easy-to-read book available to everyone, thinking to offer simple explanations on these topics.

Through a series of interviews, the professional exposes in a simple and didactic language, the origin of the main endocrine diseases, their most common symptoms, their risks and the best way to treat them.

The text is divided into twelve parts, dedicated to issues related to nutrition, obesity, diabetes, osteoporosis, short stature in children, early sexual development, menstruation disorders, infertility, erectile dysfunction, gigantism, abnormal cholesterol and triglyceride levels, metabolism of calcium, hyperthyroidism, hypothyroidism, high blood pressure and glandular tumors.

In addition, it has special sections on the most significant hormonal disorders in children, pregnant women and the elderly, and a chapter on diets and dietary advice to prevent and control different diseases.

We invite you to read these pages and enter the world of the endocrine system and its glands, responsible for the natural production of hormones that regulate our body.

The why of this book

The importance of Endocrinology

When a patient receives a diagnosis about a hormonal problem, such as diabetes or a thyroid disorder, it is common for the doctor to suggest that he consult an endocrinologist.

Faced with this scenario, many people have doubts about what this specialty is, what its function is and how it can help us.

Endocrinology is a relatively new science that emerged in the mid-twentieth century as a result of advances in medicine related to hormonal functioning.

Its focus is the endocrine system, formed by the glands responsible for the natural production of hormones that regulate our body and are responsible for our growth and development, metabolism, reproduction, sleep, lactation and aspects related to our conduct, among others.

To learn more about this specialty, we interview Mario Vega Carbó, an endocrinologist, with more than 20 years of experience.

Doctor Mario,
1. What is the main function of endocrinology?

An endocrinologist is a doctor who has studied the endocrine system and its diseases and specializes in it. Its main function is to restore the hormonal balance in the body when it is affected by various conditions or diseases.

2. What are the main endocrine glands?

The most important are the thyroid, parathyroid, pancreas, ovaries, testicles, adrenal and pituitary or pituitary, which produce most of the hormones that regulate our body. They are called endocrine glands because the substance (hormone) they produce passes into the bloodstream, and traveling in it, will reach the various tissues in which the hormone will act regulating its functions.

3. What are the most common hormonal diseases?

Among the most frequent we can mention diabetes, osteoporosis, short stature in children, early sexual development, abnormal breast growth, menstruation disorders, infertility, erectile dysfunction, obesity, overweight, gigantism, elevation of cholesterol and triglycerides , hyperthyroidism, high blood pressure, acne, excess facial hair and cancer of the glands.

4. What is diabetes mellitus?

It is one of the most common chronic diseases that endocrinologists treat. It is due to a deficit in the production of insulin in the pancreas, which prevents proper glucose metabolism, causing it to accumulate in the blood.

It is estimated that about 8 percent of the adult population suffers from diabetes and, if not treated properly, can cause heart, kidney, eye problems, polyneuropathies (peripheral nerve involvement) and severe foot ulcers .

5. What are the main symptoms of diabetes mellitus and how is it treated?

The most common symptoms are increased hunger (polyphagia), thirst (polydipsia) and urine volume (polyuria). In addition, there may be weight loss, fatigue, headaches, nausea, vomiting, tachycardia, inadequate healing, abdominal pain and blurred vision.

As for treatment, the goal is to restore normal glycemic levels (blood sugar levels), for which it may be necessary to apply an insulin substitute or insulin analogues or medications called oral antidiabetics.

On the other hand, as excessive food intake and sedentary lifestyle increase the risks of this disease, you also work on a special diet and in adapting a healthier lifestyle.

6. What are thyroid disorders?

The thyroid is the gland that is responsible for producing hormones that control metabolism, cardiovascular balance, energy consumption and body growth.

Among other problems, the thyroid can produce more or less amount of hormones in relation to those that the body needs, which is due to the appearance of nodules, enlargement and inflammation of the same (goiter) and even cancer. Its control and care is another of the main tasks of endocrinologists.

7. What other types of common inquiries do you receive?

Many of the visits we receive are linked to weight problems, both due to excess and lack, and related to sexuality. Also to drawbacks in blood cholesterol and triglyceride levels, when these are high, it is known as dyslipidemia.

8. Finally, why is consultation with an endocrinologist important?

In many cases, treatments of diabetes and high blood pressure, for example, are carried out in the first instance by a general practitioner, without consulting an endocrinologist who is the expert in hormonal issues.

This can have long-term consequences and complicate the patient's health, generating all kinds of disorders and expenses. Therefore, the early intervention of a specialist is essential for proper care and thus prevent the complications of these diseases.

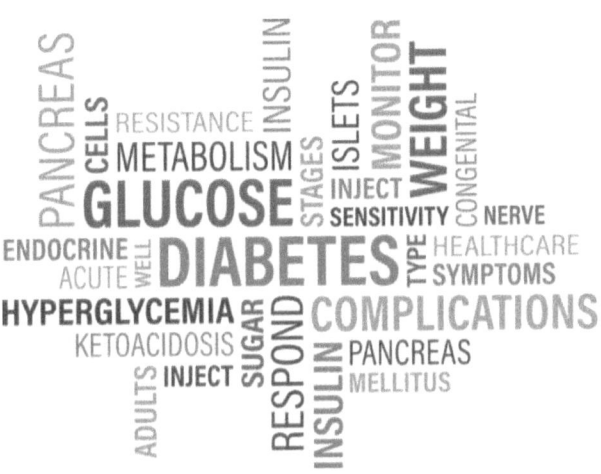

SECTION I. METABOLISM

SECTION I. METABOLISM

The first section of this book entitled *Metabolism*, clarifies the most common questions in three highly questioned and researched areas, not only among health professionals, but also among the general population.

First, we invite you to meet the answers to all your questions about *Dietetics*. This is a science that deals with the study of different types of food from the point of view of physiology and nutritional pathophysiology. In this first part you will know the main types of diet, their characteristics, advantages and disadvantages, for whom and under what situations these diets are indicated. In addition, you will find the types of diets that are recommended according to conditions or diseases in the person.

The second part of this section, invites you to know in depth Nutrition, a factor that is decisive in the emergence of numerous conditions both beneficial and harmful in the body. We will talk about dyslipidemias, psychiatric eating disorders, metabolic syndrome, and other diseases where nutrition is a key factor in its development and prevention.

In the third part of this section, we enter into pathological conditions that affect health, and that, although its genetic component is present, its development is strongly influenced by both diet and nutrition. We are talking about *Diabetes*. We will explain the most frequent types, their causes, diagnostic criteria, complications and treatment measures.

Then enjoy this first section of interviews, *Metabolism.*

Part I. DIETETICS

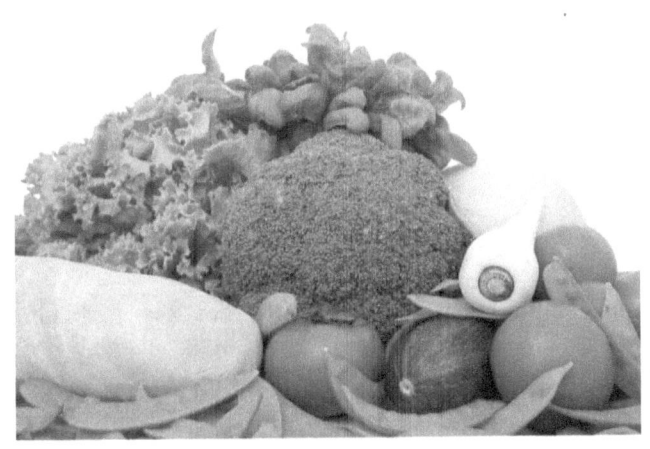

Chapter 1. Healthy Diet

A healthy and balanced diet allows the body to receive the nutrients it needs to function and grow. This includes proteins, carbohydrates, fats, vitamins, minerals and water.

To maintain a healthy weight, the eating plan must be appropriate for each person and their context.

It is estimated that an average adult should consume about 2,000 calories a day, depending on their lifestyle, their sex, their age and the activities they do.

In addition, particular aspects of each individual should be considered, such as if he suffers from hypertension, is celiac or has high cholesterol, or if he is pregnant.

Eating nutritiously is simpler than it seems. To learn more about this topic, we interview Dr. Mario Vega Carbó, a specialist in clinical endocrinology.

Doctor Mario,
What are the keys to a healthy diet?

A fundamental factor for good nutrition is variety. In that sense, it is important to include fruits and vegetables of all colors in the diet; whole grains such as oats, bread and rice; skim milk and dairy; low calorie cheese; fish, shellfish, lean meats, poultry and eggs; and nuts, beans and seeds.

On the contrary, it is key to limit salt, sugar, alcohol, saturated fats and trans fats, and processed foods.

In addition, you should also drink a lot of water and look for food alternatives that can be bought easily in stores and that fit the taste and budget of each person.

2. How do you get a good nutritional balance?

For this it is important to ingest the necessary energy, without excesses or deficits. It is estimated that between 55 and 60% of the total should be provided by carbohydrates, between 25 and 30% by fats, and between 10 and 15% by proteins.

To this we must add the consumption of vitamins, minerals, fiber and water.

In addition, it is important to distribute food throughout the day, if possible in 5 meals: breakfast, mid-morning, lunch, afternoon snack and dinner.

3. What recommendations can be given to prepare a healthy breakfast?

To start the day with energy, it is important to prepare a full breakfast that includes skim milk, fruits and whole grains, which for their greater contribution of fiber contribute to control appetite, blood cholesterol and digestion.

If you choose breads and cookies, you should choose light versions, with low fat content.

Some options may include skim milk, light brown bread toast spread with skim cheese and diet jam, yogurt with cereals and salad or fruit smoothies.

4. How can healthy lunches and dinners be prepared?

When preparing a balanced and healthy dish, it is important that half is made up of vegetables; a quarter for meat, chicken, fish or egg; and the other quarter for cereals, potatoes, sweet potatoes and cooked legumes.

Some food options are grilled chicken breast, fish fillet, grilled pork churrasquito, crepes, soy milanesas or homemade lean or lentil burger.

They can be accompanied by salads of green leaves or tomato, arugula, carrot and cucumber; baked pumpkin; or roasted eggplants.

For dessert you can consume all kinds of fruits, such as banana, apple, kiwi, orange, tangerine or pear, or light jelly.

5. What can you eat during snacks?

Snacks are essential to regulate anxiety during the day and avoid pecking between meals. It is important that they contain free or low sugar, sodium and saturated fat proposals.

Some healthy options are fruits, light yogurt with cereals or a portion of dried fruits, including almonds, nuts, hazelnuts, pistachios, chestnuts and peanuts.

6. How can you avoid eating sugar?

Based on a diet of 2,000 calories per day, it is advisable to eat less than 50 grams of sugar. To limit its consumption it is important to avoid soft drinks and commercial juices, opt for natural foods instead of industrialized ones, reduce the consumption of sweets and use sweetener in infusions.

7. Why should sodium intake be limited?

Excess sodium can cause fluid retention, high blood pressure, heart failure and long-term kidney failure, so it is recommended to consume less than 2 grams of salt per day.

8. Is vegetarian eating healthy?

Yes, it is a very healthy and recommended option. It is often mentioned that it may have nutritional deficiencies, but if the food plan is carried out correctly, it can be very complete and nutritious, and provide higher levels of antioxidants, fiber, folate and phytochemicals.

In addition, vegetarian nutrition helps reduce levels of saturated fat and blood cholesterol, and the risks of heart disease, obesity, hypertension, bad cholesterol, diabetes and certain types of cancer.

9. Who are nutritional supplements recommended for?

These supplements are used to supplement a healthy diet, but not to replace it. If a person eats properly and is in good health, they are not necessary.

However, for some cases, supplements may be useful for providing more special nutrients, for example to the elderly, pregnant women or people with eating disorders.

Chapter 2. Mediterranean diet

The Mediterranean diet is a style of food that follows the culinary customs of the countries that live in front of the Mediterranean Sea, especially Spain and Italy.

It usually reduces the consumption of meats and carbohydrates and increases that of vegetables and monounsaturated fats. It is also characterized by the use of olive oil in its preparation and for being accompanied by a glass of red wine.

Its implementation can help generate stable blood sugar levels, lower cholesterol and triglycerides and reduce the risks of developing heart disease and other health problems.

To learn more about this topic, we interview Mario Vega Carbó, an endocrinologist, with more than 20 years of experience.

Doctor Mario,
1. What is the basis of the Mediterranean diet?

It is characterized by vegetable-based meals, with only small amounts of beef and chicken, and more servings of whole grains, fresh fruits and vegetables, nuts and legumes.

The dishes usually include many fish and shellfish, and other foods with high amounts of fiber, which are prepared with olive oil and seasoned simply, without sauces or meat juices. For this, herbs and spices are used instead of salt.

Unlike traditional foods, cereals and vegetables are the basis of the dishes, while meats are the accompaniment.

Also important are pasta, rice, nuts and bread, and the grains in the region are typically whole grains and usually contain very little trans fat.

2. What foods are NOT usually used in this diet?

In the Mediterranean diet, red meat, eggs, sweets and cakes are only consumed in very small quantities or are not directly part of the food plan. In addition, butter is replaced by olive oil, which thanks to oleic acid and its vegetable fats reduces the risk of clogging arteries, and has a high content of carotenes and vitamin E.

On the other hand, this diet discourages the consumption of saturated fats and hydrogenated oils (trans fats), which contribute to heart disease.

3. Why is this diet recommended?

Usually this type of diet offers a varied, healthy and balanced nutrition, with a low content of saturated fats and sugars, and an abundance of vitamins and fibers, which makes it a healthy option for the heart and other organs of the body .

In addition, the Mediterranean diet has been associated with a lower incidence of cancer and Parkinson's and Alzheimer's diseases.

On the other hand, fish such as mackerel, lake trout, herring, sardines, albacore and salmon are important sources of Omega-3 fatty acids.

4. What are the shortcomings of the Mediterranean diet?

In many cases the levels of iron and calcium can be reduced by the low consumption of meat and dairy products.

In addition, the fats in olive oil and nuts can contribute to weight gain.

As for wine, it is advised that it only be taken during meals and in moderation.

Chapter 3. Vegetarian Diet

The vegetarian diet is a type of food based on vegetables, fruits, whole grains, peas, legumes, seeds and nuts. It may include eggs and dairy products, or not, depending on the type of vegetarianism.

On the contrary, generally no type of meat, poultry, seafood or fish is consumed. This type of diet is very healthy and recommended to prevent diseases at any age.

Many times it is mentioned that the vegetarian diet may have nutritional deficiencies, but if the eating plan is carried out correctly, it can be very complete and nutritious, and provide higher levels of antioxidants, fiber, folate and phytochemicals.

To learn more about this topic, we interview Dr. Mario Vega Carbó, a specialist in clinical endocrinology.

Doctor Mario,
1. How many kinds of vegetarian diets are there?

There are several types, but we can divide them into 6 groups:

1) Total Vegans or Vegetarians: consume only plant-based foods, not including animal protein or products derived from them, such as eggs, dairy or honey.

2) Dairy-egg-vegetarians: they follow a diet of plant foods and include dairy products and eggs.

3) Egg-vegetarians: avoid eating red meat, chicken, fish and dairy products, but they do eat eggs.

4) Dairy-vegetarians: do not consume eggs but dairy products.

5) Fish-vegetarians: avoid eating red meat and chicken, but consume fish, shellfish, eggs and dairy products.

6) Semi-vegetarian: they eat plant foods, chicken, fish, dairy products and eggs. They do not include red meat.

2. Why do people opt for a vegetarian diet?

The reasons why people opt for this type of diet are varied. Among the most common is the desire to improve health and food, concern for animal welfare, the desire to avoid excessive consumption of environmental resources and respect for the environment.

3. What are the main benefits of this type of food?

The vegetarian diet helps reduce levels of saturated fat and blood cholesterol, and the risks of heart disease, obesity, hypertension, bad cholesterol, diabetes and certain types of cancer. In addition, it increases the consumption of fiber, potassium and vitamin C.

4. Is it advisable to feed children with a vegetarian diet?

Yes. A personalized and well-planned vegetarian diet is healthy at all stages of life: infants, children, teenagers, pregnant women and older adults. In addition, following such a diet in childhood helps establish healthy eating patterns that will continue throughout life.

5. Does this diet have nutritional deficiencies?

Not necessarily. If the eating plan is done correctly, it can be very complete and nutritious. For this it is important to eat a wide variety of foods, including protein, iron, calcium, zinc, vitamin B12 and Omega-3 fatty acids.

6. How can vegetarians get these nutrients?

Proteins can be obtained from foods made from soybeans, legumes, beans, lentils, nuts, nuts, seeds and whole grains. If they consume dairy products, fish and eggs, they can also get them from there.

Iron can be consumed from dried beans and peas, lentils, legumes, broccoli, spinach, cabbage, plums, raisins, nuts, whole grains and fortified breads and cereals. In turn, eating foods high in vitamin C, such as tomatoes, cabbage, broccoli, potatoes, citrus fruits, peppers and strawberries, increases iron absorption.

As for calcium, in the case of fish-vegetarians, it can be obtained from sardines and canned salmon, or from dairy products such as milk, yogurt and cheese, for dairy-vegetarians. In addition, it is also present in dark green vegetables, such as turnip, cabbage and broccoli; oranges, figs, tofu, almonds, Brazilian nuts, sunflower seeds, white beans and fortified foods, such as cereal, orange juice and rice.

For its part, vitamin B12 is present in eggs, dairy, shellfish, salmon and tuna. Vegans can consume it from nutritional yeast and fortified foods, such as cereal and soy products.

Vitamin D can be obtained from sun exposure, egg yolk, certain fish, some cereals and margarines, and fortified foods, while Zinc is present in beans, legumes, chickpeas, wheat germ, products soy, nuts and seeds such as almonds and peanuts, seafood, yogurt and cheese.

Finally, Omega-3 fatty acids can consume them from fish rich in fat, nuts and seeds, beans, ground flaxseed and soy oils and fortified foods..

7. What other recommendations should be taken into account in this type of feeding?

Before starting a vegetarian diet, a gradual transition is recommended, in which the consumption of meat is reduced and that of fruits and vegetables is increased.

When preparing the dishes, variety is important, placing vegetables of different colors and always a source of protein. Also choose fortified foods to obtain a wide variety of nutrients.

On the contrary, it is advisable to avoid foods rich in fat, sugar and sodium, fried foods, sugary sodas, roasted nuts and with added salt, butter, margarine and refined vegetable oils.

If necessary, nutritional supplements should be added to the diet, especially in the case of vegans.

Chapter 4. Vegan Diet

The vegan diet is a type of diet based on vegetables, fruits, whole grains, peas, legumes, seeds and nuts. It does not include meat or animal proteins, or derived products such as eggs, dairy, gelatin or honey.

While this is a healthy eating option, it is important to pay special attention to diet planning to make sure you get all the necessary nutrients. In some cases, vegans may need to take supplements of vitamin B12, iron, iodine and Omega-3 fatty acids.

To learn more about this topic, we interview Dr. Mario Vega Carbó, a Cuban doctor, specialist in endocrinology.

Doctor Mario,

1. What are the advantages and disadvantages of a vegan diet?

This type of diet helps lower total and LDL cholesterol levels, serves to lose weight, reduces sugar consumption, increases antioxidant action, improves osteoarthritis and arthritis, and decreases the risks of heart disease, hypertension, diabetes and certain types of cancer

On the contrary, if the diet is very strict or not planned properly, it may be more difficult to obtain certain essential nutrients for the body.

2. What foods should be included in a vegan diet?

To be sufficient from the nutritional point of view, the diet must include a wide variety of foods. Among them fruits; vegetables; tubers such as potatoes and sweet potatoes; nuts such as almonds, hazelnuts, nuts, pine nuts and pistachios; cereals such as quinoa, millet, buckwheat, rice, amaranth, oats, polenta, pasta and couscous; ground flax, sesame, hemp and sunflower seeds; legumes such as lentils, chickpeas, peas and beans; and processed vegetable protein, such as tofu, seitan and tempeh.

3. What would be a simple example of a vegan diet?

During breakfast, vegans can eat an apple or a banana; a kiwi, orange and pineapple or apple, carrot and grapefruit smoothie; a handful of nuts; or a tomato toast, natural tofu and oregano.

In the middle of the morning you can consume a glass of vegetable milk with muesli cereals, an integral toast with salad and vegan cookies, a mango or a glass of vegetable milk with corn flakes.

Among the lunch options you can choose between a plate of lentils with rice and pumpkin; vegetable burgers with salad; peas sauteed with onion and pepper; oatmeal dumplings with tomato and natural thyme; white bean salad with onion, pepper and carrot; hummus with cucumber slices; boiled basmati rice with fried tomato or curry textured soy.

As for the snack, you can opt for a banana, a tangerine, a portion of watermelon, an apple, a pear, two peaches, sunflower seeds, almonds, hazelnuts, nuts, natural peanuts or a muesli bar.

Finally, for dinner you can consume celery and carrot grated with vegan cheese, onion and zucchini omelette, vegan chocolate custard, chickpea salad, rice and tofu with vegetables, sauteed vegetables and seitan, spaghetti with sanfaina, textured soy wrap and canned beans, caprese salad or vegan pizza.

The options are varied and depend on the particular taste and imagination in the preparation of each person.

4. What aspects require special attention in a vegan diet?

If you choose to avoid all animal foods, it is important to make sure you consume enough protein, iron, calcium, zinc, vitamins B12 and D, iodine and Omega-3 fatty acids.

If you follow a very strict diet, you should be very alert to the signs of nutrition problems, such as changes in weight, skin or hair.

It is also recommended to perform medical checks at least once a year to ensure that there are no nutritional deficits of any kind.

5. How can vegans get vitamin B12 and Omega-3 fatty acids?

Vitamin B12, necessary to produce red blood cells and prevent anemia, is found almost exclusively in animal products. The same is Omega-3 fatty acids, which improve heart health and brain function.

Therefore, it is important that vegans consume cereals and soy products fortified with them, or that they consider taking nutritional supplements. Freshly ground flax seeds, flour and flaxseed oil are also sources of Omega-3.

6. What should you keep in mind regarding iron consumption?

Iron is very important for energy and for the proper functioning of red blood cells. The absorption of this mineral is more difficult from vegetable sources, so it is necessary to eat a greater amount and accompany it with foods rich in vitamin C, which favor its digestion.

Vegans can consume it from dried beans and peas, lentils, legumes, broccoli, spinach, cabbage, plums, raisins, nuts, whole grains and enriched cereals.

Chapter 5. Hypercaloric Diet

The hypercaloric diet is a nutritional plan that aims to ingest more calories than are burned with daily activity, with the aim of gaining weight. Just as obesity is very dangerous for health, extreme thinness is too.

Gaining weight when you have a very active metabolism, a lot of physical activity is performed, there is a health problem, malnutrition, stress or other type of disorder can be very complex. Therefore, the hypercaloric diet has to be balanced and personalized, seeking not only to increase the amount of calories, but also the quality and quantity of what is eaten.

To learn more about this topic, we interviewed Cuban doctor Mario Vega Carbó, a specialist in clinical endocrinology.

Doctor Mario,
1. How is extreme thinness treated?

If the thinness is caused by a disease, it should be treated. If the patient is healthy and does not have associated pathologies, a hypercaloric diet can be prescribed and seek to reduce energy expenditure.

For this, the intake of pasta, nuts, honey, brown rice, oils, meats, fish, eggs, dairy products, fruits and vegetables is recommended, in the proportions suggested by a nutritionist.

2. How many calories should be consumed in a hypercaloric diet?

Because each person needs different amounts of calories depending on their age, physical structure, sex and activity level, there is no standard model to follow, but each one has to set their goal in a particular way.

This value must be set after a thorough nutritional study and the weight gain has to be slow and gradual.

3. What should be taken into account when planning a hypercaloric diet?

A nutritional plan that seeks to gain weight should have a caloric intake of between 20 and 50% higher than normal, gradually increasing. For this, it will be sought to increase the consumption of carbohydrates and proteins and, to a lesser extent, of fats, since they cause a greater feeling of satiety. The same is high fiber foods.

However, all planning should always be done looking for healthy nutrition, since eating junk food, sweets and other products with harmful fats or refined sugars can increase the risks of diseases such as arteriosclerosis, diabetes, high blood pressure, hypercholesterolemia and hypertriglyceridemia, among others.

4. What foods are recommended to include in a hypercaloric diet?

Among the caloric foods that are healthy and nutritious we can mention avocado, goat cheese, soybeans, black olives, salmon, nuts, dark chocolate, fresh coconut, banana, hazelnuts, raisins, Pumpkin seeds, barley, chickpeas, olive or sunflower oil, eggs, honey, mayonnaise and butter.

The meats that are recommended to eat are white, while fruits and vegetables are recommended to eat cooked and not raw. As for dairy products, it is advisable to include the integers. Yogurt can be accompanied with nuts, seeds, brewer's yeast, cocoa powder, jam or honey, while powdered milk can be used to enrich the puree. On the other hand, pasta, rice, cereals and potatoes can be consumed daily.

5. What foods are recommended to avoid in a hypercaloric diet?

While they may be high in calories, some foods are not healthy, so it is best to avoid them. Among them we can mention sodas and sugary drinks, alcohol, industrial pastries, fried snacks, sausages, cookies, precooked pizzas and ultraprocessed sauces.

On the other hand, the temperature of the food you eat should not be very high, since the hotter they are, the more they satisfy.

Similarly, before the main course it is not recommended to eat salads or soups, since they decrease appetite and cause you to eat less.

It is also important not to skip meals and add one or two snacks between them. It is better to distribute the intake in 5 or 6 shots throughout the day, than to make 2 or 3 very copious.

6. What other aspects should be taken into account to accompany this diet?

Along with the diet, it is important to control stress, which in many cases is the main factor of weight loss. For this you can practice relaxation techniques or yoga.

With regard to physical exercise, it is beneficial for health and helps to whet your appetite and build muscle mass. However, in cases of extreme thinness it is recommended to follow moderate training routines, such as gentle bodybuilding, avoiding aerobic exercises that activate the metabolism and burn fat.

For its part, vitamin supplements are not advisable, since in constitutional thinness there are usually no nutritional deficiencies or malnutrition.

Finally, if necessary, medications can be given to stimulate appetite.

Chapter 6. Low calorie diet

The hypocaloric diet is a nutritional plan that aims to eat fewer calories than are burned with daily activity, with the aim of losing weight. For this, the first thing that is done is to set a reference level of calories, based on the basal metabolism and the degree of physical wear of the person.

Then a menu system is organized that is below that number, so that the body is forced to consume calories from adipose tissue, reducing its volume.

To learn more about this topic, we interview Mario Vega Carbó, an endocrinologist, with more than 20 years of professional experience.

Doctor Mario,
1. How many calories should be consumed in a hypocaloric diet?

The main objective of this diet is to consume fewer calories than are used during the day. Because each person needs different amounts depending on their age, physical structure, sex and activity level, there is no standard model to follow, but each one has to set his caloric goal in a particular way.

For this it is advisable to consult with a specialized nutritionist to study each case, define a personalized diet and the objectives to follow.

2. What types of foods are usually included in these types of diets?

Most include a wide variety of fruits and vegetables, since they have high nutritional power and low caloric density.

Low-calorie foods include carrots, strawberries, asparagus, celery, broccoli, zucchini, watermelon, cantaloupe, mushrooms, cauliflower, cucumber, eggplants, tomatoes, spinach, cherries, watercress, blueberries, squash, turkey breast, pear, lettuce, kiwi, artichokes, orange, grapefruit, fresh cheese, olives, natural yogurt, apple, Plum, pineapple, arugula, peach, salmon and tuna.

3. What foods are you trying to avoid?

Among the foods that are usually avoided in this diet are fried potatoes, red meat, pasta, pizza, margarine, refined vegetable oils, fast foods, ultraprocessed products, fried foods, soft drinks, Soft drinks and alcohol.

4. What should be taken into account when planning a hypocaloric diet?

It is important that the plan be balanced and includes all food groups. To do this you must have a good amount of protein, some lipids to cover the contribution of fat-soluble vitamins and essential fatty acids, fiber and microcomponents.

In this way, it is sought that the low caloric content does not restrict certain nutrients from the diet.

5. What are the limitations of this type of food?

The problem with this diet is that over time the metabolism adapts to the caloric decrease. For a matter of survival, the body to receive fewer calories also consumes less.

The body also reduces energy expenditure, so physical activity tends to decrease, since we are more tired and more lazy. For this reason the weight loss is getting smaller, because there is a progressive decrease in the consumption of calories contained in our reserves.

In many cases, when the diet is abandoned, by consuming more calories the body, which has become accustomed to working with less, stores excess fat, which causes it to regain weight.

6. For whom is the hypocaloric diet not recommended?

This diet is not recommended for people with heart disease, recent stroke, psychiatric illnesses or a history of eating disorders such as bulimia or anorexia, infections, treatments that cause protein loss, ketosis-prone diabetes and in pregnant and nursing women.

7. Why are "miracle" hypocaloric diets that become fashionable not recommended?

These magical diets are very dangerous, because they mostly do not have any medical or scientific endorsement and do not usually contemplate all the essential nutrients.

In addition, they are the cause of patients fail in their attempts to lose weight, get discouraged and fall back into routines harmful to their health.

Chapter 7. Ketogenic Diet

The ketogenic diet or keto diet is a type of nutrition low in carbohydrates and very high in fat, which causes a change in the energy source and metabolic state.

Glucose is the main fuel of muscles, brain and other tissues of the body. When there is a shortage of blood sugar, the body creates small molecules called ketones, to use as energy. These chemicals are produced in the liver, burning fat. When too few carbohydrates and moderate amounts of protein are consumed, insulin levels are reduced and the body begins to function almost exclusively with the fuel provided by ketones. This causes you to burn a lot of fat, which helps you lose weight and offers other potential health benefits.

To learn more about this topic, we interview Mario Vega Carbó, an endocrinology specialist, who works as an endocrinologist at the Vega & Vado Office.

Doctor Mario,
1. How is a ketogenic diet composed?

It is made up of 65 and 75 percent fat, between 15 and 25 percent protein and between 5 and 10 percent carbohydrates.

In this case, by limiting the amount of carbohydrates and metabolized proteins, energy is obtained from the fat consumed and stored in the body.

2. What foods should be eaten on this diet?

The foods allowed are those fatty and with some protein. Among them we can mention vegetables with few carbohydrates, such as spinach, cucumber, cauliflower, broccoli, asparagus, cabbage, tomatoes and onions; high-fat fish, such as salmon, sardine, mackerel, trout, tuna, dove, and swordfish; meats and sausages, such as chicken, turkey and fatty meats; the eggs; the Mayo; fatty dairy products, such as milk cream, butter, goat cheese, cheddar, mozzarella or sugar-free yogurt; nuts and seeds, such as nuts, almonds, pumpkin and chia seeds; and olive, coconut or avocado oils.

As for the drink, the ideal is water, although you can also drink coffee, tea and mate, preferably without any sweetener.

3. What foods should not be eaten in the ketogenic diet?

To achieve ketosis, the most important thing is to avoid eating carbohydrates. Ideally, keep your consumption below 40 grams per day.

Among the foods that should be limited are fruits, especially fig, grape, mango, cherry, banana, tangerine, orange and apple; starchy vegetables and tubers; bread, pasta, flour, pizza and rice; the cereals; legumes; sweets and cakes; low-fat dairy products; sugary soft drinks, juices and alcohol; processed foods and prepared foods.

4. What are the benefits of this type of food?

Among its benefits, it stands out that it allows you to lose weight faster than diets based on consuming little fat and many proteins. In addition, the circulation of ketone bodies in the body generates a greater absence of hunger, which helps reduce intake.

On the other hand, for those with diabetes, it reduces blood sugar levels, improves insulin sensitivity and decreases body fat and obesity.

Meanwhile, in some cases of childhood epilepsy, this diet also reduces the frequency of seizures, while reducing sugar consumption may help reduce the risk of cancer.

5. What inconveniences can this diet bring?

Among its main disadvantages are the low contribution of vitamins, minerals and fiber, by restricting the consumption of fruits and vegetables.

Among other symptoms, this can lead to constipation, indigestion, fatigue, difficulty concentrating, headache and insomnia. In addition, it is also common to suffer from bad breath due to the high production of ketone bodies.

On the other hand, this form of nutrition is not advisable for people with liver or heart problems, as it can lead to the development of arrhythmias. Finally, by restricting a large amount of food, it is not usually sustainable in the long term

Chapter 8. DASH diet to lower blood pressure

The DASH diet, "Dietary Approaches to Stop Hypertension," is a type of diet to help reduce blood pressure. It is a low sodium option that includes many fruits, vegetables, whole grains, dairy and lean proteins.

Its implementation can reduce the risks of heart attack, stroke, osteoporosis and kidney stones, and helps control diabetes and improve cholesterol levels. In addition, it also serves to lose weight.

To learn more about this topic, we interview Mario Vega Carbó, an endocrinology specialist, who works as an endocrinologist at the Vega & Vado Office.

Doctor Mario,

1. What is high blood pressure and what are its possible consequences?

Blood pressure is the force exerted by the blood that circulates against the walls of the arteries. When it increases, hypertension occurs, which is a condition suffered by a third of the adult population.

If left untreated, it can cause serious complications, such as heart attack, stroke and kidney and visual damage.

2. How does the DASH diet work and what types of foods does it include?

This diet lowers hypertension by reducing the amount of sodium consumed per day and adding a variety of foods rich in potassium, calcium, magnesium and fiber.

Their dishes include many vegetables, fruits, low-fat dairy products, whole grains, legumes, seeds, nuts, vegetable oils, fish, poultry and lean meats. Potassium, present in potatoes, spinach and bananas, helps control blood pressure.

3. What foods are avoided in the DASH diet?

In this diet, salt, saturated fats and total fats are avoided, reducing the consumption of red meat, whole dairy products, fried foods, sweets and sugary and alcoholic drinks.

4. What is the recommended sodium intake?

It is generally recommended to reduce your consumption to 2,300 milligrams a day. If the patient already suffers from hypertension, suffers from diabetes or kidney disease or is over 50 years old, the ideal is to consume less than 1,500 milligrams per day.

5. How can you reduce salt intake?

To reduce its consumption, it is recommended to season foods with herbs and spices, lemon, lime orange or vinegar instead. Also avoid canned foods or rinse them in water, and check the labels of products that are purchased to see the sodium content.

Other tips are to reduce foods and condiments that have a lot of salt, such as pickles, olives, sausages, mustard and tomato and soy sauces; and do not add it when cooking rice, pasta or hot cereal.

6. How many servings of each food should be consumed per day on this diet?

It is estimated that 6 to 8 servings of grains (bread, cereals, rice, pasta), 4 to 5 servings of vegetables (tomatoes, carrots, broccoli, sweet potatoes, vegetables), 4 to 5 servings of fruits (banana, orange, apple, pear, kiwi, watermelon, tangerine, strawberry), 2 to 3 servings of dairy products (milk, yogurt, cheese), less than 6 servings of lean meats, poultry and fish, and 2 to 2 3 servings of fats and oils.

In addition, 4 to 5 servings of nuts, seeds and legumes (almonds, sunflower seeds, beans, peas, lentils) and less than 5 servings of sweets (jelly, jam, sorbet, lemonade, ice creams) can be eaten per week. fruit, candies, low-fat sweet cookies).

7. What advice can be given to someone who wants to implement the DASH diet?

The first thing that can be told is that you do not try to change your diet overnight, but instead do it gradually. Then you should start thinking of meat as a part of the meal and not as the main course. On the contrary, you should stop seeing the vegetables as a garnish and understand that well accompanied can be the basis of food.

Meanwhile, to start eating more fruits, you can add them to breakfast cereal or oatmeal or choose them as a dessert for lunch or dinner, or as a snack option.

8. Does the DASH diet offer all the necessary nutrients?

Yes. When it is well planned and personalized, it is a healthy diet for both adults and children. Being low in saturated fat and high in fiber is a highly recommended eating style for everyone by providing all the nutrients.

9. What other aspects are important to accompany this diet?

In addition to taking care of food, for a better control of blood pressure, regular exercise is also recommended, maintaining an adequate body weight, drinking plenty of water, not smoking and controlling stress.

On the other hand, if the person takes medications to treat hypertension, they should continue taking them as soon as they have the DASH diet.

Chapter 9. Carbohydrate counting to control Diabetes

Carbohydrate counting is a meal planning technique that aims to control the level of blood glucose.

It is specially designed for people with Diabetes and involves keeping track of the foods consumed each day.

Carbohydrates are one of the main nutrients present in food, and include sugars, starches and fiber.

Some are healthy, such as those that come from fruits, vegetables and whole grains, and others not so much, such as those found in foods and beverages with added sugars.

To learn more about this topic, we interview Dr. Mario Vega Carbó, an endocrinology specialist, with more than 20 years of experience.

Doctor Mario,
1. How does carbohydrate counting work and what is it used for?

Foods that contain carbohydrates can raise blood glucose, as the body quickly converts them into sugar. Counting the amount consumed per day, it is possible to set a maximum limit that allows keeping the levels of this substance in the body controlled.

Many of the foods that contain carbohydrates are nutritious and a fundamental part of a healthy diet. The goal is not to eliminate them from food, but to seek to eat the right amount.

2. How is this count done?

Carbohydrates are counted per grams. In order to carry out this measurement it is necessary to know what foods contain them and learn to calculate how many grams are eaten in each serving, in order to obtain a total daily amount.

Your doctor can teach you to determine the values or you can suggest a special diet based on the glucose levels you want to reach.

3. What foods contain carbohydrates?

Carbohydrates are present in a large amount of food. Among them we can mention grains, such as bread, noodles, pasta, crackers, cereals and rice; fruits, such as apples, bananas, mangoes, melons and oranges; dairy products, such as milk and yogurt; legumes, such as beans, lentils and peas; sweets, such as cakes, cookies, candies and other desserts; juices, sodas and sports drinks; and vegetables, such as potatoes, corn and peas.

4. What foods do not contain them?

Red meat, fish, poultry, most cheeses, eggs, nuts and oils do not contain carbohydrates.

5. How many carbohydrates should be consumed per day?

The ideal amount depends on each person, taking into account their lifestyle, their sex, their age, the activities they perform and whether or not they suffer from certain diseases.

On average, it can be estimated that carbohydrate consumption for most people should be between 45 and 60 percent of total daily calories. A gram of carbohydrates provides about 4 calories. For a diet of 1,600 calories per day, one could suggest, for example, about 200 grams of carbohydrates, which would account for 50 percent of total calories.

For most adults with Diabetes, a diet of around 135 grams per day is recommended, but each person must have their own carbohydrate goal.

6. How can you calculate the amount of carbohydrates?

To do this you will have to review the labels of nutritional information of the foods that are normally consumed, to know the amount of carbohydrates per serving. It is also possible to obtain this information in books or websites, by consulting a nutritionist or using scales or measuring cups.

As an example, and to have as a base, there are approximately 15 grams of carbohydrates in a small fruit, half a cup of canned fruit, a slice of bread, half a cup of oatmeal, a third of a cup of noodles or rice and 5 cookies salty

As the person becomes familiar with the food and its grams, the count will become easier.

7. How is it possible to know if carbohydrate counting is being effective?

Ideally, check blood glucose levels periodically, to see if they are high, normal or low. If they are very high, the patient may have to make changes in their eating plan or lifestyle.

Chapter 10. Glycemic Index Diet

The diet based on the glycemic index is a nutritional plan that is governed by the way in which food influences the level of blood sugar.

What is generally sought is to consume those that contain carbohydrates that are less likely to cause increases in the amount of glucose in the body. This diet can be very useful for losing weight and preventing or controlling chronic ailments such as diabetes or hypercholesterolemia and cardiovascular diseases.

The glycemic index is a classification system that assigns a number to food and serves as a tool to make better food choices.

To learn more about this topic, we interview Mario Vega Carbó, an endocrinology specialist, who works as an endocrinologist at the Vega & Vado Office.

Doctor Mario,
1. How is the glycemic index measured?

Usually this figure is obtained by comparing how much a food raises the level of blood sugar in relation to pure glucose, represented by the number 100. The values are divided into three categories: low glycemic index, ranging from 1 to 55 ; medium, ranging from 56 to 69; and tall, 70 or more.

2. What foods are in each category?

Among those with low glycemic index are green leafy vegetables, most fruits, raw carrots, chickpeas, lentils and bran cereals. In the middle category are sweet corn, bananas, raw pineapple, raisins, oatmeal cereals and rye bread.

Meanwhile, within the high we can mention rice and white bread, potatoes and honey.

3. What effects does the glycemic index have on appetite?

It is estimated that foods with a high glycemic index cause a rapid increase in blood sugar and, therefore, generate an increase in appetite quickly. On the contrary, it is believed that those who have a low level delay this feeling of hunger, which causes them to eat less. However, scientific studies on this subject did not yield decisive results on this issue.

4. What are the limitations of this tool?

The glycemic index does not reflect the amounts and portions that should be consumed for each food. For example, some have a high value, but few digestible carbohydrates, so you should eat a lot of them to significantly raise sugar levels.

On the other hand, liquids and prolonged cooking increase its absorption rate, while high fat or fiber contents decrease it. In short, its influence on blood glucose also depends on other factors, such as the mode of preparation, processing and combination with other foods.

5. How is this problem resolved?

To remedy this difficulty, the concept of "glycemic load" was developed. It is a numerical value that indicates the change that occurs in blood sugar levels by ingesting a usual portion of a food, which allows a better forecast of its effects.

The glycemic load is also divided into three categories: low (1 to 10), medium (11 to 19) and high (20 or more).

6. What are the main factors that should be taken into account in a healthy diet of a diabetic?

Some keys are: to limit foods with high sugar content; eat small portions throughout the day; pay special attention to the amount of carbohydrates ingested and seek to maintain the same proportion on a daily basis; consume a wide variety of whole foods, fruits and vegetables; eat less saturated fat; and avoid salt and alcohol.

7. For a person with diabetes, which control method is safer, carbohydrate counting or glycemic index?

It is generally estimated that the carbohydrate count in the diet allows better control of the blood sugar level than the glycemic index. But well applied, both methods are effective.

Chapter 11. Diet and dyslipidemia

Hypercholesterolemia and hypertriglyceridemia increase the risk of heart and circulatory diseases, heart attacks, strokes and liver or kidney problems.

Both conditions involve an increase in fats that circulate in the blood and are usually related to being overweight, an unhealthy diet and lack of physical exercise. A balanced diet, with low intake of saturated fats, is essential to prevent atherosclerosis and decrease blood pressure and insulin resistance.

To learn more about this topic, we interview Mario Vega Carbó, an endocrinology specialist, who works as an endocrinologist at the Vega & Vado Office.

Doctor Mario,
1. What are the keys to a diet of a patient with dyslipidemia?

As a first step it should be low in calories and fat, especially saturated ones, and you should also avoid sugar, refined carbohydrates and alcohol consumption. It is important to replace meats with healthier options, such as olive oils and fish such as mackerel or salmon, and increase the consumption of complex carbohydrates with high fiber content. In addition, to supplement the diet you should exercise regularly, drink plenty of water, eliminate overweight and quit smoking.

2. What foods are recommended in these cases?

For this diet you should choose skim milk products, poultry and lean meats without visible fat or skin, and consume plenty of fruits, vegetables and salads.

Preference should also be given to blue fish (sardines, anchovies, tuna, salmon and mackerel) over red meat and substitute egg yolks for egg whites. Legumes should be made with low fat and for flavoring, herbs, mustard, vinegar or lemon can be used.

In addition, whole wheat bread, refined or whole grain cereals, rice, pasta, flour and semolina are also allowed, while sugar can be replaced by saccharin.

3. What foods should be avoided in this diet?

Avoid whole milk and dairy products and foods rich in simple carbohydrates, such as sugar, honey, jellies, candies, fruits in syrup, jams, compotes and pastry products, pastries and pastries.

Nor should you eat pre-cooked foods, such as fried fish, breaded chicken, croquettes, snacks, lasagna, stews and pizzas, or creamy ice cream. In addition, you should avoid beef, beef, pork and lamb, sausages, french fries, butter, margarine, mayonnaise and ketchup, and dried foods.

On the other hand, the consumption of alcohol, soft drinks and commercial juices should be restricted.

4. What are the recommended types of cooking?

Steaming and steaming (boiled or poached), grilled, grilled, grilled, baked or microwave, or papillote are recommended.

On the contrary, fritters, breaded, battered, stews and stews should be avoided.

In addition, the use of extra virgin olive oil in the preparation of the dishes and control the amount of salt for cooking is advised.

5. What other aspects should be taken into account in this diet?

For people with abnormal cholesterol or triglyceride levels it is important to read the labels of the products they buy.

When they indicate that they were "made with vegetable fat", without clarifying the type, most likely they have been prepared with palm or coconut oil, which are not advisable for these patients.

On the other hand, it is recommended to avoid foods that contain trans fatty acids, hydrogenated fats and sodium-rich ones.

Chapter 12. Diet for elevated uric acid

Gout is a type of arthritis that occurs when uric acid builds up in the blood and causes inflammation in the joints.

It is characterized by sudden and intense attacks of pain, in which the affected area swells, reddens and heats for no apparent reason.

The most common occurs in the big toe, which can be very annoying and manifest during the night, causing the person to wake up suddenly from the discomfort.

Following a diet that limits the production of uric acid and increases its elimination can help control the disease.

To learn more about this topic, we interviewed Cuban doctor Mario Vega Carbó, a specialist in clinical endocrinology.

Doctor Mario,
1. What is uric acid?

It is an organic compound that is formed when the metabolism disintegrates purines, which are substances found in some foods and beverages.

Purines are necessary to regenerate the body's cells and their excess is eliminated in the urine in the form of uric acid.

When it stays in the bloodstream, it creates crystals in the joints that produce inflammation and a lot of pain.

2. How can a proper diet help in the treatment of gout?

Eating certain foods and beverages, and avoiding others, can help lower uric acid levels in the blood.

While the diet does not cure the disease or replace medications, it can decrease recurrent attacks and the progression of joint damage.

It also helps to lose weight and avoid obesity, which increases the risks of suffering from this disease.

3. What foods should be included in this diet?

Among the recommended foods are fruits, vegetables and whole grains that provide complex carbohydrates.

Within fruits, cherries, apples, strawberries, raspberries, blueberries and red fruits in general are especially advised. Also citrus fruits, such as orange, lemon, grapefruit, lime or tangerine.

As for vegetables, the ones that help lower uric acid the most are artichokes, onions, pumpkins, celery and carrots.

Fish and meat can be consumed in moderate doses, with chicken, turkey, rabbit, sole, hake and fresh cod being the most recommended.

On the other hand, dairy products should be low in fat and skim milk.

Other foods that can be included in the diet are potatoes, nuts, olive oils from sunflower or corn seeds, and cereals, such as rice, wheat, and products made from them.

As for drinks, in addition to water, coffee consumption is recommended, which could help reduce the risks of gout.

If you want to drink alcohol, wine may be a good option.

4. What foods and drinks should be avoided?

In this diet it is important to avoid high-fructose corn syrup foods and the saturated fats present in red meats such as veal, pork, ox or lamb; poultry meats; sausages such as sausages or sausages; and high-fat dairy products.

On the other hand, the liver, kidney, gizzards, anchovies, crustaceans, salmon, sardines and tuna have a high purine content so they should not be consumed. As for vegetables, asparagus and spinach are discouraged.

In addition, it is important to limit sugary foods, such as sweetened cereals, bakery products, industrial pastries and sweets, and dehydrated foods, such as envelope soups. Also soybean oil and lard.

As for drinks, it is recommended to avoid alcohol, especially beer and spirits, sugar-sweetened beverages and naturally sweet fruit juices.

5. What should you eat and drink during a gout attack?

In these cases it is important to drink a lot of water; limit red meat, fish and sugar, and eat protein in moderation.

To help lower uric acid quickly you can consume low-fat milk and dairy products, eggs, cereals, fruits and vegetables that are low in purines. Also avoid alcoholic drinks, fruit juices and sugary drinks.

6. What other recommendations are important?

During this diet it is advisable to eat small portions about 5 or 6 times a day and drink plenty of water to maintain good hydration and favor the elimination of uric acid through the urine.

In addition, it is recommended to eat in moderation and exercise regularly to avoid being overweight.

Finally, it may also be necessary to take vitamin C supplements, which helps lower uric acid levels.o.

Chapter 13. Diet in case of renal lithiasis

Renal lithiasis, also known as "stones" in the kidneys, is a condition caused by the presence of urinary tract stones.

It originates when the urine has a high concentration of mineral salts that are not diluted correctly.

Its most frequent symptoms are severe pain in the lower back, blood or the removal of sand in urination, sweating, nausea and vomiting when pain crises occur.

A proper diet, such as the DASH diet already discussed in another chapter, can help prevent kidney stones

To learn more about this topic, we talked with Mario Vega Carbó, an endocrinology specialist, who currently works as an endocrinologist at the Vega & Vado Office.

Doctor Mario,
1. What can be done to prevent renal lithiasis?

The most important thing is to always keep the body well hydrated. In that sense, it is advisable to drink between 2 and 3 liters of water per day to keep the urine diluted, which makes it difficult to form stones. In contrast, dark yellow urine is a sign that you are not drinking enough fluid.

In addition, it is also recommended to lead a healthy life and exercise, since obesity and sedentary lifestyle increase the possibility of generating lithiasis.

As for the diet, the key is to avoid salt and sodium, sugars, alcohol and excess meat and animal proteins. These include beef, chicken, pork, fish and eggs. In addition, coffee, tea and soft drinks should also be reduced.

On the contrary, a low fat diet and eating lemons and oranges, whose citrate prevents stone formation is recommended

2. How many types of kidney stones are there?

The calculations can be divided into 4 types. The most frequent, between 75 to 80 percent, are formed by calcium oxalate, while the remaining 20 to 25 percent correspond to uric acid, struvite and cystine. Individual treatment depends on the type of calculation.

3. In the case of calcium oxalate calculation, what diet should be followed?

If the patient had such a calculation, it is recommended that he reduce the amount of salt and sodium in the diet, limiting it to less than 2,400 milligrams a day.

It is generally not advisable to significantly lower calcium intake, as this can cause bone loss and osteoporosis. It is advisable to eat only 2 or 3 servings a day of foods such as milk, cheese, yogurt and tofu.

As for oxalate, foods such as peanuts, tea, instant coffee, beets, beans, rhubarb, blackberries, raspberries, strawberries, chocolate, grapes, dark leafy vegetables, semolina, nuts, tofu, sweet potatoes and pulled beer should be limited.

4. In the case of uric acid calculation, what diet should be followed?

In this case it is recommended to avoid alcohol; the anchovies; the asparagus; brewer's yeast or baking powder; the cauliflower; the sauces; the fungi; the oils; organ meats, such as liver, kidney or gizzards; Sardines and spinach.

It is also advised to limit the consumption of animal protein in each meal and fatty foods such as dressings, ice cream and fried foods.

On the contrary, it is good to include enough carbohydrates, lemons and oranges in the diet. Also replace meat with plant-based foods that are high in protein, such as legumes, soy foods, nuts or dried fruits, and sunflower seeds.

5. How can cystine and struvite stones be avoided?

Drinking a lot of liquid, especially water, is the best thing to do to avoid these types of stones.

In the case of cystine stones, it is also recommended to limit methionine source foods, such as eggs, cheeses, fish, nuts and beans.

6. How can you reduce salt intake?

To reduce its consumption it is recommended to season foods with herbs and spices, lemon, lime orange or vinegar instead.

Also avoid canned foods or rinse them in water, and check the labels of products that are purchased to see the sodium content.

Other tips are to reduce foods and condiments that have a lot of salt, such as pickles, olives, sausages, mustard and tomato and soy sauces; and do not add it when cooking rice, pasta or hot cereal.

7. Can vitamin or mineral supplements generate the appearance of stones?

Vitamins B have not been shown to have a harmful effect for people with kidney stones. However, the use of vitamin C and D, fish liver oils and calcium-containing mineral supplements may increase the likelihood of forming stones. Therefore before using them it is recommended to consult with the dietitian.

Chapter 14. Diet for chronic kidney disease

Chronic kidney disease involves progressive loss of kidney function. These two organs are responsible for filtering the blood and eliminating waste and excess water from the body through the urine.

The main causes of this medical condition are diabetes and high blood pressure. Many times it has no symptoms until its consequences are severe. When the kidneys lose the ability to remove wastes and fluids, the patient must undergo dialysis or an organ transplant. A proper diet can help control and prevent its damage.

To learn more about this topic, we interview Mario Vega Carbó, an endocrinology specialist, who works as an endocrinologist at the Vega & Vado Office.

Doctor Mario,
1. How can a change in diet help these patients?

Everything we eat and drink affects our health. Maintaining an adequate weight and following a balanced diet can help control blood pressure and diabetes, and prevent kidney disease.

In addition, the limitation of liquids and the consumption of foods low in protein, potassium, phosphorus and other electrolytes can prevent damage to these organs from progressing.

2. What is the purpose of this diet?

It seeks to maintain a balance in the levels of electrolytes, minerals and fluid in the body.

In addition, in those people who need dialysis, it aims to reduce the accumulation of waste and limit fluids, which is very important since these patients urinate very little.

3. What are the main nutritional suggestions?

Usually in these cases low-protein diets are recommended, since they make the kidneys work hard and can damage them.

Some foods low in protein are fruits, vegetables, bread, pasta and rice. On the contrary, red meat, chicken, fish and eggs should be avoided.

To replace these nutrients you can consume more carbohydrates as a source of energy. However, healthy options should be sought, avoiding sugars and soft drinks.

As for fats, monounsaturated and polyunsaturated ones are recommended, such as olive, peanut and corn oil, which help protect the heart.

On the contrary, the saturated ones (red meat, butter, milk and its derivatives) and trans (fried, cakes, cookies) that can raise the level of cholesterol and the risks of heart disease should be avoided.

4. What should be done with phosphorus, calcium and potassium?

The kidneys are also responsible for balancing the salts and minerals that circulate in the blood, such as calcium, phosphorus, sodium and potassium.

When these organs do not work properly phosphorus levels can be too high and lower calcium levels, generating weaker bones.

Therefore, this diet usually limits phosphorus-rich foods, such as milk, yogurt and cheese. In addition, the patient may need to take calcium and vitamin D supplements to control the balance between these two chemicals in the body.

As for potassium, when the kidneys do not work well it can also accumulate and generate abnormal heart rhythms. In these cases it is recommended to avoid oranges, kiwis, bananas, melon, plums, asparagus, avocado, potatoes and tomatoes, among other foods rich in this chemical.

5. Why is it important to limit sodium intake?

Sodium limitation helps control hypertension, prevents increased thirst and prevents the body from retaining extra fluid. To reduce its consumption it is recommended to season foods with herbs and spices, lemon, lime orange or vinegar instead.

Also avoid canned foods or rinse them in water, and check the labels of products that are purchased to see the sodium content.

6. How should the consumption of liquids in this diet be managed?

As I said before, when the patient is on dialysis it is necessary to limit their consumption between sessions to avoid accumulation in the body. If this is not controlled, excess fluid can be generated in the heart and lungs and make breathing difficult, which requires immediate medical assistance.

To reduce its consumption it is advisable to avoid salty foods and cool off during hot days.

7. What other nutritional advice can be given to patients with chronic kidney disease?

Generally when this condition is advanced, patients usually have anemia and need to consume more iron. Some foods rich in this mineral are liver, blood sausage, nuts, legumes and green leafy vegetables.

On the other hand, in addition to following a healthy diet, they are advised to control the portions, eat slowly and avoid excesses.

Chapter 15. Diet for Gastritis and Gastroesophageal Reflux

Gastritis is an inflammation of the mucous lining of the stomach, which causes pain in the upper abdomen, nausea and, sometimes, vomiting.

For its part, reflux is a condition in which stomach acid returns to the esophagus, irritating its lining and causing acidity and regurgitation of food and liquids.

Due to their symptoms and complications, these ailments usually cause lack of appetite and desire to eat.

Following a proper diet can facilitate digestion and avoid this type of discomfort.

To learn more about this topic, we talked with Mario Vega Carbó, an endocrinology specialist, who currently works as an endocrinologist at the Vega & Vado Office.

Doctor Mario,
1. What guidelines should people with gastritis or reflux follow?

These types of patients are advised to avoid the consumption of alcohol and copious, heavy or spicy foods, which may aggravate their symptoms.

They are also advised to eat slowly, in small quantities, chew food well and divide the intake into 4 or 5 meals a day.

In addition, it is important to reduce foods and high-fat cooking, and not eat foods at extreme temperatures, or very cold or very hot, as they can enhance irritation.

2. What types of foods are recommended for these patients?

In this diet it is important to include many fruits and vegetables, which provide antioxidants, B vitamins and vegetable fiber. Also rice and potatoes, and legumes in soft cooking.

As for dairy products, skimmed or semi-skimmed milk, fresh cheese and light or skimmed yogurts are recommended.

For its part, white meat is ideal, such as skinless chicken or turkey, and white fish. Foods rich in Omega 3 fatty acids, such as salmon or mackerel, have an anti-inflammatory function, so it is good to include them.

To drink the best is always the water, and you can also drink soft defrosted broths and digestive infusions such as fennel, chamomile or lemon balm.

3. What types of foods are not recommended?

In this diet you should avoid foods rich in salt or sugar, fatty dairy products, immature or acidic fruits, citrus fruits, pastries, pastries, sausages, ice cream and beef or beef.

Also spicy seasonings, fatty sauces, stews, fried foods, chocolate, breads that include whole milk and carminatives, such as fennel, mint, basil, coriander, carrot, nut Nutmeg or sage.

On the other hand, some people may have intolerance to flatulent vegetables (artichoke, cabbage, cauliflower, broccoli, garlic, cucumber and onion) or acidic foods such as tomatoes.

As for drinks, in addition to alcohol, tea, coffee and soda should be avoided.

4. What type of cooking is recommended for these cases?

Steaming, boiling, papillote, microwave or oven cooking are recommended. On the contrary, you have to avoid grilled and fried foods.

5. What other aspects are important to prevent these ailments?

Other recommendations include not smoking, maintaining a healthy weight and managing stress, as it increases gastric acids. Also do not wear tight clothes and do not lie down or go to sleep after finishing eating, but wait 2 or 3 hours.

As for liquids, the ideal is to consume them between meals and not during them, to avoid increasing the volume of the stomach.

Finally, it is advisable to raise the head of the bed about 10 centimeters to achieve a minimum inclination of the entire trunk, to prevent the risk of reflux.

Chapter 16. Diet for fatty liver and cirrhosis

The liver is the body's metabolic center and is responsible for assimilating nutrients from food, storing energy and eliminating and filtering toxic substances.

Among the diseases that can affect it, one of the most common is that of fatty liver, which can be alcoholic or non-alcoholic, depending on whether or not it is related to its consumption.

When the liver ailment becomes chronic and irreversible, it results in cirrhosis, which causes scars and nodules in its tissues that make the organ function with difficulty.

Today obesity is the main cause of this condition, surpassing even alcohol. A diet that helps you lose weight can reduce fat, inflammation and fibrosis in the liver.

To learn more about this topic, we consulted Dr. Mario Vega Carbó, an endocrinology specialist, who is in charge of the Vega & Vado Office.

Doctor Mario,
1. How does obesity influence the development of non-alcoholic fatty liver?

When a person gains weight accumulates excess fat in different parts of the body including the liver. As it grows, it produces an inflammation in the organ that, if maintained over time, can cause death of part of the liver tissue.

Each time this gland suffers an injury, it tries to repair itself and, in that process, generates a scar that hinders its functioning. When 70 percent of the liver is in this state, cirrhosis appears, whose only solution is transplantation.

2. What are the symptoms of fatty liver?

In general it is a silent disease that has few or no symptoms. When they appear, the patient may feel fatigue or pain in the upper right side of the abdomen.

3. How can a diet help control this medical condition?

Weight loss through a combination of healthy diet and exercise can help prevent this disease, in addition to protecting the liver and improving its functioning.

4. What are the recommended dietary changes?

These patients are advised to avoid fat consumption almost completely, since they are responsible for the inflammation of the liver.

In addition, they should moderate carbohydrate intake and increase that of fruits, vegetables and legumes, as they are a natural source of vitamins and minerals that the body needs to function.

On the other hand, they should avoid salt, which worsens the accumulation of fluids and swelling in the liver, sugars and alcohol. They are also advised to limit portion sizes and eat foods that help improve the purification of the organ, such as artichoke and spirulina.

5. What types of fats are there and which are the most recommended?

The main types of fats are 4: the saturated ones, found in red meat, butter, vegetable fats and milk and their derivatives; the trans, present in commercially baked cookies and cakes and in fried foods such as donuts and French fries; monounsaturated, which are in olive, peanut and canola oils; and polyunsaturated, found in corn and rope oils, some types of nuts and fatty fish such as salmon or mackerel. In this diet, the ideal is to replace saturated and trans fats with monounsaturated and polyunsaturated fats, especially omega-3 fatty acids.

6. What other nutritional advice can be given to these patients?

A recommended diet for patients with fatty liver or cirrhosis is the Mediterranean, which is characterized by vegetable-based meals, with only small amounts of beef and chicken, and more servings of whole grains, fresh fruits and vegetables, nuts and legumes .

It usually reduces the consumption of meats and carbohydrates and increase that of vegetables and monounsaturated fats, which helps to lose weight.

On the other hand, it is advisable to add low-glycemic foods to your diet, such as green leafy vegetables, most fruits, raw carrots, chickpeas, lentils and bran cereals; and avoid high places, such as rice, white bread, potatoes and honey.

Also that they take vitamin supplements, especially B, C and E complex, which act as protectors against liver inflammation.

Finally, when cooking, they are recommended olive oil and avoid other fats.

Chapter 17. Diet for irritable bowel FODMAP

Irritable bowel or colon syndrome is a chronic functional disorder of the digestive tract that causes abdominal pain and swelling and gas. People with this medical condition can alternate between periods of constipation and diarrhea. The causes of this condition are not entirely clear. It can appear after a bacterial intestinal infection, by parasites, or be a consequence of high levels of stress and nervousness.

The FODMAP diet, which is based on excluding certain foods that are difficult to absorb from the nutritional plan, is intended to alleviate its symptoms.

To learn more about this topic, we interview Mario Vega Carbó, an endocrinologist, with more than 20 years of experience.

Doctor Mario,
1. What is the FODMAP diet?

The name FODMAP refers to the English meaning of oligosaccharides, disaccharides, monosaccharides and fermentable polyols ("Fermentable Oligosaccharides, Disaccharides, Monosaccharides And Polyols").

All these are carbohydrates that are characterized by not being digested completely by the intestine, but they move towards the colon, where they cause gases that cause abdominal distention. Therefore, this diet seeks to eliminate them from the food plan, in order to avoid these consequences.

2. How is the process of implementing this diet?

In a first stage all foods are eliminated with fermentable carbohydrates, with the aim of achieving digestive stability. Then, once an improvement of the symptoms is achieved, small amounts of these foods can be introduced gradually to check the individual tolerance to each of them.

Based on this, a nutritional plan is established as varied, complete and balanced as possible to continue over time, limiting only those that cause serious disorders.

3. What foods should be avoided in the FODMAP diet?

Among foods with fermentable carbohydrates that should be limited are milk and its milk derivatives such as cheese and yogurt; cereals of wheat, barley, rye, oats and brown rice; garlic, artichoke, eggplant, onion, cabbage, asparagus, lettuce, pepper, leek and beet; olives, avocado, cranberry, cherry, plum, raspberry, strawberry, apple, mango, peach, melon, blackberry, pear, watermelon and grape; all legumes except soy; almonds and hazelnuts; sausages, cold cuts, hamburgers and sausages of pork, veal, turkey or chicken; the butter; and sugar, chocolate and honey.

In addition, it is recommended to avoid excess fiber, especially if you suffer from diarrhea, and products that contain gluten. Also the pastries, candies, cookies, custards, ice cream, sauces, broths, soft drinks and alcohol.

4. What foods are allowed in this diet?

Among the foods for free consumption are dairy products with or without low lactose content; cereals of corn, wheat and refined rice, and quinoa; chard, zucchini, squash, spinach, cucumber, tomato and carrot; coconut, kiwi, lemon, orange, tangerine, passion fruit, pineapple and banana; the nuts; the soy; seafood, mollusks, white and blue fish, white and red meats; the eggs; Olive and sunflower oil and margarine. On the other hand, it is recommended to increase water consumption.

5. How long is it advisable to follow the FODMAP diet?

The first phase of the diet, which is the most restrictive, is recommended to be followed for no more than 6 weeks until digestive stability is achieved. It is not advisable to continue it in the long term to avoid nutritional deficiencies, since it limits many products that are considered basic. Then it is important to progressively introduce other foods according to individual tolerance.

6. For what other purposes can this diet be used?

In addition to the irritable bowel, the FODMAP diet can help treat ulcerative colitis, Crohn's disease and other intestinal discomforts.

7. What other aspects are important during this treatment?

In addition to taking care of food, to improve irritable bowel syndrome, regular exercise, drinking plenty of water and controlling stress through relaxation techniques or yoga are also recommended.

Chapter 18. Biliary Protection Diet

The gallbladder is a bag-shaped organ in which the bile produced by the liver accumulates. This liquid helps digestion and the breakdown of fats present in food into fatty acids that can be absorbed.

A proper diet can prevent symptoms of colic and biliary dyspepsia, and prevent stone formation.

In addition, it also allows a better recovery of patients after a cholecystectomy, a surgical intervention in which the organ is removed when it is infected, inflamed or blocked by lithiasis.

To learn more about this topic, we consulted Dr. Mario Vega Carbó, an endocrinology specialist, who works at the Vega & Vado Office.

Doctor Mario,
1. What are the main nutritional recommendations to protect the gallbladder?

First of all, you should try to limit the fat in all its forms, consuming a maximum of about 40 grams per day, preferably of vegetable origin. In addition, the diet should be rich in carbohydrates (rice, pasta, potatoes, legumes and bread), in fruits and vegetables.

Among other foods, hot and mild infusions of tea and chamomile are recommended; skim milk in small quantities; well-cooked vegetable broth soups; porridge, lentil and corn porridge; mashed potatoes or legumes; beef, rabbit, chicken, turkey or ram; the lean ham; and low-fat white fish.

2. What other foods are recommended in this diet?

To those already mentioned we can add skim milk, natural yogurt, fresh cheese, white or toasted plan, white rice, simple pasta (not egg), Maria-type cookies and roasted or compote fruits.

On the other hand, to protect the gallbladder it is also advised to eat slowly, in small amounts, chew well and divide the intake into 4 or 5 daily meals.

3. What foods should be avoided?

In this diet you should avoid fatty meats, such as lamb, pork, chicken and all sausages; the chocolate and the quince jam; blue or canned fish; the seafood; hard or fried eggs; fatty and fermented cheeses; the nuts; vegetable margarines and butters; Alcohol and soft drinks.

Also flatulent foods (cabbage, cauliflower, broccoli, whole sifted legumes, cucumber and raw onion) or spicy, pastries, pastries and pastries, especially industrial, and copious meals.

As for milk and its derivatives, they should be skimmed.

4. What type of cooking is recommended?

Those with low fat incorporated, without frying and without heating above 100 degrees are recommended. Some options are steaming, water, baked, grilled, grilled, grilled or wrapped in vegetable or aluminum foil.

On the other hand, olive oil is preferable to that of other seeds, such as sunflower, corn and soy. In addition, it is recommended to avoid stews and stews, and eliminate sauces.

5. How can biliary lithiasis be prevented?

To prevent stone formation it is important not to skip meals and maintain a healthy weight, reducing the number of calories ingested and doing regular physical activity.

In the case of needing to lose weight, the loss should be done slowly since if it is carried out quickly it can increase the risks of lithiasis.

As for the diet, it must be low in fat, low in cholesterol and high in fiber. It should prioritize foods of plant origin, which have few calories, less fat and a lot of fiber.

Chapter 19. Diet for the control and prevention of thyroid diseases

The thyroid is one of the most important glands in the body and its activity influences metabolism and most of the body's functions, such as heart rate and blood pressure.

That there are normal levels of its hormones in the body is essential for healthy growth and development in childhood, and for the functioning of the brain throughout life. Among the most common problems that can affect the gland are hypothyroidism, hyperthyroidism and goiter. A proper diet can help control and prevent this type of ailments.

To learn more about this topic, we interview Mario Vega Carbó, a specialist in clinical endocrinology.

Doctor Mario,
1. What nutritional guidelines can be followed to prevent thyroid damage and hypothyroidism?

First, it is important to reinforce the consumption of foods with iodine and selenium, which help the gland to function properly. Iodine is present in fish, seaweed, lobsters, tuna, turkey breast, sardines, seafood, bread, eggs, cow's milk, cheeses, yogurt, ice cream, iodized table salt and soy products. For its part, selenium is obtained in cashew seeds and nuts. As for fats, the consumption of those of good quality should be increased, such as those provided by avocado, olive or canola oil, quinoa, salmon and nuts in general.

On the other hand, it is also good to eat a lot of antioxidant glutathione, which strengthens the thyroid's immune system. This is found in asparagus, broccoli, garlic, grapefruit and peach, and can also be consumed by supplements. In addition, it is recommended to consume quality probiotics and fermented foods.

2. What foods should be avoided?

On the one hand you should stop using stimulants such as caffeine, alcohol and sugar, which increase stress, which can be harmful to the thyroid. In addition, care should be taken with goitrogens, substances present in cruciferous vegetables and some fruits. These have the ability to block the absorption and use of iodine, slowing thyroid activity, and may favor the development of goiter.

3. What are the most common goitrogens?

Among the foods that have this substance are broccoli, Brussels sprouts, millet, mustard, cabbage, cauliflower, radishes, kale, peaches, peanuts, turnip, spinach, almonds, Cranberries, strawberries and watercress.

4. Should these foods be eliminated from the diet?

Many of these foods are rich in vitamins and minerals, in addition to antioxidants, so it is not advisable to definitely remove them from the diet. The important thing is not to eat them raw, so you have to cook them beforehand to reduce the goitrogen effect.

5. What kind of meats are most recommended?

It is preferable to consume white meat such as chicken or fish, which have more protein.

6. What foods affect the absorption of thyroid hormone?

Soy and the foods and supplements that contain it can decrease the amount of hormone absorbed by the body. In addition, coffee and certain foods enriched with dietary fiber can interfere with the absorption of levothyroxine.

7. In what cases is it advisable to follow a diet high or low in iodine?

As I mentioned earlier, iodine helps the gland to function properly and is a necessary element for the production of thyroid hormone. Its deficiency can produce an enlarged thyroid (goiter) and hypothyroidism.

On the contrary, people with hyperthyroidism should control their intake, since their consumption can make symptoms worse.

Similarly, a diet low in this mineral may be recommended to increase the effectiveness of a radioactive iodine treatment.

8. What should be taken into account in a diet for hyperthyroidism?

This diet should seek to increase the consumption of some foods that reduce thyroid activity and avoid those that encourage it. To block the absorption and use of iodine, foods with goitrogens mentioned above can be consumed.

Also, those foods high in caffeic and chlorogenic acids, which reduce thyroid activity. Among them we can mention celery, orange, lemon, carrot, plum, eggplant and grapes.

In addition, dairy products and other foods rich in calcium and iron are recommended. Also an increase in protein and calorie intake to counteract catabolism. On the contrary, in addition to foods with iodine, exciting drinks and fatty meats should be avoided.

Meanwhile, spirulina dietary supplement is contraindicated if you have hyperthyroidism.

Chapter 20. Diet for Polycystic Ovary Syndrome

Polycystic Ovary Syndrome is a common disorder in women of reproductive age, who have an elevated level of androgen-like hormones in their body.

Its main signs include irregular menstruation, excessive hair growth in areas of male distribution, severe acne and infertility. In addition, this condition usually involves other metabolic disorders such as hyperinsulinemia, insulin resistance, high cholesterol and triglyceride levels, and eating disorders.

A special diet and regular physical activity can help reduce your symptoms.

To learn more about this topic, we interview Mario Vega Carbó, an endocrinologist with more than 20 years of experience.

Doctor Mario,
1. How can a proper diet control this condition?

Obese women are more likely to develop Polycystic Ovary Syndrome and in them the symptoms of the disease are usually more severe. Therefore, a diet that allows to maintain an adequate and healthy weight is important to prevent and mitigate its signs.

On the other hand, in women who have insulin resistance, controlling levels of this hormone through food can help restore ovarian function, menstrual cycles and fertility.

2. What is the diet for Polycystic Ovary Syndrome?

In general, for these cases, a low carb diet is recommended that allows weight loss and blood glucose control, improving insulin resistance. For this, the ideal is to consume those that have a low glycemic index and are rich in proteins and healthy fats with anti-inflammatory action.

3. What types of foods are usually included in this diet?

Among foods that have a low glycemic index are green leafy vegetables, most fruits, raw carrots, chickpeas, lentils and bran cereals. In addition, the diet usually includes white meats without preservatives, veal liver, blue fish, whole wheat flour and other high-fiber foods.

Within the consumption of protein, the ideal is that it is 50 percent animal and the other 50 vegetable, being able to find the latter in legumes, soybeans, quinoa, nuts and seeds.

4. What foods are usually reduced in these cases?

In this diet, refined flours, rice, white bread, potatoes, honey and foods and drinks with a lot of sugar, which have a high glycemic index, are usually avoided.

It is also important to reduce dairy, cereals with gluten, vegetable oils, cookies, cakes and desserts, fast foods, industrial pastries and ultra-processed products.

5. What other aspects are important in this diet?

These people are recommended to eat small portions throughout the day, maintain regular feeding schedules and not spend more than 4 hours without ingesting anything, as this can favor the decompensation of blood sugar and insulin levels.

In addition, they are also advised to include in each meal a source of low-fat protein, which helps control appetite. Some options are cooked egg, fish or chicken.

Finally, if necessary, women with this syndrome may be prescribed magnesium supplements, chromium picolinate, Omega-3 fatty acids and flaxseed to supplement the diet.

Chapter 21. Gluten-free diet for celiac people

A gluten-free diet is a food plan that excludes this protein and is especially designed for people with celiac disease. Gluten is a substance present in wheat, barley and rye, which can also be found in vitamins, supplements, hair and skin products, dentifrices and lipsticks.

When a celiac consumes it, it causes the immune system to damage and inflame the small intestine, generating diarrhea, abdominal pain, anemia and constipation, among other symptoms.

To learn more about this diet, we consulted Dr. Mario Vega Carbó, an endocrinology specialist, in charge of the Vega & Vado Office.

Doctor Mario,
1. What foods are usually included in a gluten-free diet?

When planning this diet it is important to pay special attention to both the ingredients of the food and its nutritional content.

Among those that can be consumed without problems are fruits and vegetables, beans, seeds and nuts in their natural, unprocessed form; the eggs; fresh veal or pork, poultry, fish and seafood; and most low-fat dairy products.

On the other hand, among the cereals, starches and flours allowed are amaranth, arrowroot, buckwheat, corn, flax, millet, quinoa, rice, sorghum, soybeans, tapioca.

Meanwhile, sweeteners include jellies; the jams; Honey; peanut butter; corn starch; brown, white or icing sugar; and as spices and herbs seasonings; the salt; the pepper; the olives; mustard and distilled vinegars.

2. What foods are not allowed?

In this diet you should avoid all foods and beverages that contain wheat, barley, rye and, in some cases, oats.

All wheat derivatives such as Grahan or yeast flour, the scab, the farro, the kamut, the spelled and the semolina should also be excluded.

In addition, unless indicated that they are gluten free, beer is also not recommended; bread; sausages; the patents; melted, grated or spread cheeses; cakes and pies; the candies; the cereals; the communion hosts; sweet cookies; French fries; the malt; Pasta; hotdogs and canned meat and fish; the sauces; chocolate and cocoa; The Ice creams; salad dressings; seasoned rice mixes; soups or broths and poultry marinated with oils or fats.

3. How can you tell if a food or drink has gluten?

When buying processed foods you should read the labels of the products carefully, since there is indicated if they contain wheat, barley, rye or triticale, any derived ingredient or if they were processed with them.

4. What effects does this diet have on coeliacs and for how long should it be followed?

Celiac disease has no cure, so the gluten-free diet must be strictly followed throughout life.

Food care usually works in most patients, who achieve an improvement in symptoms after two weeks, serological normalization between 6 and 12 months and recovery of intestinal villi around 2 years.

5. What benefits does this diet have for non-celiac people?

While some people claim that this diet can improve overall health, help you lose weight and increase energy and athletic performance, there is not enough medical or scientific evidence to confirm it.

On the other hand, this diet is useful for those who have a gluten sensitivity not related to celiac disease or wheat allergy.

6. What risks can this type of food bring?

Many of the foods that contain gluten provide important vitamins and other nutrients, such as iron, calcium and fiber that must be replaced by others. On the contrary, many of those who do not have this protein have higher fat and sugar content, so healthy alternatives should be chosen.

7. What other precautions should celiacs follow with food?

If you have doubts about whether or not a food has gluten, it is advisable not to eat it. As for manufactured, processed or packaged products, labels should be carefully controlled, while those produced by hand or those in which their ingredients cannot be checked, it is recommended to discard them.

Chapter 22. Lactose free diet

The lactose-free diet is a food plan that excludes this sugar present in the milk of mammals and other dairy products.

It is especially designed for those people who have intolerance to this substance, which usually occurs when the small intestine does not produce enough of the enzyme lactase.

This creates difficulty digesting milk sugar, producing gas, bloating, cramping and diarrhea. Eating a lactose-free diet is not difficult, although many times dairy products are very present in our diet, so it is necessary to take special care.

To learn more about this topic, we consulted Dr. Mario Vega Carbó, an endocrinology specialist, with more than 20 years of experience.

Doctor Mario,
1. What are the main foods that have lactose?

Among the foods that have this substance we can mention the mammalian milk, evaporated, condensed and the milk cream; the butter; cream; the cheese; the yogurts; The Ice creams; the flan; rice pudding; the mousse; and milk chocolate.

In addition, other products that may contain lactose are margarine, creams, soups, purees, bread, sausages, pre-cooked dishes, meat fritters, salad dressings, cakes and pies, enriched cereals, cookies, chocolate substitutes, alcoholic beverages, toothpaste, vitamin supplements and some medications.

2. What foods are allowed in this diet?

Lactose-free foods include natural fruits, nuts, fish and shellfish, cereals, eggs, honey, marmalade, potatoes, rice, pasta, vegetables, legumes, white meat and red, and soy drinks, coconut and oatmeal.

3. How can you tell if a food contains lactose?

When you buy food you should read the labels of the products carefully, since there it is indicated if they contain lactose or not. In many cases this substance is added to foods such as breads, sauces and snacks so it is important to review each particular item.

4. Can this diet include milk and adapted products without lactose?

Yes, adapted lactose-free milks and products, such as cheeses, creams, butters, yogurts and custards, can be consumed without problems.

To these foods are added lactase artificially, which generates that it no longer contains lactose, but glucose and galactose, which are sugars that the body can digest without problems.

These products keep all the nutrients of the original food, so they are highly recommended for people with intolerance to this substance.

5. How can people with lactose intolerance consume dairy products without later having digestive discomfort?

On the one hand there are the adapted products without lactose that I mentioned before.

Another option is to look for the most tolerated dairy and consume them in very small doses throughout the day. Most people with low lactase levels can drink up to half a cup of milk without symptoms.

Dairy products that are easier to digest include milk butter, hard cheeses such as Swiss or cheddar, fermented products such as yogurt, goat milk, and soy or rice formulas for young children.

It is also possible to take a medicine with the enzyme lactase, which helps digest more lactose without being bothered.

6. What are the precautions to be taken in this diet?

If it is decided to eliminate dairy products completely, it is important to look for alternative foods that are rich in the same nutrients calcium, vitamin D, riboflavin and other proteins to avoid deficiencies.

Calcium, for example, can be obtained from sardines and canned salmon; prawns; dark green vegetables, such as turnip, cabbage and broccoli; oranges; figs; tofu, almonds; brazilian nuts; sunflower seeds; and white beans. If necessary, you can take calcium supplements with vitamin D.

7. What happens if a lactose intolerant person consumes it?

When this occurs, the person may have a series of unpleasant symptoms such as swelling, diarrhea, nausea and gas, which will decrease their intensity as the body eliminates undigested lactose.

Part II NUTRITION

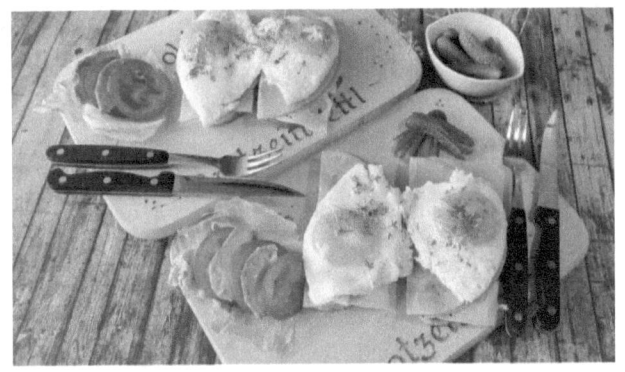

Chapter 23. Endocrine disruptors

"Invisible" contaminants that affect our health"

We live with them daily. Endocrine disruptors are present in the air, on the ground, in water, in beverages, in food, in cleaning and personal hygiene items, in insecticides and in a large number of other products. The worst part is that, without our knowledge, they seriously affect our body and our health, and also that of our children.

We are talking about endocrine disruptors, a series of chemical or biological substances, usually produced by man, that alter the glands responsible for the natural secretion of hormones that regulate our body.

Among other consequences, this can cause neurological and behavioral changes, interfere with thyroid function, affect reproductive health, weaken the immune system and alter sexual development. In addition, it can increase the risks of diabetes, obesity and certain types of cancer.

To learn more about this topic, we interviewed Cuban doctor Mario Vega Carbó, a specialist in clinical endocrinology.

Doctor Mario,
1. What is the endocrine system and what is its function?

The endocrine system is the set of organs and tissues responsible for secreting hormones, which are released into the bloodstream to regulate some of the functions of our body, such as the speed of growth, metabolism, development of sexual organs and aspects of our behavior It is one of the three most important systems of integration and regulation of our body, along with the nervous and immune systems.

2. What are endocrine disruptors and how do they affect us?

Endocrine disruptors are substances capable of altering the hormonal balance and regulation of the endocrine system, which can cause harmful effects on health.

They can interfere, either by increasing, blocking or decreasing the chemical signals of hormones, sending confusing messages to the body and generating consequences of all kinds.

For example, it can cause disorders related to women's reproductive health, such as breast cancer, infertility, precocious puberty; disorders of male reproductive function, such as prostate cancer, decreased semen quality, congenital malformations; metabolic disorders such as diabetes or obesity; neurological diseases such as behavioral changes, attention deficit hyperactivity disorder, autism and Parkinson's; Thyroid cancer and cardiovascular disorders.

3. In addition to all these effects, what would be the most serious of this situation?

The most serious of all is that the sequelae of endocrine disruptors on the body are usually cumulative and irreversible. In addition, its impacts can be imperceptible during one generation and transmitted to the next without having manifested itself pathologically. In this way, someone who has never been exposed to these substances can also suffer its consequences.

On the other hand, endocrine disruptors are also harmful to the environment and wildlife.

4. Where are these substances present?

Endocrine disruptors are present everywhere and we live with them daily in our homes, at work, at school and on the street. You can find them in food, pesticides, personal hygiene and cleaning products, construction and decoration materials, air fresheners, paints, cosmetics, insecticides, toys, clothes, appliances and electronic devices.

The catalog of chemical substances that alter the endocrine system is very wide and grows day by day.

5. What can we do to avoid exposure to endocrine disruptors?

In principle, try to avoid products made with polycarbonate or polyvinyl chloride, and reduce the consumption of canned foods, processed foods and packaging with PVC film. In addition, it is preferable to consume fresh fruits and vegetables than frozen.

It is also advised to use glass bottles and containers, to avoid plastic materials that can release BPA or phthalates, and avoid heating plastics with food.

On the other hand, it is necessary to dispense with the use of anabolic, non-stick in the kitchen and insecticides in the home and control the composition of cosmetics and detergents. In children and babies, use bisphenol A-free pacifiers and avoid plastic toys that contain plasticizers. In all cases, always try to consume organic products.

6. What other preventive measures can we take at the society level?

In addition to the control and elimination measures of these substances by governments, it is essential that research on their effects on health and the environment is continued in order to take preventive actions.

Chapter 24. Extreme Thinness and its dangers

According to the conventional aesthetic patterns of our time, thinness is usually considered attractive and a beauty canon. However, just as obesity is very dangerous for health, extreme thinness is too.

Thinness is a condition that occurs when a person's body weight is lower than what would correspond to him according to his age, sex and size. Some of the causes that can cause it are poor nutrition, the use of drugs such as alcohol, smoking, mental and nutritional problems, inherited factors and other underlying diseases.

To learn more about this issue, we interview Cuban doctor Mario Vega Carbó, an endocrinology specialist.

Doctor Mario,
1. What is considered extreme thinness?

It is generally considered that someone suffers from this disorder when their Body Mass Index (BMI) is below 18. The BMI is calculated by dividing the weight of a person by the meters of height squared (kg / m2).

2. What are the main causes of thinness?

In some cases it can be caused by physical and genetic issues, such as a scarcer adipose tissue than usual, which means that the body does not have the ability to accumulate large amounts of fat, or an accelerated metabolism.

It can also be a consequence of another disease, such as diabetes, some types of cancer or HIV; an addiction to alcohol, drugs or smoking; the consumption of certain medications; a chronic infection or excessive use of laxatives.

Other possible reasons are too low diets, eating disorders such as anorexia and bulimia, stress and anxiety situations and mental or psychiatric problems.

3. What damage can this disorder cause?

Low potassium levels can cause muscle cramps and pain and, in severe cases, brain inflammation. Insufficient protein and nutrient shortages can also damage the immune system and make people more prone to infections and disease.

In addition, extreme thinness can lead to fertility problems, irregular menses, erectile dysfunction, risky pregnancies, osteoporosis, arrhythmias and anemias, among other disorders.

4. What are your main symptoms?

Some signs are brittle and dull hair, pale skin and mucous membranes, peeling skin, eye problems, white spots on teeth, the appearance of wounds and swelling of the lips and concave nails. Also fatigue, weakness, exhaustion, low blood pressure, palpitations and low blood sugar levels.

5. What is the treatment of extreme thinness?

If it is caused by another disease, it should be treated. If the patient is healthy and does not have associated pathologies, a nutritious diet rich in calories can be prescribed and seek to reduce energy expenditure.

In these cases the consumption of pasta, nuts, honey, brown rice, oils, meats, fish, eggs, dairy products, fruits and vegetables is recommended, in the proportions suggested by a nutritionist.

Physical exercise is beneficial to health and helps to whet your appetite and build muscle mass. However, people with extreme thinness should follow moderate training routines. In cases where necessary, medications can be given to stimulate appetite.

Finally, if the reason is an eating disorder or a psychological problem, they should be treated by a special therapist.

Chapter 25. Celiac Disease or Celiac Disease

Celiac disease is a disease of the immune system in which people cannot consume gluten because it damages and inflames their small intestine.

Gluten is a protein present in wheat, barley and rye, which can also be found in vitamins, supplements, hair and skin products, dentifrices and lipsticks.

This medical condition affects each patient differently. Your symptoms may manifest in the digestive system or in other parts of the body. Some people may have diarrhea and abdominal pain, others feel irritated or depressed and others show no sign.

To learn more about this condition, we consult Dr. Mario Vega Carbó, a specialist in clinical endocrinology.

Doctor Mario,
1. What are the causes of Celiac disease?

Celiac disease is a fairly common inherited condition. Patients usually have anti-endomysial antibodies with atrophy of the intestinal villi. It is estimated that infant feeding practices, infections, environmental agents and bacteria in the intestines can contribute to their appearance.

In some cases the condition is activated after surgery, pregnancy, childbirth, a viral infection or intense emotional stress.

2. How is this disease diagnosed?

Its diagnosis is usually complicated, because its same symptoms are also present in many other diseases.

To detect it, it is necessary to analyze the patient's family history, perform blood tests, serological studies and, in some cases, examine a small sample of small intestine tissue.

3. Who are more likely to suffer it?

Celiac disease can affect anyone. However, it usually occurs more frequently in people with a family member who already has the condition. Those with type 1 diabetes, Down or Turner syndrome, autoimmune thyroid disease, rheumatoid arthritis, primary biliary cirrhosis, microscopic colitis, psoriasis, vitiligo, epilepsy or adrenal insufficiency are also more likely.

This condition can manifest itself at any time in life, being diagnosed to the same extent in both adults and children.

4. What are its main signs?

If a celiac eats gluten, this triggers an immune response in the small intestine. Over time this damages the lining of the organ and prevents the absorption of some nutrients. The disease often causes severe diarrhea, heavy bowel movements, fatigue, weight loss, bloating, gas, abdominal pain, nausea, vomiting and constipation, although symptoms vary from person to person.

In children, insufficient absorption of nutrients can affect growth and development, causing short stature and late puberty.

5. What other symptoms may occur?

In addition to intestinal symptoms, Celiac disease can cause deterioration of tooth enamel, canker sores, headache and joint pain, spleen problems, irregular menses, hair loss and nervous system injuries..

Another very common sign is dermatitis herpetiformis, a skin disease that causes itching and blisters. This rash may appear on the elbows, knees, torso, scalp and buttocks.

On the other hand, Celiac disease can also cause irritability, depression and attention and concentration problems.

6. What is the treatment of this medical condition?

Celiac disease has no cure. The treatment consists of following a strict gluten-free diet for life. This involves avoiding wheat, barley, rye, bulgur, flour and whole-wheat flour, malt, semolina and triticale. Food care usually works in most patients, who achieve an improvement in symptoms after two weeks, serological normalization between 6 and 12 months and recovery of intestinal villi around 2 years.

Those who do not respond to therapy may have other conditions, such as bacteria in the intestine, problems in the pancreas or irritable bowel syndrome. If the intestine is severely damaged, there is a steroid treatment that reduces inflammation and medications that suppress the immune system.

On the other hand, if Celiac disease caused a significant nutritional deficiency, the intake of vitamins and mineral supplements will be necessary.

7. What other damage can this disease cause?

By preventing the absorption of some nutrients, Celiac disease can cause malnutrition and, therefore, anemia and a decrease in body weight.

Also loss of calcium, vitamin D and bone density, generating rickets, osteoporosis, infertility and more chance of having abortions.

On the other hand, intestinal damage can cause lactose intolerance, increased risk of some types of cancer, liver disorders and neurological problems, such as seizures.

8. What other recommendations should be taken into account?

In addition to eating a proper diet, patients should also be aware of the hidden gluten in certain medications and non-food products, such as vitamin supplements, lipsticks, mouthwashes and toothpastes.

Chapter 26. Anorexia nervosa

Anorexia nervosa is an eating and emotional disorder that causes people to lose more weight than is considered healthy.

In general, those who suffer from it have a distorted perception of their figures, become obsessed and reject food systematically. The condition is usually accompanied by provoked vomiting, starvation, excessive exercise, extreme weight loss and, in the case of women, disappearance of menstruation. These patients also use improperly laxatives, diuretics and dietary supplements to try to lose weight.

To learn more about this topic, we interview Mario Vega Carbó, a specialist in endocrinology, nutrition and family medicine, who works as an endocrinologist at the Vega & Vado Office.

Doctor Mario,
1. What are the causes of anorexia nervosa?

There is no exact cause that explains this ailment, but it is estimated that it is the result of a combination of biological, hormonal, psychological, social and emotional factors. While it is more common in women during adolescence, anorexia can also affect men and people of any age.

2. What are your main symptoms?

These people usually have a lower weight than what is considered normal for their age and height. Your physical symptoms may include yellow or dry skin, fatigue, insomnia, dizziness and fainting, dry mouth, extreme sensitivity to cold, thin or brittle hair, constipation and abdominal pain.

In addition, there may be low blood pressure, dehydration, irregular heartbeat, swelling of the arms or legs, osteoporosis, loss of body fat, muscle atrophy and dental erosion.

On the other hand, these patients often present with confusing or slow thoughts, depression, irritability and emotional and behavioral problems associated with an unreal perception of body weight and an intense fear of gaining weight.

They can also spend a lot of time without feeding and, when they do, they cause vomiting to expel it. Therefore, they usually go to the bathroom immediately after meals, while others refuse to eat in front of other people.

Other signs are to follow very strict diets, skip meals and exercise excessively.

3. How is this disease diagnosed?

Faced with its symptoms, tests are usually done to determine the cause of weight loss, rule out other medical conditions and assess the damage that the disease has caused.

This usually includes a physical examination, bone density tests, blood and urine tests, electrocardiographies, kidney, liver and thyroid function tests, and a psychological evaluation, among other studies.

4. What is your treatment?

The therapy should be followed by a multidisciplinary team that includes doctors, nutritionists and mental health professionals.

The main challenge is to get the patient to understand that he has a serious problem that needs attention. Most people with anorexia often deny that they suffer from an eating disorder and therefore do not seek help until the damage is serious.

In the first place, the patient will seek to recover weight and follow healthy eating habits, with routines and schedules marked for eating.

On the other hand, to treat depression or anxiety, certain medications may be prescribed. In cases of severe malnutrition, psychiatric problems or situations in which there is a danger to life, hospitalization and intravenous or tube feeding may be necessary.

In addition, support groups and individual and family therapy can also be an important part of treatment.

5. What complications can anorexia nervosa bring?

This medical condition can cause a decrease in bone mass; an increased risk of infections; anemia; heart, gastrointestinal, kidney, thyroid gland and seizure problems.

In addition, malnutrition and dehydration can cause serious and irreversible damage to different organs.

On the other hand, anorexia can even be fatal, as a result of arrhythmias or an electrolyte imbalance.

As for psychological and emotional disorders, there may be obsessive and compulsive behaviors, depression, anxiety, personality changes, suicidal thoughts and self-harm.

Chapter 27. Bulimiaa

Bulimia is an eating disorder of neurotic origin that is characterized by periods of compulsive eating, followed by others of guilt and discomfort in which vomiting is caused or laxatives or diuretics are consumed to prevent weight gain. It is usually observed in young women, although it can also occur in men and people of any age.

The limitation of self-imposed food leads the bulimic to a strong state of anxiety and the pathological need to ingest large amounts of food. Many patients suffering from this disease also suffer from anorexia. Bulimia is a serious and life-threatening condition.

To learn more about this topic, we interview Mario Vega Carbó, a specialist in endocrinology, nutrition, who works as an endocrinologist at the Santa Fe Medical Center and the Vega & Vado Office.

Doctor Mario,
1. What are the causes of bulimia?

The causes involved in the onset of bulimia are numerous and sometimes difficult to determine. In its origin, biological, hormonal, psychological, emotional and social factors participate that distort the patient's vision of himself. Usually this condition manifests itself after having made numerous harmful diets without medical control. In addition, it is estimated that half of the cases of anorexia lead to bulimia.

2. What are your main symptoms?

Bulimics often see themselves as overweight, but often have a normal weight, so it is possible that people around them do not detect anything unusual. Some common behaviors are spending a lot of time exercising, going to the bathroom immediately after eating, losing control during the binge and then forcing vomiting or using laxatives or diuretics, fasting or skipping meals, or refusing to eat in front of other people. The cycles of compulsive intake and subsequent purging manifest at least twice a week.

On the other hand, these patients may present weakness; headache; sores, scars or calluses on the knuckles or hands; dental erosion; dizziness menstrual irregularities and inflammation of the face, arms and feet.

3. What is the treatment of bulimia?

The goals of therapy are to correct the eating and psychological disorders of the ailment. To do this, they work together with a multidisciplinary team that includes doctors, nutritionists and mental health professionals.

First, it seeks to avoid vomiting, normalize metabolic functioning and that the patient follow a balanced diet and healthy eating habits.

In addition, treatment usually includes the combination of psychotherapy with antidepressants, family collaboration and participation in support groups.

4. What complications can this ailment bring?

Bulimia is a chronic disease and many patients continue to have some symptoms even with therapy. On the other hand, repetitive vomiting can cause permanent damage to the esophagus, throat inflammation and severe tooth decay.

Other complications include dehydration, constipation, hemorrhoids, heart problems and damage to the pancreas.

As for psychological and emotional disorders, there may be obsessive and compulsive behaviors, negative self-esteem, depression, anxiety, personality changes and relationship problems.

5. What is the difference between bulimia and anorexia?

These diseases differ in that in anorexia there are usually no bingeing or overfeeding, but a strict restriction of food, so over time the purges disappear through vomiting.

Instead, the bulimic suffers a feeling of lack of control over the food that he later blames.

On the other hand, by gradually reducing food, in the anorexic, weight loss is evident, while in bulimic changes are not usually as marked.

As for the personality, the anorexic is usually obsessive, perfectionist and rigid, and usually does not eat anything outside the self-established. For its part, the bulimic is impulsive and has no self-control, and usually eats food improvisedly.

Chapter 28. Hypercholesterolemia or high cholesterol

Hypercholesterolemia is a disorder in which excessively high levels of cholesterol are present in the blood. Cholesterol is a natural body fat that serves to form new cells and certain hormones. It does not dissolve in the blood, but accumulates and circulates through the veins and arteries with the help of proteins that carry lipids.

When it is elevated, fatty deposits may form in the blood vessels. This increases the chances of clogged arteries, heart attacks, strokes and other complications of the circulatory system. Hypercholesterolemia can be caused by genetic disorders, although it is usually caused by other factors, such as an unhealthy lifestyle and certain diseases.

To learn more about this topic, we interview Mario Vega Carbó, an endocrinology specialist, who currently works as an endocrinologist at the Vega & Vado Office in Managua, Nicaragua.

Doctor Mario,
1. What are "good" and "bad" cholesterol?

Cholesterol circulates in the blood attached to proteins and the combination of both is called lipoprotein. LDL or "bad" cholesterol is a low density lipoprotein that carries its particles throughout the body. It accumulates in the walls of the arteries, and can cause hardening and narrowing. For its part, HDL or "good" cholesterol is responsible for collecting its excess and bringing it back to the liver.

2. What causes Hypercholesterolemia?

This condition is usually related to being overweight, an unhealthy diet and lack of physical exercise. In addition, Diabetes, kidney disease, Polycystic Ovary Syndrome, hypoactive thyroid gland, pregnancy, certain inherited disorders and some medications can also cause it.

100

3. Who has more risks of having it?

Obese people, those who do not exercise, smokers and those over 50 have a higher risk of suffering from it. Also those who eat many saturated fats and trans fats, red meats and whole dairy products and those who suffer from the aforementioned diseases.

4. How is this disease detected?

Hypercholesterolemia is detected by a blood test that measures the levels of cholesterol, triglycerides and other fats. Your diagnosis may also require a blood glucose test to check for diabetes and tests for kidney and thyroid function.

Normal values of LDL or "bad" cholesterol between 70 to 130 mg / dL, HDL or "good" cholesterol are considered if it is greater than 50 mg / dL and total cholesterol if it is less than 200 mg / dL.

As this condition has no symptoms, it is important to carry out periodic checks, at least once every 4 years if normal results are obtained. In case the levels are high, the doctor's instructions should be followed.

5. What is the treatment of Hypercholesterolemia?

The first step is to instill in the patient healthy lifestyle habits. This includes exercising regularly and maintaining adequate body weight. Also follow a low-salt diet that limits animal fats, and is rich in fruits, vegetables and whole grains, in addition to not smoking or drinking alcohol.

On the other hand, there are several types of medications that help lower cholesterol levels, such as statins, bile acid fixing resins and cholesterol absorption inhibitors.

Tolerance to these drugs varies from person to person and may have side effects, such as muscle and stomach aches, reversible memory loss, confusion, constipation, nausea, diarrhea and increased blood sugar.

6. What other disorders can Hypercholesterolemia cause?

This medical condition can cause the arteries to harden due to the accumulation of fat and other substances in their walls. Over time this can block them and cause a heart attack or stroke.

Chapter 29. Hypertriglyceridemia or high triglycerides

It is known as hypertriglyceridemia at the high level of triglycerides in the blood. These are the most common type of fat in the body and come from food. Its function is to store energy for times when you are not eating.

Regular intake of more calories than burned can cause hypertriglyceridemia. The excess of triglycerides in the blood increases the risks of suffering from heart disease, diabetes, overweight or liver or kidney problems.

To learn more about this topic, we interview Mario Vega Carbó, an endocrinology specialist with more than 20 years of experience.

Doctor Mario,
1. What is the difference between triglycerides and cholesterol?

Cholesterol is a natural body fat that serves to form new cells and certain hormones. Instead, triglycerides are ingested with meals and used for energy. The two are similar in that they cannot dissolve in the blood, but they accumulate and circulate through the veins and arteries with the help of proteins that transport lipids.

2. How are triglycerides measured?

Triglycerides are measured with a simple blood test, with 12 hours of fasting. Ideally, they are below 150 milligrams per deciliter (mg / dl).

Between 150 and 199 mg / dl, they are at the limit of developing problems. Above 200 mg / dl are already considered high and, when they approach or exceed 500 mg / dl, very high. The risks of cardiovascular disease increase as the level rises.

3. What causes excess triglycerides?

High levels may result from obesity, high cholesterol, smoking, excessive alcohol consumption, metabolic syndrome and other diseases such as diabetes mellitus, hypothyroidism and liver or kidney problems.

They may also be due to the intake of certain medications, such as birth control pills, beta-blockers, diuretics, steroids and certain drugs to treat breast cancer and the Human Immunodeficiency Virus.

On the other hand, in some cases they may be a consequence of genetic defects combined with environmental factors.

4. How is hypertriglyceridemia treated?

Opting for a healthy lifestyle generally helps normalize blood triglyceride levels. This includes eating foods low in fat and calories, avoiding sugar, refined carbohydrates and alcohol consumption.

It is important to replace the saturated fats found in meats with healthier options, such as olive oils and fish such as mackerel or salmon. Also exercise regularly, drink plenty of water, eliminate overweight and quit smoking.

If changes in lifestyle are not enough, the doctor may prescribe some medication such as statins, fibrates, omega-3 fatty acids and niacin to help normalize the level in the blood. If there is another disease that causes hypertriglyceridemia, it must be treated.

5. What other complications can this disorder bring?

Hypertriglyceridemia can contribute to hardening of the arteries or thickening of the arterial walls, which increases the chances of suffering from strokes, heart attacks and heart disease. Also, when levels are too high, this can cause acute inflammation of the pancreas.

Chapter 30. Dyslipidemias

Dyslipidemia is a disorder in which excessively high levels of blood fat concentration occur. This condition, which includes cholesterol and triglycerides, usually has no symptoms. Its appearance increases the chances of clogged arteries, heart attacks, strokes and other complications of the circulatory system.

Dyslipidemias are classified as primary, when they are due to genetic disorders and are familiar; and secondary, when they are caused by other factors, such as lifestyle and certain diseases.

To learn more about this topic, we interview Mario Vega Carbó, an endocrinology specialist and in charge of the Vega & Vado Office in Managua, Nicaragua.

Doctor Mario,
1. What causes dyslipidemia?

In adults this condition is usually related to being overweight, an unhealthy diet and lack of physical exercise. In addition, Diabetes, kidney disease, Polycystic Ovary Syndrome, hypoactive thyroid gland, pregnancy, certain inherited disorders and some medications can also cause it.

2. How is this condition detected?

Dyslipidemia is detected by a blood test that measures the levels of cholesterol, triglycerides and other fats. Your diagnosis may also require a blood glucose test to check for diabetes and tests for kidney and thyroid function. As this condition has no symptoms, it is important to carry out periodic checks, at least once every 4 years if normal results are obtained. In case the levels are high, the doctor's instructions should be followed.

3. What is the treatment of dyslipidemia?

The first step is to instill in the patient healthy lifestyle habits. This includes eating low-fat foods, exercising regularly and maintaining adequate body weight, as well as not smoking or drinking alcohol. On the other hand, there are several types of medications that help lower cholesterol levels (statins) and triglycerides (fibrates and niacin). Tolerance to these drugs varies from person to person and may have side effects, such as muscle and stomach aches, constipation, nausea and diarrhea.

4. What other recommendations can people with this condition follow?

For these patients it is also advised to distribute the food in 4 main meals and 2 snacks, and moderate the portion sizes.

Similarly, reduce the consumption of foods with a high content of saturated fats, sugar and salt; and eat at least 2 fruits and 3 servings of vegetables a day.

In addition, they are recommended to incorporate legumes, whole grains, seeds and dried fruits to the diet.

5. What other disorders can cause dyslipidemia?

This medical condition can cause the arteries to harden due to the accumulation of fat and other substances in their walls. Over time this can block them and cause a heart attack or stroke.

In addition, dyslipidemia may increase the risk of developing pancreatitis, a condition that causes severe abdominal pain and can be fatal.

Chapter 31. Obesity, a serious chronic disease that grows year by year

The data is increasingly alarming. In the world it is estimated that about 40 percent of adults are overweight and about 15 percent are obese. Among children and adolescents the figures are even more worrisome and specialists believe that it is one of the most serious public health issues of the 21st century.

Per year, about 3 million people die as a result of obesity and overweight, which cause an increase in cardiovascular and respiratory diseases, diabetes, musculoskeletal disorders and some types of cancer.

To learn more about this problem, we interview Dr. Mario Vega Carbó, an endocrinology specialist with more than 20 years of experience.

Doctor Mario,
1. What is obesity and how is it defined?

Obesity is a chronic disease that is characterized by excessive accumulation of fat in the body, which produces a clear increase in risk to the health of the person. Someone is considered obese when the percentage of fat exceeds 25 percent of body weight in men and 33 percent in women.

2. What are the main causes that cause it?

The origin and reason of obesity are due to a multitude of factors. It is important to understand that it is not a consequence only that the person eats a lot and has no willpower to lose weight. There are also social, cultural, economic and hereditary components that influence its diagnosis and proliferation.

3. What would be those other elements that must also be taken into account when analyzing this problem?
There are genetic factors, which are involved in 40-75 percent of the causes of obesity; age, which is associated with nutritional disorders and

physical inactivity; menopause; sedentary lifestyle; pharmacological treatments; stress; sleep problems and neurological, endocrine and psychiatric diseases. Of course, nutrition and physical activity are also very important, but as I said, they are not the only thing to analyze.

4. What role does the environment play in these cases?

The environment surrounding the patient is very important. It is essential that people have the possibility to choose a healthy way of life, with access to healthy food and places with spaces for exercise. Mainly in the case of children, their diet and physical habits depend on the environment and what it teaches them.

5. What is the recommended treatment for obesity?

Being a chronic disease, which is often not recognized as such, its treatment is complex. The first thing to do is to adopt a healthy diet in which the intake of fats, sugar and salt is reduced, and increase the consumption of fruits, vegetables, legumes, whole grains and nuts.

You should also do physical activity on a regular basis, which exceeds 150 minutes divided into at least 5 days a week. In the most extreme cases it may be necessary to prescribe medications and even get surgery.

On the other hand, it is important that the treatment be carried out by a multidisciplinary team that includes endocrinologists, nutritionists, obesity experts and psychologists to improve its effectiveness and attack all fronts.

6. In recent years, all kinds of miraculous diets have proliferated that generally do not produce the results they promise. What can you tell us about these diets?

These magical diets are very dangerous, because they mostly have no medical or scientific endorsement. They are also the cause of patients fail in their attempts to lose weight, get discouraged and fall back into routines harmful to their health.

7. What are gastric bypass and gastric sleeve?

They are two surgeries that restrict food intake by reducing the size of stomach and small intestine use. This produces a feeling of satiety with a lower consumption of food and a decrease in the production of insulin from the pancreas.

These treatments are increasingly used because they do not change the quality of life of patients after the intervention and because they achieve the greatest long-term weight loss.

8. Finally, what would you recommend to a person suffering from obesity?

The first thing I would say is that obesity is the second cause of preventable death derived from personal habits, surpassed only by smoking. That is why I would advise you to deal with specialists and not give up if you had previous bad experiences.

I would also seek to understand that changes in habit must be long term, since in most cases, when treatment is abandoned, weight is recovered. This is a disease that you have to take care of for life.

Chapter 32. Morbid Obesity and its risks

It is considered Morbid Obesity when a person has 45 kilos or more over their appropriate weight with a body mass index (BMI) of more than 40. It is a dangerous condition that, in addition to decreasing life expectancy, causes disability and social exclusion problems.

On the other hand, this condition contributes to the development of other chronic diseases, such as high blood pressure, diabetes, hypercholesterolemia, heart conditions and some types of cancer.

Morbid obesity is the most serious form of overweight. Education and the acquisition of healthy habits early are the best way to prevent it.

To learn more about this topic, we interview Dr. Mario Vega Carbó, an endocrinology specialist with more than 20 years of experience.

Doctor Mario,
1. What are the main causes of Morbid Obesity?

This disorder is usually due to a sum of elements. In addition to excessive calorie intake, genetic, environmental, psychological, social and cultural factors are also involved.

Family predisposition, sedentary lifestyle, lack of exercise, poor diet, low self-esteem, stress, sleep problems and depressive states can be some possible causes. Also the consumption of certain medications and the presence of other diseases, such as hypothyroidism and other endocrine and neurological disorders.

2. How does a person become so obese?

This is not a process that occurs from one day to the next, but is generally a problem that comes from childhood. A boy who was obese during childhood is more likely to be during adulthood. It is estimated that 60 percent of people who begin adolescence with overweight maintain it for the rest of their lives.

On the other hand, who suffers from Morbid Obesity has surely tried different diets, exercises or medications without result for several years, until reaching this extreme situation.

3. What other health complications causes this medical condition?

This condition usually increases diabetes risks; hypertension; heart, lung and neurological problems; certain types of cancer, such as breast and colon cancer; osteoporosis; hypoxemia and sleep apnea.

On the other hand, it also tends to generate low self-esteem, depression and social and behavioral problems.

4. How is Morbid Obesity treated?

Usually, in these situations where diet, exercise and medications have not achieved results, the only possible treatment is bariatric surgery.

Gastric Bypass and Gastric Sleeve, for example, are two surgical interventions that restrict food intake by reducing the size of stomach and small intestine use. This produces a feeling of satiety with less food consumption and a decrease in the production of insulin from the pancreas.

These treatments are increasingly used because they do not change the quality of life of patients after the intervention and because they achieve the greatest long-term weight loss.

On the other hand, they also favor the normalization of blood glucose and cholesterol levels, and the reduction of blood pressure and sleep apnea.

5. Can anyone undergo bariatric surgery?

No. It is generally only recommended for people between 18 and 60 years of age with excessive obesity, who have a low surgical risk, who have tried to combat obesity with traditional methods (exercise and diet) without succeeding HAVING THEM FULFILLED AT THE FOOT OF

THE LETTER, and / or that present risk or diseases derived from complications of obesity (diabetes, hypertension, for example).

It is important that these candidates do not present psychiatric illnesses or addictions and that they assume the commitment to continue with the treatment after the intervention.

6. How is Morbid Obesity prevented?

In recent years, obesity has progressively increased to become a serious public health problem. Education and the acquisition of healthy lifestyle habits since childhood are essential to try to prevent it.

7. What other aspects must be taken into account during this medical condition?

In addition to physical and health problems, people who suffer from this condition are often subject to discrimination and social stigma. Many times they are rejected by their own family, they find it difficult to get a job, they have trouble moving and end up locked in their own illness.

In these cases, to guarantee the success of the treatment, the support of the environment is essential. In addition, if necessary, therapeutic follow-up is also recommended.

Chapter 33. Obesity drugs: Orlistat and Phentermine

The adoption of a healthy and balanced diet, together with the practice of regular exercise, are the first measures usually taken to treat obesity.

In severe cases, it is possible the doctor also recommends adding to this plan the use of prescription drugs to lose weight. They are generally used when the body mass index is greater than 30 or when there are other associated complications, such as diabetes, high cholesterol, high blood pressure or heart disease.

The most commonly used medications are Orlistat and Phentermine. However, these are not advisable for all patients.

To talk about this topic, we interview Mario Vega Carbó, an endocrinologist with more than 20 years of experience.

Doctor Mario,
1. How do weight loss medications work?

Most of these drugs, among which Phentermine is found, decrease appetite and increase feelings of fullness. Orlistat, however, works by preventing the intestines from absorbing certain fats from food.

2. Are these medications effective?

In most cases yes, they help to achieve greater weight loss. Different studies show that patients who use these drugs lose about 5 percent more of the total body weight in a year, than those who do not use them. In addition, they also help prevent weight recovery after treatment.

However, it is important to clarify that these drugs are used as part of a global plan in obese people, along with a proper diet and exercise practice. They are not recommended as a shortcut for normal patients who want to lose a few kilos.

3. How are these drugs used?

Orlistat comes in capsules that are usually taken orally three times a day, along with meals. It is usually used for 2 or 3 months and then rests for a month.

Phentermine, meanwhile, is sold in the form of tablets and a single daily dose is taken in the morning, or three times a day 30 minutes before meals. Most people take this drug for 3 to 6 weeks.

The duration of treatment will depend on each particular case, depending on the response to the medicine and its results.

4. What should be done if you forget to take a dose?

In the case of Orlistat, if it hasn't been more than an hour since the meal, it can be taken at that time. If more time has elapsed, you should let go and continue with the normal schedule. In both cases, you should not take a double dose to make up for the one you forgot.

5. What are the negative effects of these medications?

Orlistat usually causes flatulence and soft stools, so it is advisable to follow a low-fat diet during use. In addition, it blocks the absorption of some vitamins, so it is recommended to take multivitamins.

Other side effects that can cause are pain in the rectum and stomach, irregularities in menstrual periods, anxiety, vomiting and nausea. In severe cases, there may be difficulty breathing or swallowing, yellowing of the skin or eyes, dark urine and liver damage.

For its part, Phentermine can cause diarrhea, constipation, an increase in heart rate and blood pressure, drowsiness or insomnia and nervousness.

On the other hand, if used improperly, it can cause dependence, causing effects similar to those of amphetamines. Therefore, it should not be used more than the indicated dose or for longer than prescribed.

6. What other precautions should be taken before using these drugs?

Before starting the treatment it is important to inform the doctor about any other medication, vitamin or supplement that is being used, so that it evaluates whether the combination can be harmful.

You should also notify if you have other conditions, such as eating disorders, diabetes or kidney or heart problems; if you are pregnant or planning to conceive in the short term; if you are breastfeeding or if you have received an organ transplant.

Finally, these medications should be stored in a suitable place, at room temperature and out of reach of children.

Chapter 34. Metabolic Syndrome and associated disorders

Metabolic Syndrome is called a series of disorders that occur together and increase the risks of suffering from heart or kidney disease, a stroke or Diabetes.

Among them are high blood pressure, high blood sugar levels, excess body fat around the waist and abnormal cholesterol and triglyceride levels. Metabolic Syndrome is increasingly common and can cause serious damage to health. A proper diet, regular exercise, weight loss and certain medications can help treat it.

To learn more about this topic, we interview Mario Vega Carbó, an endocrinologist with more than 20 years of experience.

Doctor Mario,
1. What causes Metabolic Syndrome?

In many cases the cause of this disorder is insulin resistance. It causes the body's cells not to respond normally to this hormone and that glucose cannot enter them with the same ease, causing it to accumulate in the blood. It is also associated with overweight, obesity, lack of physical activity and sedentary lifestyle.

2. Who has more risks of suffering it?

Old people; the obese; those with a history of family members with diabetes; those who suffered from diseases such as non-alcoholic fatty liver, polycystic ovary syndrome or sleep apnea; Those with high blood pressure and high triglyceride levels and low HDL cholesterol are more likely to suffer from it.

3. What are your main symptoms?

The factors associated with the Metabolic Syndrome do not usually show obvious signs. The most visible is the excess body fat around the waist. In case of high blood glucose level, there may be an increase in hunger, thirst and the need to urinate. Other common symptoms are fatigue, headaches and abdominal pain, nausea, vomiting, tachycardia, areas of darkened skin and blurred vision.

4. How is this disease detected?

The following parameters are taken into account to diagnose Metabolic Syndrome:

- That the patient's waist measures at least 89 centimeters in the case of women and 102 centimeters in the case of men.
- That triglyceride levels are above 150 mg / dl.
- That the levels of HDL or "good" cholesterol are less than 50 mg / dL.
- That the blood pressure is 130/85 millimeters of mercury (mmHg) or more.
- That fasting blood glucose is 100 mg / dl (5.6 mmol / l) or more.

5. What is the treatment of Metabolic Syndrome?

The therapy to be applied will depend on the underlying reason that causes this condition. In the case of insulin resistance it is necessary to modify the lifestyle, exercise regularly and control body weight. It is also important to adopt a balanced diet, with lower consumption of saturated fats.

On the other hand, arterial hypertension, blood sugar level and hypercholesterolemia should be controlled and, if necessary, take specific medications for this purpose. Similarly, there are drugs that help solve insulin resistance, such as metformin, glitazones, exenatide and liraglutide.

6. What other complications can this disorder bring?

If not controlled correctly, it can cause heart disease and stroke; Mellitus diabetes; eye, hearing, dental and skin problems; kidney damage; loss of sensation; Nerve injury and severe foot ulcers. Also inconvenient to digest food, slow healing, sleep apnea and erectile dysfunction.

7. How can Metabolic Syndrome be prevented?

To avoid this disorder it is essential to lead a healthy life. This includes controlling weight and eating a well-balanced diet with fewer calories, refined carbohydrates and saturated fats, and more fruits, vegetables, lean proteins and whole grains.

Also do physical activity for at least 30 minutes on most days, limit salt and avoid smoking and excessive alcohol consumption.

Finally, it is also important to take care of emotional health. In that sense, it is advised to practice meditation to free the mind from worries, do yoga and other relaxing activities.

Chapter 35. Non-Alcoholic Fatty Liver Disease

Nonalcoholic Fatty Liver Disease (EHGNA) is a condition in which the accumulation of fat in this organ is not caused by excessive alcohol consumption. It is usually related to overweight and obesity. Some medications, such as calcium channel blockers, can also cause it.

On the other hand, people with Diabetes Mellitus, high cholesterol and triglycerides, high blood pressure, polycystic ovary syndrome, sleep apnea and intestinal diseases have a higher risk of suffering from it. When EHGNA is severe, it can cause liver failure and cirrhosis.

To learn more about this condition, we talked with Mario Vega Carbó, an endocrinology specialist in charge of the Vega & Vado Office in Managua, Nicaragua.

Doctor Mario,
1. What are the symptoms of EHGNA?

Usually people who have this condition have no symptoms. In some cases there may be an enlarged liver, fatigue and pain in the upper right part of the abdomen. If there is liver damage, there may be loss of appetite, nausea, confusion and itching. Also gastrointestinal sacred, dilated spleen and accumulation of fluid and abdominal swelling.

From the physical you can see an enlarged chest, red palms and a yellowish color in eyes and skin.

2. How is this disease diagnosed?

Usually this condition is detected during routine blood tests that are performed to check liver function. To confirm the diagnosis, ultrasound, MRI, computed tomography and biopsy of a sample of liver tissue may be necessary to detect signs of inflammation and scarring.

3. What is your treatment?

The therapy seeks to manage risk factors and advise the patient to lead a healthy life that helps take care of his liver. This includes weight loss, following a low salt diet, avoiding alcohol, performing regular physical activity and reducing cholesterol and triglyceride levels.

In addition, vaccines against hepatitis A and B can be applied to protect the patient from harmful viruses that affect this organ.

On the other hand, if there are other diseases that increase the risks of EHGNA, these should be treated. For example control diabetes. Some medications, such as metformin and vitamins E and D help decrease weight and body fat.

4. What complications can this condition bring?

This disease can cause an increase in abdominal fat, high blood pressure and decrease the ability to consume insulin. In severe cases, it can lead to non-alcoholic liver steatosis, where inflammation of the liver can progress and cause cirrhosis and liver failure.

If necessary, liver transplantation may be an option in complex situations.

5. Why is this disease talked about so much today?

Along with obesity, EHGNA has become the most common liver disease in children and adolescents. That is why the importance of preventing their symptoms and encouraging healthy lifestyle habits from childhood.

Chapter 36. Acanthosis Nigricans or Pigmented Acanthosis

Acanthosis Nigricans or Pigmented Acanthosis is a rare skin condition characterized by dark and thick spots on different areas of the body.

It is usually suffered by obese people or with diabetes and, in some cases, it can also be a sign of a cancerous tumor in an internal organ, such as the stomach or liver. This skin disorder usually appears around the joints and in areas with many folds, such as the armpits, elbows, knees, groin and lateral sides of the neck. Acanthosis Nigricans is not contagious.

To learn more about this topic, we interview Mario Vega Carbó, an endocrinology specialist, who works at the Vega & Vado Office in Managua, Nicaragua.

Doctor Mario,
1. What causes this condition?

The exact etiology is not known, but it usually appears in people with high insulin levels, usually associated with being overweight and with diabetes. It can also be related to genetic disorders, such as Down and Alström Syndromes, and some cancers of the digestive system, liver, kidney and bladder.

On the other hand, ovarian cysts, underactive thyroid or problems with the adrenal glands can cause it. The same some medications and supplements, such as niacin, birth control pills, prednisone and other corticosteroids.

2. What are your symptoms?

Acanthosis nigricans appears progressively and, except for skin changes, does not produce any symptoms. The skin becomes dark, thick and velvety. In some cases the patient may experience itching (itching) and bad smell in the affected area.

3. How is this condition diagnosed?

Just by observing the skin, it can detect Acanthosis Nigricans. In a few cases, a biopsy may be necessary. If the cause of the ailment is unclear, to make an accurate diagnosis, blood tests can be performed to measure sugar and insulin levels, endoscopies and x-rays.

4. What complications can this condition bring?

People with acanthosis nigricans have a higher risk of diabetes, this is a sign of insulin resistance.

5. What is your treatment?

In most cases Acanthosis Nigricans only causes changes in appearance and does not require a specific treatment. Sometimes the spots disappear by themselves. If these are very noticeable, moisturizing creams and lotions containing ammonium lactate, tretinoin or hydroquinone can be used to help lighten the skin.

If the condition is a consequence of a disorder or disease, it must be treated. For example, if it is related to obesity, losing weight will improve your symptoms. The same stop taking medications that may be causing it.

6. What other recommendations can patients follow?

To reduce and prevent Acanthosis Nigricans, it is recommended to maintain an adequate weight, exercise frequently and follow a healthy diet. If the spots are very noticeable, patients may suffer from lack of self-esteem, shame and depression due to the change in appearance, so it is advisable to accompany the treatment with psychological and family support.

Chapter 37. Acrocordones and skin lumps

Acrocordones are abnormal non-cancerous formations, which manifest through small fleshy stems that protrude from the skin. They usually appear on the neck, forearms, armpits, groin and eyelids, and are usually small, soft and slightly dark in color.

They are usually harmless and painless, although they can become irritated and bleed through contact with clothing. Acrocordones are very common, they appear more in men than in women, especially after 40 years of age, and are not contagious. In most cases they do not require treatment, but can be easily removed for aesthetic reasons or to avoid discomfort.

To learn more about this topic, we interview Mario Vega Carbó, an endocrinology specialist, with more than 20 years of experience.

Doctor Mario,
1. Why do acrocordons arise?

It is believed that these small lumps are caused by the accumulation of collagen in the thickest parts of the skin or by repeated friction. They can also be developed by the use of steroids.

2. Who are more susceptible to suffer them?

People with diabetes mellitus or obesity have a greater tendency to suffer them since the accumulation of fat softens the skin and increases the wrinkles of the body, facilitating its development.

Similarly, pregnant women and those with a family history with this condition are also more likely to have it. The same people with acromegaly and Polycystic Ovary Syndrome.

3. Can Acrocordones become evil?

No, these lumps are benign and usually do not continue to grow or change color. However, since its appearance is similar to that of other conditions, such as nevus or soft tissue tumors, it is important that the diagnosis be made by a dermatologist.

4. What is your treatment?

Acrocordones are harmless and sometimes fall off on their own. However, they can be eliminated for aesthetic reasons or because they cause some discomfort.

Cryotherapy, electrosurgery, laser therapy or scalpel removal are some of the procedures used for this purpose. They usually do not require anesthesia or hospitalization and are performed in a few minutes.

5. Are acrocordones the same as warts?

No. Warts are lesions caused by the Human Papillomavirus and usually appear when the immune system is low. Although they may appear visually similar, when caused by a virus, warts can be spread from one person to another through sexual contact or blood transfusions.

On the other hand, being two different conditions, anti-wrinkle liquids sold in pharmacies are not useful for treating acrocordones.

6. What other aspects should be taken into account of this condition?

An abnormal outbreak of acrocordones may indicate that the person is suffering from diabetes. Therefore, in these cases it is recommended to perform the necessary tests to detect the disease.

The term Hyperinsulinemia indicates a condition in which insulin levels in the blood are higher than normal.

Insulin is the hormone produced by the pancreas, responsible for regulating sugar (glucose) in the body and its use as a source of energy in the cells. Hyperinsulinemia can occur when the body is not able to administer blood glucose effectively.

Another cause may be a tumor in the pancreas, known as Insulinoma, or a congenital problem. Over time, severe hyperinsulinemia can lead to diabetes mellitus, which if left untreated causes heart and kidney disease, eye disorders, polyneuropathies and severe foot ulcers.

To learn more about this topic, we interview Mario Vega Carbó, an endocrinologist with more than 20 years of experience.

Doctor Mario,
1. What are the symptoms of Hyperinsulinemia?

This condition itself does not produce any symptoms, but an excess of insulin can cause a reduction in blood sugar levels, which is known as hypoglycemia.

This can cause hunger, anxiety, dizziness, tremor, sweating, difficulty speaking, headache, confusion, seizures and loss of consciousness, among other signs.

2. Why is this condition?

Hyperinsulinemia is usually a sign of another problem. The most common is an insulin resistance, which causes the body's cells not to respond normally to this hormone. This means that glucose cannot enter them with the same ease, causing it to accumulate in the blood. Another cause, much less frequent, is a tumor in the pancreas.

On the other hand, this condition can occur from birth as a result of diabetes in the mother, poor fetal growth or suffocation when giving birth.

In addition, too high an insulin dose in a person with diabetes may also be the reason for Hyperinsulinemia.

3. What can cause insulin resistance?

Although in most cases the specific reason is unknown, there are a number of factors that influence its appearance. These include hereditary components, obesity, physical inactivity, consumption of saturated fats and diets rich in sodium, sedentary lifestyle, hypertension, arteriosclerosis, Alzheimer's, cholesterol and high triglycerides, certain types of cancer and some medications such as cortisone.

4. What is the treatment of hyperinsulinemia?

The therapy to be applied will depend on the underlying reason that causes this condition. In the case of insulin resistance it is necessary to modify the lifestyle, exercise regularly and control body weight. It is also important to adopt a balanced diet, with lower consumption of saturated fats. Blood hypertension and hypercholesterolemia should be controlled and, if necessary, take specific medications for this purpose.

Similarly, there are drugs that help solve insulin resistance, such as metformin, glitazones, exenatide and liraglutide.

In the event that hyperinsulinemia is a consequence of insulinoma, the tumor can be removed with surgery, which usually resolves the problem. If there are many tumors, it will be necessary to remove part of the pancreas.

5. What is the relationship between Hyperinsulinemia and Diabetes?

Over time, insulin resistance could generate diabetes. As the sensitivity to this hormone decreases, the pancreas will seek to generate more, to maintain normal blood sugar levels.

When the pancreas no longer has the ability to secrete insulin, it can cause glucose intolerance that results in diabetes.

6. What are the main symptoms of Diabetes and how is it treated?

The most common signs are increased hunger, thirst and the need to urinate. In addition, there may be weight loss, fatigue, headaches, nausea, vomiting, tachycardia, inadequate healing, abdominal pain and blurred vision.

As for the treatment, the objective will be to restore normal glycemic levels, for which it may be necessary to apply an insulin substitute or insulin analogs or oral antidiabetics. In addition, the patient must lead a healthy life.

Chapter 39. Insulinoma and Hypoglycemia

Insulinoma is a rare tumor in the pancreas, which generates an excessive production of insulin in the blood. This hormone is responsible for regulating glucose levels in the body and its use as a source of energy in cells.

A high amount of insulin can cause sugar values to fall too low, resulting in hypoglycemia. Insulinoma is usually small - less than 2 centimeters - and benign (non-cancerous) in most cases.

To learn more about this topic, we interview Mario Vega Carbó, a clinical endocrinologist with more than 20 years of experience.

Doctor Mario,
1. What causes an Insulinoma?

In the vast majority of cases, these are tumors that have a sporadic origin. Only a small proportion are hereditary and associated with genetic syndromes, such as multiple endocrine neoplasia (NEM) type I.

2. Who has more risks of suffering it?

Insulinoma usually appears between 40 and 50 years, more frequently in women. The reported incidence is 3-10 cases per million people. Patients with certain genetic syndromes also have a higher risk of suffering them.

3. What are your main symptoms?

Its signs are usually related to the development of hypoglycemia and may include anxiety, weakness, hunger, confusion, blurred vision, headache, dizziness, sweating and palpitations. Associated with frequent food intakes, progressive weight gain in recent months.

In more severe cases there may be loss of consciousness, seizures and coma.

4. How is an Insulinoma detected?

In view of its symptoms, a blood test is usually performed to measure glucose, insulin, C-peptide and proinsulin levels, and body response tests to glucagon injection. In addition, computed tomography, magnetic resonance imaging, transabdominal ultrasound, endoscopic ultrasound or other examinations in search of the tumor can be performed.

5. What is your treatment?

Therapy consists of surgical removal of Insulinoma. If there are many tumors, it may be necessary to remove part of the pancreas.

In very rare situations, if there are many insulinomas or if they continue to reappear, the entire gland is removed. If this occurs, when the body stops producing insulin, the patient should apply hormone substitutes for life.

If for some reason the person cannot undergo surgery, certain medications help decrease insulin production and avoid hypoglycemia. Among them are diazoxide, calcium channel blockers, somatostatin analogues and streptozotocin.

6. What are the expected results of this therapy?

The cure rate with surgery is almost 100 percent of cases.

7. What other complications can this disease cause?

A severe hypoglycemic reaction can cause seizures, brain damage and even death.

On the other hand, the few cases in which total excision of the pancreas occurs can lead to diabetes and metabolic problems. In turn, if Insulinoma is cancerous, it can spread to other organs and be fatal.

Chapter 40. Gout: what it is and how it is treated

Gout is a type of arthritis that occurs when uric acid builds up in the blood and causes inflammation in the joints. It is characterized by sudden and intense attacks of pain, in which the affected area swells, reddens and heats for no apparent reason.

The most common occurs in the big toe, which can be very annoying and manifest during the night, causing the person to wake up suddenly from the discomfort. There are two types of gout: the acute one, which only affects one joint and is usually very painful; and the chronicle, in which repetitive episodes occur that can occur in different parts of the body. It is estimated that between 1 and 2 percent of the population suffer from it.

To learn more about this issue, we interview Cuban doctor Mario Vega Carbó, an endocrinology specialist.

Doctor Mario,
1. What is the cause of the drop?

This disease occurs when a lot of uric acid builds up in the fluid around the tissues. This causes crystals to form, which causes the joint to swell and raise the temperature. The high level of uric acid may be due to excess production or because the body has some difficulty getting rid of it. It can also be given by the intake of certain medications, such as hydrochlorothiazide and other diuretics, that interfere with their natural elimination.

2. Who are more likely to suffer from this condition?

It is believed that Gout can be hereditary. Its appearance is more frequent in men and the risks of suffering it increase with age. People who drink alcohol or have hypertension, diabetes, obesity, anemia, leukemia, osteoarthritis and kidney disease are also more likely to suffer from it. The same happened to those who had surgery or recent trauma.

3. What are your symptoms?

Its main signs are pain, swelling, redness and warming of one or more joints. The most affected are usually those of the big toe, knees, ankles, elbows and wrists.

The discomfort usually appears suddenly and at night, with great intensity. Some patients may also develop a fever and, over time, uric acid deposits may form bumps under the skin, known as tofo.

4. How is this condition detected?

When your symptoms occur, synovial fluid tests and uric acid tests in blood and urine, and joint x-ray are usually done to confirm the diagnosis.

5. What is your treatment?

To relieve pain, the intake of nonsteroidal anti-inflammatory drugs, such as ibuprofen, is recommended. A higher than normal dose may be needed, which should be prescribed by the doctor. In very intense cases, corticosteroids, such as prednisone, can be injected into the inflamed joint. In addition, colchicine, rest and local application of ice are also effective in reducing discomfort.

On the other hand, if it is confirmed that uric acid levels are very high, allopurinol, febuxostat, lesinurad or probenecid will be prescribed daily to prevent crystal formation.

6. What can happen if it is not treated properly?

Gout can cause damage and loss of joint movement, causing the person to feel pain and other symptoms most of the time. It can also generate kidney stones and deposits in the kidneys.

7. What else can be done to improve the forecast?

Leading a healthy life, exercising, drinking plenty of fluids and eating well can help prevent attacks.

It is recommended to avoid alcohol (especially beer), red meat, poultry, shellfish and sugar-sweetened beverages.

On the contrary, it is advised to maintain an adequate weight, drink coffee, consume dairy products and cherries and take vitamin C supplements.

Chapter 41. Hemochromatosis and excess iron in the body

Hemochromatosis is an inherited condition that causes excessive accumulation of iron in the body. This anomaly causes the mineral to be stored in the tissues, especially in the liver, heart and pancreas, damaging the organs.

This can generate different diseases, such as cancer, irregular heart rate, diabetes, arthritis and cirrhosis. In many patients, the accumulation of iron is so excessive that the skin becomes dark. To lower your levels, it is necessary to draw blood from the body on a regular basis.

In order to learn more about this topic, we interview Mario Vega Carbó, an endocrinology specialist with more than 20 years of experience.

Doctor Mario,
1. How often does this disease occur and what are its causes?

Hemochromatosis is a genetic disease that affects 1 in 250 people. It is characterized by an increase in iron absorption as a result of the mutation of a gene. In order for the condition to occur, it is necessary to inherit the gene from both the mother and the father.

2. What is the amount of normal iron present in the body?

In healthy individuals, the total amount is about 2 to 4 g and remains at those levels throughout life. In the case of people suffering from Hemochromatosis, this figure varies between 20 and 40 g.

3. What are the symptoms of this disease?

Its main signs are joint pain, osteoporosis, chronic tiredness, lack of energy and sexual desire, abdominal discomfort, weight loss and other disorders associated with heart disease and diabetes. However, some people with Hemochromatosis never have symptoms.

4. Who are more likely to suffer from them?

These signs are more frequent in men between 40 and 60 years and in women over 50, being the men more likely to suffer from the disease. The reason is that women lose a considerable amount of blood each month with menstruation and also during childbirth if they get pregnant. Excessive alcohol consumption contributes to the progression of symptomatic hemochromatosis.

5. How is this disease diagnosed?

Through a blood test it is possible to determine the amount of iron in the body. On the other hand, a test can also be performed to determine if the defective gene that causes it is present. Usually, along with these studies, an analysis of liver function is usually performed to detect liver damage.

Once the disease is diagnosed, it is important to make an evaluation of the rest of the family due to its hereditary nature.

6. What is your treatment?

Hemochromatosis is controlled with frequent phlebotomies, that is, with blood drawn. This reduces the body's iron levels because the mineral is stored in the red blood cells.

In the beginning of the treatment, one or two extractions per week are usually necessary and, when the values are normalized, it is carried out with wider intervals, every two or three months. This must be maintained for life.

For those who cannot undergo a blood draw, either because they suffer from anemia or cardiac complications, there are medications to eliminate excess iron.

7. What are the expected results?

If therapy is started before the organs are damaged, complications associated with this disease can be avoided.

In that sense, frequent phlebotomies can stop the progression of deterioration in the liver in its initial phase, allowing a normal life expectancy. However, if there are already signs of cirrhosis, there is a high risk of cancer, even achieving normalize iron levels, since this is irreversible.

In the case of diabetes caused by damage to the pancreas, it usually improves with treatment. On the other hand, blood draws also help relieve symptoms of tiredness, abdominal pain and darkening of the skin.

8. What other care can be taken to improve the disease?

Patients suffering from Hemochromatosis are advised to avoid supplements containing iron and vitamin C, drink alcohol and eat raw fish and shellfish.

PART III DIABETES

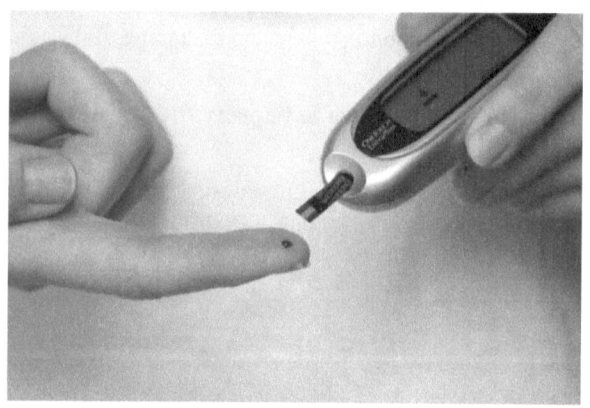

Prediabetes is a disorder in which the level of sugar (blood glucose) is higher than normal, but without reaching the limit levels to make the diagnosis of diabetes mellitus.

This condition can occur in both adults and children and, if left untreated, can cause long-term damage to the heart, blood vessels and kidneys, among other organs. Lifestyle changes can help regulate the level of sugar in the body and prevent its evolution.

To learn more about this topic, we interview Mario Vega Carbó, an endocrinologist, with more than 20 years of experience.

Doctor Mario,
1. What are the causes of Prediabetes?

The exact cause is unknown, but family history, genetics and excess fat in the body seem to play an important role. Most of the glucose in the body comes from the food we eat. Then insulin, a hormone generated by the pancreas, transports it to the cells, for use as a source of energy.

People with prediabetes do not process sugar properly and it accumulates in the bloodstream causing negative health effects.

2. What are the symptoms of this condition?

In general, prediabetes has no signs. When it is advanced, there may be a darkening of the skin in certain parts of the body and an increase in hunger, thirst and the need to urinate.

In addition, there may be weight loss, fatigue, headaches, nausea, vomiting, tachycardia and blurred vision. If this occurs, the patient is at serious risk of having diabetes.

3. How is this condition detected?

In the absence of symptoms, to diagnose prediabetes it is necessary to perform a blood test to measure the level of sugar.

4. Who has more risks of having it?

As in the case of diabetes mellitus, those over 45, those who are obese and overweight, those who do not perform physical activation, those who suffer from high blood pressure or Polycystic Ovary Syndrome, and those who have cholesterol " good "(HDL) low, high triglycerides and family history with this disease, are more likely to suffer.

5. What is your treatment?

Opting for a healthy lifestyle generally helps normalize blood sugar levels. This includes eating foods that are low in fat and calories, and high in fiber. Also exercise regularly, drink plenty of water, eliminate overweight, quit smoking and avoid drinking alcohol.

On the other hand, if necessary, the doctor may prescribe some medication to control the levels of glucose, cholesterol, triglycerides and high blood pressure.

6. What other complications can prediabetes bring?

People with this condition have a higher risk of developing diabetes mellitus in the next 10 years. In addition, they also increase the chances of suffering from heart disease, blindness, kidney failure, neurological damage and stroke.

Chapter 43. Type 2 Diabetes Mellitus

Type 2 Diabetes Mellitus is a chronic disorder that prevents proper glucose metabolism, causing it to accumulate in the blood. This can be caused by a deficit in the production of insulin in the pancreas that is preceded by a resistance of the cells to the action of this hormone.

Insulin is responsible for regulating sugar in the body and its use as a source of energy in muscles and other tissues.

It is estimated that about 8 percent of the adult population suffers from diabetes and, if not treated properly, can cause heart and kidney disease, eye problems, polyneuropathies and severe ulcers in the extremities, mainly in the lower limbs. Although it has no cure, it can be controlled with proper diet, regular exercise, weight loss, medications and treatment.

To learn more about this topic, we interview Mario Vega Carbó, an endocrinologist with more than 20 years of experience.

Doctor Mario,
1. What is insulin resistance and what causes it?

Insulin resistance causes the body's cells not to respond normally to this hormone. This means that glucose cannot enter them with the same ease, causing it to accumulate in the blood. Although in most cases the specific reason for the cause is unknown, there are a number of factors that influence its appearance.

These include hereditary components, obesity, physical inactivity, consumption of saturated fats and diets rich in sodium, sedentary lifestyle, hypertension, arteriosclerosis, Alzheimer's, cholesterol and high triglycerides, certain types of cancer and some medications such as cortisone.

2. What is the relationship this has with Diabetes?

Over time insulin resistance could generate it. As the sensitivity to this hormone decreases, the pancreas will seek to generate more, to maintain normal blood sugar levels. When the pancreas no longer has the ability to secrete insulin, it can cause glucose intolerance that results in diabetes.

3. Who has more risks of having it?

Most people with this disease are overweight or obese, since increasing fat makes it difficult for the body to use insulin in the right way. In addition, family history, genetics, a low level of physical activity and a poor diet increase the risks of suffering from it.

Similarly, having suffered diseases such as prediabetes, gestational diabetes and Polycystic Ovary Syndrome, are risk factors for diabetes.

Another factor to take into account is age, since the possibilities grow as you get older, especially after your 45th birthday. However, type 2 diabetes mellitus is increasing significantly among children, adolescents and young adults.

4. What are your main symptoms?

Diabetes usually develops slowly and initially the person may have no signs. When it is more advanced, there may be an increase in hunger, thirst and the need to urinate.

Other common symptoms are bladder, kidney or skin infections; fatigue; headaches and abdominal pain; nausea, vomiting; tachycardia; inadequate healing; areas of darkened skin, usually in the armpits and neck; and blurred vision.

5. How is it detected?

In view of its symptoms, an analysis of the patient's medical history, a physical examination and the level of glycemia, glycosylated hemoglobin and blood lipids are usually performed.

It is also possible that urine, osmolarity, heart rate, blood pressure and other tests to confirm the diagnosis may be carried out.

6. What is your treatment?

The goal of therapy is to restore normal glycemic levels, for which it may be necessary to apply an insulin substitute or insulin analogs or oral antidiabetics.

On the other hand, as excessive food intake and sedentary lifestyle increase the risks of this disease, you also work on a special diet and in adapting a healthier lifestyle.

In that sense, it is important to control the weight and consume a well-balanced diet with fewer calories, refined carbohydrates and saturated fats, and more fruits, vegetables and fibers. Also do physical activity on a regular basis and avoid smoking and consuming excess alcohol.

In addition, the patient must learn to measure his blood sugar level using a glucometer and perform periodic checks. Based on these results, the treatment will be adjusted according to the needs to maintain an appropriate range.

If necessary, the doctor will prescribe injectable or oral medications that help regulate the level of sugar, such as metformin, sulfonylureas, meglitinides or thiazolidinediones. Insulin administration may also be necessary.

7. What other complications can Diabetes bring?

Among the problems related to Diabetes that require immediate attention are Hyperglycemia, Hyperglycemic Hyperosmolar Syndrome, Diabetic Ketoacidosis and Hypoglycemia.

On the other hand, if not controlled correctly, it can cause heart disease and stroke; eye, hearing, dental and skin problems; kidney damage; loss of sensation; Nerve injury and severe foot ulcers that may even lead to amputation. Also, inconveniences to digest food, slow healing, sleep apnea, Alzheimer's and erectile dysfunction.

8. What other aspects should be taken into account during this disease?

Living with diabetes can be very stressful and cause depression and distress. That is why it is also important to take care of emotional health. It is advised to practice meditation to free the mind from worries, do yoga and other relaxing activities. If necessary, psychological and therapeutic support is recommended.

On the other hand, it is important that these patients wear a bracelet or special card that indicates their condition, to alert others in emergency situations.

Chapter 44. MODY Diabetes

The mature age diabetes that occurs in the young is known as MODY by its acronym in English ("Maturity Onset Diabetes of the Young"). It is a type of condition with characteristics of Diabetes Mellitus, whose onset usually occurs in adulthood, but which in this case arises before the age of 25.

It is not related to the trend observed in recent times, in which the disease appears in the child population as a result of obesity, the result of inadequate diet and lack of physical exercise. In general, patients with MODY Diabetes are not overweight.

To learn more about this topic, we consulted Dr. Mario Vega Carbó, specialist in clinical endocrinology.

Doctor Mario,
1. What characterizes MODY type diabetes?

This type is characterized by appearing before age 25, being mostly hereditary (transmitted strongly from parents to children), having a slow and progressive evolution, and presenting a deficit in insulin secretion.

This does not usually start with high concentration of ketone bodies in the urine and is not related to obesity.

2. What is the cause of this disease?

It is usually a monogenic disease, which is the result of mutations in a single gene that affects the maturation of pancreatic beta cells, insulin producing.

This differs from types 1 and 2, which are usually caused by several genes, in addition to lifestyle factors. At least 13 genes that can cause MODY diabetes are known. Most of them are transcription agents that are involved in embryonic development.

This medical condition appears more frequently in children and adolescents, who generally have a lower capacity to produce insulin. In very few cases, the problem is a severe resistance to this hormone.

3. How is MODY Diabetes detected?

In many cases, patients with MODY are misdiagnosed with Type 1 or 2 Diabetes, which causes them to receive inadequate treatment. For its correct detection it is essential to analyze the family history, the age of onset, the degree of hyperglycemia and the absence of pancreatic autoantibodies.

On the other hand, blood glucose and insulin levels tests and genetic tests and several antibodies can contribute to the diagnosis.

4. How is this condition treated?

The therapy will depend on the type of MODY and its symptoms. Some people can control the disease with proper diet and regular physical exercise. Others will need to take diabetes medications, either insulin or some oral antidiabetic.

While the initial response to oral antidiabetics is usually good, some MODY subtypes are more predisposed to require insulin as the disease progresses. Occasionally, patients should also follow treatments for related conditions, such as kidney or gout cysts.

5. What other aspects should be taken into account during this disease?

As with other types of diabetes, the patient must learn to measure glycemic levels and follow a personalized diet that helps control the disease.

If MODY Diabetes is confirmed, it is important to detect family members at risk, for their ability to be inherited.

Chapter 45. LADA Diabetes

Latent Autoimmune Diabetes in Adults, or LADA by its acronym in English ("Latent Autoimmune Diabetes in Adults"), is a type of late onset condition, which is usually diagnosed in people over 30 years.

Also known as type 1.5 diabetes, it is a genetic autoimmune disorder, in which the immune system mistakenly attacks the pancreas and destroys the cells that produce insulin, as does type 1 (Juvenile Diabetes). In this case, progress is made slowly and progressively, which sometimes causes it to be confused with type 2 diabetes.

To learn more about this topic, we interview Mario Vega Carbó, an endocrinologist with more than 20 years of experience.

Doctor Mario,
1. What are the special characteristics of this type of diabetes?

LADA Diabetes has some characteristics of type 1 and others of type 2. Some specialists even consider it a variant of Juvenile Diabetes, since it is also of autoimmune origin, it is not hereditary and there is presence of antibodies in the blood. However, it varies in the age at which it appears, in which its progression is much slower and in which no ketone is seen in the blood or urine.

With regard to type 2 diabetes, he agrees that it occurs in adults between 30 and 50 years old and that the patient continues to produce insulin at first.

On the contrary, it differs in a low level of C-peptide and increased levels of antibodies against pancreatic islets.

2. What are the symptoms of LADA Diabetes?

The symptoms are similar to those of type 1 and 2 diabetes: increased hunger, thirst and the need to urinate; feeling tired; blurry vision; headache; irritability and mood swings

3. How is this disease detected?

In view of its signs, an analysis of the patient's medical history, a physical examination and the levels of glycemia, glycosylated hemoglobin and blood lipids are usually performed. Also tests of several antibodies, such as islet cell (ICA), glutamic acid decarboxylase (GAD) and anti-insulin (IAA).

Since it usually appears in adults, many times its symptoms are confused with type 2 diabetes. It is estimated that between 10 and 15 percent of the diagnoses of this condition are actually LADA type diabetes.

To confirm that this condition is involved, the patient must be over 30 years old, present at least one of the antibodies corresponding to type 1 diabetes and not have been treated with insulin in the first six months after detection.

4. What is the treatment of LADA Diabetes?

As with type 2 diabetes, patients with LADA may initially use oral medication, exercise and eat a balanced diet to control the disease. However, over time the pancreas will stop producing insulin completely, as in type 1, and the injection of the hormone will be necessary.

The process between one stage and another can take months and even years after diagnosis. Medications for high blood pressure and for lowering cholesterol may be prescribed.

5. What complications can LADA diabetes bring?

As with types 1 and 2, those diagnosed with LADA have a higher risk of circulatory and heart disease; nerve injuries, kidney damage, eyes and feet, skin and mouth infections, and pregnancy complications.

Chapter 46. Other specific types of Diabetes

Glucose is the body's main source of energy. This sugar comes from the food consumed and insulin is responsible for regulating its entry into the body's cells.

When blood glucose levels are high, a chronic and irreversible metabolic disease known as diabetes is generated.

This can be divided into 4 large groups: type 1 or autoimmune; type 2; Gestational and other specific types of diabetes. In type 1 diabetes the pancreas does not produce enough insulin. In type 2, which is the most common, there is usually a resistance to this hormone and the body does not use it properly. As for gestational diabetes, it is the one that appears during pregnancy.

Within the category "other specific types of diabetes", all types that are triggered as a complication or symptom of genetic syndromes, surgeries, medications, malnutrition, infections and other health conditions are included.

To learn more about this topic, we interview Mario Vega Carbó, an endocrinologist with more than 20 years of experience.

Doctor Mario,
1. What percentage of cases of this disease correspond to these other specific types of diabetes?

It is estimated that this type represents between 1-2% of the total cases.

2. What genetic alterations and endocrinopathies can cause these types of secondary diabetes?

Among the genetic syndromes that can lead to diabetes are Klinefelter, Turner, Down, Prader-Willi, Laurence-Moon-Biedl and Wolfram.

Meanwhile, endocrinopathies include Cushing's syndrome, acromegaly, thyroid diseases or thyroidepathies, tumors that produce hormones such as glucagon or somatostatin, pheochromocytoma, primary hyperaldosteronism, carcinoid syndrome, autoimmune polyglandular syndromes and syndrome. of polycystic ovary.

3. Why can these endocrine pathologies lead to diabetes?

This is because there are hormones with properties opposite to the action of insulin, such as cortisol, growth hormone, glucagon and adrenaline; and others that inhibit its secretion, such as aldosterone and somatostatin.

4. What diseases of the pancreas and medications can lead to other types of diabetes?

Among the first are chronic pancreatitis, whether induced by drugs, viruses or vesicular lithiasis; pancreatic carcinoma, hemochromatosis; cystic fibrosis and pancreatectomy (surgical removal of the pancreas).

As for medications, some of them are corticosteroids, thiazide diuretics, nicotinic acid, estrogens, oral contraceptives, pentamidine and psychoactive drugs.

5. How are these types of secondary diabetes treated?

The therapy will depend on the cause of the disease and its symptoms. Some people can control it with proper diet and regular physical exercise. Others will need to take diabetes medications. If it is a consequence of another medical condition, it must be treated. If the cause is a medication, it can be substituted for another.

Chapter 47. Acute Complication of Diabetes

Diabetes is a chronic disorder that prevents proper glucose metabolism, causing it to accumulate in the blood. If not properly controlled, this can lead to serious problems in the heart, eyes, kidneys, nerves and feet.

In addition, some acute complications of this disease can appear quickly and put the patient's life at risk. Among these serious situations are Hypoglycemia, Hyperglycemia, Coma Hyperosmolar and Ketoacidosis.

To learn more about this topic, we interview Mario Vega Carbó, an endocrinologist with more than 20 years of experience.

Doctor Mario,
1. What is hypoglycemia and what acute complication can it cause?

Hypoglycemia is a disorder in which blood sugar levels are below normal. It usually occurs in patients taking diabetes medications in larger doses than necessary. This causes a lot of insulin and low blood sugar. If it is not resolved quickly, hypoglycemia can worsen rapidly and cause epileptic seizures and brain damage.

2. How is hypoglycemia treated?

Faced with its symptoms, therapy seeks to correct low blood sugar. This may include drinking juices, eating food and taking glucose tablets. In severe cases, an injection of glucagon, a hormone that quickly raises sugar, may be necessary.

3. What is Hyperglycemia and what serious disorders can it cause?

Hyperglycemia is a condition in which blood sugar levels are above normal. When they are very high for a prolonged period of time, they can cause two serious disorders: Hyperosmolar Hypoglycemic State and Diabetic Ketoacidosis.

4. What is the Hyperosmolar Hypoglycemic State and what acute complications can it generate?

It is one of the most serious metabolic disorders that occur in patients with diabetes and involves a very high level of blood sugar, extreme dehydration and decreased consciousness.

Generally this condition occurs in older people who do not have the disease controlled. It can also be triggered by acute infections or the consumption of medications such as corticosteroids or diuretics. If left untreated, severe dehydration can cause seizures, coma and ultimately death.

5. What is your treatment?

In general, the first thing that is done is to correct the loss of fluid by administering a physiological solution intravenously. This improves blood pressure, urine output and circulation. Then, the high glucose level is treated with the administration of insulin.

6. What is Diabetic Ketoacidosis?

This is another serious complication of diabetes that occurs when the body produces high levels of ketones, acids present in the blood.

Ketones are chemicals that the body creates at the time it burns fat to use as energy. That happens when there is not enough insulin to use glucose, the main source of fuel for muscles and other tissues.

7. What complications can this condition bring?

Diabetic ketoacidosis can cause a buildup of fluid in the brain, heart attack and kidney failure, among other serious diseases. That is why it is important that, in the face of your symptoms, urgently seek attention.

8. How is Diabetic Ketoacidosis treated?

First, it seeks to correct the high level of glucose in the blood with insulin and replace lost fluids and electrolytes.

If there is a bacterial infection, fight with antibiotics. If another disease is causing this condition, it must also be treated.

9. How can these acute complications of diabetes be prevented?

People with this disease have to do blood glucose self-tests to regularly monitor blood levels. It is essential that they take the prescribed medication correctly and that they do not modify insulin doses without medical supervision.

On the other hand, it is important that they follow a balanced diet, that they exercise regularly, that they maintain an adequate weight and that they avoid alcohol and tobacco.

Chapter 48. Diabetic Hypoglycemia and its complications

Hypoglycemia is a disorder in which blood sugar levels are below normal. On the contrary, diabetes is a disease in which they are too high.

Insulin is responsible for regulating blood glucose in the body and its use as a source of energy in muscles and other tissues. During the treatment of diabetes, substitutes or analogs of this hormone are usually applied to restore normal sugar levels. If a very high dose is used, this may cause the values to fall too low, resulting in Diabetic Hypoglycemia.

To learn more about this topic, we interview Mario Vega Carbó, an endocrinologist with more than 20 years of experience.

Doctor Mario,
1. What are the causes of hypoglycemia?

This disorder usually occurs in patients taking diabetes medications in larger doses than necessary. This causes a lot of insulin and low blood sugar. Another cause may be a tumor in the pancreas, known as Insulinoma.

In addition, it can also appear when you do not eat enough, if you skip or delay meals, if you drink excess alcohol or exercise more than usual.

2. What are your main symptoms?

The normal blood sugar level is between 70 and 99 mg / dL. When it is between 55 and 70 mg / dL, the patient is considered to have mild hypoglycemia and may present with hunger, perspiration, nervousness and tremor.

When it is between 40 and 55 mg / dl, it is considered Moderate Hypoglycemia and there may be dizziness, drowsiness, confusion, difficulty speaking, anxiety and weakness.

When it is less than 40 mg / dl, it is considered Severe Hypoglycemia and can present confusing thinking, seizures, loss of consciousness and coma.

3. What is your treatment?

The therapy will seek to correct low blood sugar. This may include drinking juices, eating food and taking glucose tablets. In severe cases, an injection of glucagon, a hormone that quickly raises sugar, may be necessary.

If hypoglycemia is the result of an Insulinoma, the tumor can be removed with surgery, which usually resolves the problem. If there are many tumors, it will be necessary to remove part of the pancreas.

4. What other complications can this ailment cause?

If it is not resolved quickly, hypoglycemia can worsen rapidly and cause epileptic seizures and brain damage. In some cases, this disorder can occur while the person sleeps. Its symptoms are excessive sweating, nightmares, tiredness, irritability and disorientation on waking.

5. How is Diabetic Hypoglycemia prevented?

To avoid this disorder, it is recommended to regularly measure glucose levels and maintain a fixed schedule for meals. Also follow the medical therapy indicated for the control of diabetes and take the medications at the time and at the indicated doses.

If you are going to practice physical activities, it is advisable to drink liquid and eat before. In addition, people at risk of hypoglycemia are advised to always have glucose tablets or candies on hand. Also that they measure their glucose levels before driving or operating any machine.

Finally, it is important that these patients wear a bracelet or special card that indicates their condition, to alert others in emergency situations. It is good to alert family members, friends and coworkers about hypoglycemia and how to act in a crisis.

Chapter 49. Hyperosmolar Hyperglycemic State

Hyperosmolar Hyperglycemic State is one of the most serious metabolic disorders that occur in patients with Diabetes. It implies a very high level of sugar (glucose) in the blood, extreme dehydration and decreased consciousness.

This condition usually occurs in older people who do not have the disease controlled. It can also be triggered by acute infections or the consumption of medications such as corticosteroids or diuretics. If left untreated, severe dehydration can cause seizures, coma and ultimately death.

To talk about this topic, we interview Dr. Mario Vega Carbó, a specialist in clinical endocrinology.

Doctor Mario,
1. What are the symptoms of a Hyperglycemic Hyperosmolar State?

When the blood sugar level rises, the body tries to remove the excess in the urine, so one of its signs is having to go to the bathroom very often. Other symptoms include excessive thirst, the need to drink plenty of fluids, dry mouth and chapped lips, fever and dark urine.

The patient may also feel weak, have drowsiness or confusion, nausea, weight loss, decreased vision, hallucinations and weakness on one side of the body. The signs can get worse for days or weeks and cause problems with movement, speech impairment, seizures and coma.

2. What other factors can trigger this condition?

In addition to uncontrolled Diabetes, Hyperosmolar Hyperglycemic State can be caused by an acute infection or other coexisting diseases, such as a heart attack, stroke or recent surgery. Also, it can be a consequence of drinking little liquid, consuming many foods with carbohydrates and sugar, or heart or kidney failure.

In addition, certain medications that decrease the effect of insulin on the body or that increase fluid loss can trigger it.

3. How is the Hyperosmolar Hyperglycemic State detected?

In view of its symptoms, an analysis of the patient's medical history is usually performed and blood glucose level, fever, heart rate and blood pressure are measured.

It is also possible that urine, osmolarity, BUN, sodium and creatine levels, chest x-ray, electrocardiogram, and CT scan of the head are performed to confirm the diagnosis.

4. What is your treatment?

Usually the first thing that is done is to correct the loss of fluid by administering a physiological solution intravenously. This will improve blood pressure, urine output and circulation. Then the high glucose level is treated with the administration of insulin.

5. What other complications can Hyperosmolar Hyperglycemic State bring?

If this condition is not treated, it can cause a shock in which the body does not receive sufficient blood flow, causing damage to different organs. In addition, it can generate clot formation, cerebral edema and an increase in the level of acid in the blood.

6. How can it be prevented?

Hyperglycemic Hyperosmolar State only occurs when Diabetes is not well controlled. That is why it is recommended to measure blood sugar on a regular basis and take the medications prescribed by the doctor. In addition, it is advisable to drink liquid frequently.

Chapter 50. Diabetic Ketoacidosis

Diabetic Ketoacidosis is a serious complication of diabetes that occurs when the body produces high levels of ketones, acids present in the blood.

Ketones are chemicals that the body creates at the time it burns fat to use as energy. That happens when there is not enough insulin to use glucose, the main source of fuel for muscles and other tissues. This complication usually occurs in people with type 1 diabetes. When ketones accumulate in the blood, it becomes more acidic. A high level can be toxic and life-threatening.

To learn more about this topic, we interview Mario Vega Carbó, an endocrinology specialist who works as an endocrinologist at the Vega & Vado Office in Managua, Nicaragua.

Doctor Mario,
1. What can trigger Diabetic Ketoacidosis?

In general, this complication occurs when there is an uncontrolled blood sugar level for a long period of time. It can also be a consequence of insufficient food, an insulin reaction, an infection, an injury, a serious illness, a physical or emotional trauma, a heart attack, surgery, certain medications, such as corticosteroids and some diuretics, and consumption excessive alcohol or drugs, especially cocaine.

In many cases ketoacidosis may be the first symptom that appears in people with type 1 diabetes that has not been detected. In cases where it was already diagnosed, it can be triggered when the patient stops taking the medications or when a higher dose is required.

2. What are your main symptoms?

People with Diabetic Ketoacidosis may have a decreased state of consciousness, shortness of breath, dry mouth and skin, redness of the face, frequent urination, excessive thirst, headache and abdominal pain, fatigue, fruity breath , muscle stiffness, nausea and vomiting.

3. How is this condition diagnosed?

In the face of its symptoms, a physical examination and a ketone test are usually performed using a blood or urine sample. In order to complete the diagnosis, arterial blood gas, chest x-ray, electrocardiogram, metabolic tests and measurement of blood pressure and glucose levels can also be carried out.

4. What is your treatment?

First, it will seek to correct the high level of blood glucose with insulin and replace lost fluids and electrolytes. If there is a bacterial infection, it will be fought with antibiotics. If another disease is causing this condition, it must be treated.

If the patient has diabetes, he can be taught to detect high sugar levels and ketone accumulation through household glucometers that analyze blood and urine.

5. What complications can Diabetic Ketoacidosis bring?

This condition can cause a buildup of fluid in the brain, heart attack and kidney failure, among other serious diseases. That is why it is important that, in the face of your symptoms, urgently seek attention.

Chapter 51. Diabetic Neuropathy and its complications

Diabetic Neuropathy is nerve damage that occurs as a result of Diabetes. High blood sugar (glycemia) and decreased blood flow can affect the nerves of the entire body, mainly those of the legs and feet.

It is estimated that half of diabetics suffer from such disorders. In general they are a consequence of a lack of control in the disease. In some people their symptoms are mild, but in others they can be very painful and cause serious damage.

To learn more about this topic, we interview Mario Vega Carbó, an endocrinology specialist with more than 20 years of experience.

Doctor Mario,
1. What are the symptoms of this condition?

Diabetic neuropathy develops slowly and initially the person may have no signs. When it is more advanced, the symptoms depend on the nerves that are affected. In the feet and hands, there may be tingling, burning or pain in the fingers. Also loss of sensation, which does not cause blisters, cuts or contact with something too cold or hot.

In the digestive system, there may be problems digesting food, gastric acidity, inconvenience to swallow, nausea, constipation, diarrhea and vomiting. When it affects the heart and blood vessels, there may be a feeling of dizziness and increased heart rate, even while at rest.

In addition, there may be loss of balance and coordination; increased sweating; sexual problems, such as erectile dysfunction and vaginal dryness; and bladder, with urinary tract infections or urinary retention or incontinence.

2. Who has more risks of suffering from Diabetic Neuropathy?

Any person with Diabetes can suffer from it, but those who do not control the disease, those who have kidney problems or overweight, those who smoke and those over 50 have a higher risk of suffering from it.

3. How is this disease detected?

A physical exam is performed to assess muscle strength, reflexes, sensitivity to touch and changes in skin and hair. Possibly nerve conduction and tilt tests, electromyography and a gastric emptying study are carried out to confirm the diagnosis.

4. What is your treatment?

Diabetic neuropathy has no cure, but actions can be taken to reduce its progression, relieve its symptoms and control complications arising from it. Among other initiatives, it is possible to prescribe medications for pain in the feet, legs or arms; for nausea, vomiting or other problems with digestion; and for erectile dysfunction and vaginal dryness.

On the other hand, it is important to treat Diabetes by eating healthy foods, exercising regularly, losing weight and taking the drugs or insulin prescribed by the doctor. Also, checking blood sugar levels and taking care of and checking feet frequently.

5. What other complications can this ailment bring?

Diabetic neuropathy can increase the risks of urinary tract and kidney infections, joint damage, sudden drops in blood pressure and foot ulcers that can even reach an amputation. Other problems are sexual and digestive.

On the other hand, this medical condition can hide the symptoms of a chest pain that warns of a disease or heart attack, so precautions should be taken.

Chapter 52. The Diabetic Foot and the possibilities of amputation

Over time, excess blood sugar can damage nerves and cause sensation in the feet to be lost. This can cause lesions, cuts, blisters or sores to be perceived and that they result in ulcers and infections.

On the other hand, the deterioration in the blood vessels caused by Diabetes can also cause the feet to not receive enough blood and oxygen and make healing and healing more difficult. In severe cases, this can even lead to an amputation.

To learn more about the subject, we interview Dr. Mario Vega Carbó, an endocrinology specialist with more than 20 years of experience.

Doctor Mario,
1. What is this disorder?

Diabetic foot is a condition that occurs as a result of maintaining glucose levels higher than normal.

It is characterized by a decrease in sensitivity and blood circulation, which can increase the risk of serious ulcers.

2. What are your main symptoms?

Some signs related to this disorder are redness, increased temperature, callused areas that do not improve and lesions that do not heal. It is important to pay special attention to ingrown toenails, blisters, plantar warts, open or bleeding sores, unpleasant smell, discoloration of the foot, swelling and ulcers that do not improve.

3. Who has more risks of suffering from this ailment?

The risks increase as the disease progresses. It is estimated that 15 percent of diabetics have at some time such injuries on their feet.

High blood glucose levels, peripheral neuropathy, poor blood circulation, impaired vision, kidney disease, high blood pressure, smoking and corns and deformities increase the chances of getting them.

4. What is the treatment of diabetic foot?

At the lowest sign of ulcer, it is recommended to seek immediate attention. An injury that does not heal and damages tissues and bones may eventually require the amputation of a finger, foot or part of the leg.

The treatment usually first seeks to relieve plantar pressure, by resting or using splints. Then the callus and dead tissue are removed, the wound is cleaned and the infection is treated with antibiotics. The use of hydrogel dressings as debriders may be recommended to facilitate healing. On the other hand, it is important to control and treat diabetes, platelet aggregation, hypertension and dyslipidemia to avoid complications.

5. In what cases is an amputation necessary?

When the condition causes severe tissue loss or a fatal infection, amputation may be the only option. In these cases the damaged tissue is removed by surgery.

6. How can this disorder be prevented?

The best way to prevent diabetic foot is by properly controlling the disease with a healthy diet, regular exercise, blood sugar control and compliance with the prescribed medication regimen.

On the other hand, it is also advisable to do a neuropathic and vascular study to measure sensitivity and visit the podiatrist or a traumatologist regularly to inspect and care for the feet. In case of calluses, bunions or warts, it is recommended not to remove them on their own and go to a specialist.

7. What care can we perform at home?

Those with this disease are advised to observe the feet every day, looking for chafing, wounds, blisters, swelling or redness. The areas that should be looked more closely are the tip of the big toe, the inside of the rest of the toes, the heel, the sole and the outside of the foot. When cutting the nails, straight cuts should be made, avoiding leaving corners that can cause injuries.

In addition, it is important to wash your feet daily, keep them clean, dry them well, hydrate them with appropriate creams and protect them from cold and heat. It is advisable to wear comfortable shoes, synthetic socks that do not squeeze and avoid walking barefoot.

Chapter 53. Diabetic Retinopathy and Eye Problems

Diabetic Retinopathy is a complication of diabetes that affects eyesight. It occurs when high blood sugar damages the blood vessels of the retina, the light-sensitive tissue located in the back of the eye.

Initially it may have no symptoms, but over time it can cause severe damage and even blindness. Blood vessels may swell and lose fluid or close and prevent blood from flowing. Diabetic Retinopathy affects both eyes.

To learn more about this problem, we interview Dr. Mario Vega Carbó, an endocrinology specialist.

Doctor Mario,
1. Who is affected by Diabetic Retinopathy?

Anyone with type 1 or type 2 diabetes can suffer from this disorder. The longer you have the disease and the less you are controlled, the greater the chances of getting it. Pregnancy, high blood pressure, high cholesterol and tobacco use can also increase the risks. All patients with diabetes have a complete eye exam at least once a year.

2. What are your symptoms?

Usually this condition does not offer any early warning signs. When it is more advanced, the patient may have blurred vision and altered colors, and dark or empty areas.

Blood vessels can drip blood and leave small spots that float in sight. These may disappear without treatment, but the bleeding usually reappears, so it is important to turn to the doctor at the first symptom. The earlier it is treated, the more chances of success the therapy will have.

163

3. How is Diabetic Retinopathy detected?

A complete vision analysis includes tests of visual acuity, examination with dilation of the pupils and tonometry to measure the pressure of the eye, which allow to detect if there are dripping blood vessels, inflammation or detachment of the retina, and abnormalities of the optic nerve.

If necessary, fluorescein angiography and optical coherence tomography can also be performed to confirm the diagnosis.

4. What is your treatment?

If diabetic retinopathy is mild, blood sugar levels, blood pressure and cholesterol should be monitored to delay the onset and progression of the condition. In more advanced cases, a laser surgery treatment, known as retinal photocoagulation, will be necessary. It helps reduce abnormal blood vessels and is more effective if done before bleeding begins.

If the bleeding is already severe, a vitrectomy, a surgical procedure in which blood is removed from the center of the eye, can be performed. If there is macular edema, which involves inflammation and fluid accumulated in the part of the eye responsible for central vision, it should also be treated with laser focal surgery.

5. Are these surgeries effective?

Yes, treatments are effective in reducing vision loss, especially when treated on time. However, they do not cure diabetic retinopathy so patients will always be at risk of new bleeding and may need to repeat therapies on more than one occasion.

6. What other complications can this disorder cause?

Diabetic retinopathy can cause vitreous hemorrhage, retinal detachment, glaucoma and vision loss.

7. How can it be prevented?

By taking good care of blood sugar levels, cholesterol and blood pressure, and carrying out periodic eye checks, the risks of serious conditions are reduced

Chapter 54. The Heart and Diabetes

People with diabetes have higher risks of heart disease. This is because excess blood sugar can cause damage to many parts of the body, including blood vessels. Your obstruction can cause a heart attack, stroke and other serious problems.

It is estimated that patients with diabetes are more than twice as likely to have coronary heart disease, heart failure and heart disease as those who do not.

To learn more about the subject, we interview Dr. Mario Vega Carbó, an endocrinology specialist with more than 20 years of experience.

Doctor Mario,
1. What is the relationship between diabetes and heart problems?

Diabetes is one of the main cardiovascular risk factors. It can cause abnormal cholesterol and triglyceride levels and contribute to hardening of the arteries or thickening of the arterial walls, which increases the chances of suffering from strokes, heart attacks and heart disease.

When blood flow is blocked, the heart, lungs and kidneys do not receive the same amount of blood and their functioning becomes abnormal.

In addition, diabetes damages the peripheral nerves, affecting the heart rate and hiding the symptoms of a chest pain that warns of a disease or attack. It decreases the body's ability to fight infections or pathogens and heal wounds.

2. What other factors increase the risk of heart disease?

Along with diabetes, obese people with excess body fat around the waist, those with high blood pressure, abnormal cholesterol and triglyceride levels, and a history of family members with heart disease are more likely to suffer from them.

3. What are the most frequent heart diseases related to diabetes?

The most common are coronary heart disease, heart failure and diabetic cardiomyopathy. Coronary heart disease occurs when the arteries that supply blood to the heart muscle harden and narrow. As this progresses less blood flows through the arteries, which can lead to chest pain or a heart attack.

Heart failure, meanwhile, is a condition in which the heart cannot pump the amount of blood the body needs. This causes symptoms to occur throughout the body. Meanwhile, cardiomyopathy is a disease of the heart muscle that usually causes an increase in the size of the heart or makes it thicker and stiffer than normal.

4. What are the previous signs of a heart attack?

The person may feel pain or discomfort in the chest; shortness of breath; sweating indigestion; sickness; dizziness; tiredness or fatigue If chest pain continues after resting, it may be the sign of a heart attack. In many cases, as diabetes affects the peripheral nerves, symptoms do not appear.

5. How are heart problems related to diabetes treated?

Therapy includes medications to treat heart damage, to lower blood sugar levels and control disease, for blood pressure and to normalize cholesterol and triglycerides.

The doctor may also recommend taking aspirin daily to prevent blood clots from forming in the arteries. The treatment includes the adoption of healthy lifestyle habits, such as a balanced diet, the practice of regular exercise, drinking a lot of water, eliminating overweight, quitting smoking and avoiding alcohol consumption.

6. How can the damage caused by Diabetes be prevented?

The best way is to properly control the disease with healthy lifestyle habits, blood sugar control and compliance with the prescribed medication regimen.

Chapter 55. Diabetes and kidney disease

Diabetic Nephropathy is a kidney disease that occurs over time in people who have diabetes. It is a consequence of the damage that excess blood glucose causes in the nephrons, the basic structural and functional unit of the kidney, and the blood vessels.

When this occurs, the task of removing waste and additional fluids from the body is affected. If the Nephropathy is not treated, it can lead to kidney failure, a life-threatening condition. The best way to prevent this disease is to lead a healthy lifestyle and control diabetes and high blood pressure.

To learn more about this topic, we interview Mario Vega Carbó, an endocrinologist, with more than 20 years of experience.

Doctor Mario,
1. What is the main function of the kidneys?

The kidneys are responsible for filtering waste and excess fluids in the form of urine. They are also responsible for balancing the salts and minerals that circulate in the blood, such as calcium, phosphorus, sodium and potassium. They help control blood pressure and produce hormones that are important for generating red blood cells and keeping bones strong.

2. What causes Diabetic Nephropathy?

As a result of elevated blood sugar levels and high blood pressure, nephrons and blood vessels become damaged over time, affecting the normal functioning of the kidneys.

3. Who has more risks of having it?

People with uncontrolled diabetes, obese, smokers and those with high blood pressure, high cholesterol or a family history of kidney problems are more likely to suffer from it.

4. What are the symptoms of Diabetic Nephropathy?

Usually this condition shows no signs until the damage is severe. Over time the patient may experience fatigue, malaise, headache, swelling of the feet and ankles, increased need to urinate, irregular heartbeats, loss of appetite, difficulty breathing, stomach pain, persistent itching, insomnia and confusion .

5. How is this disease detected?

Urine tests are usually done to check the protein levels in it. If they are elevated, this may mean that the blood vessels of the kidneys are damaged and fail to filter the nutrients that the body needs properly. Also, blood and blood pressure tests, and imaging tests and kidney biopsy are performed to confirm the diagnosis.

6. What is your treatment?

The therapy seeks to control and delay the damage caused by the disease. To do this, you must maintain blood pressure and stabilized sugar levels and adopt a healthy lifestyle. This includes following a balanced diet, practicing regular exercise, drinking lots of water, eliminating overweight, quitting smoking and avoiding alcohol consumption.

Medications to lower cholesterol, control calcium and phosphate balance, and reduce the level of protein in the urine may also be necessary.

Before consuming any new drug or vitamin, it is important to notify the doctor to see if it can affect the kidneys. It is advised to avoid nonsteroidal anti-inflammatory drugs such as Ibuprofen and maintain normalized vitamin D levels.

7. What is kidney failure and how is it treated?

When Diabetic Nephropathy causes serious damage, this can cause the kidneys to stop working. If this happens, waste accumulates in the body and renal failure occurs. Its symptoms are nausea, vomiting, weakness, shortness of breath and confusion, and may lead to seizures and coma.

In this case, a dialysis treatment is necessary, in which a machine is used to remove waste from the blood. Another option is to perform a kidney transplant.

8. What other complications can this disease bring?

Diabetic Nephropathy can cause fluid retention and generate swelling in the arms and legs, high blood pressure and pulmonary edema.

In addition, it can cause irreversible damage to the kidneys, blood and heart vessel disease, anemia, foot ulcers, erectile dysfunction, diarrhea and other problems.

On the other hand, during pregnancy it can bring risks to the mother and the developing fetus.

Chapter 56. Surgery in the diabetic patient

When a person with diabetes needs to undergo surgery, either because of a complication of the disease or for other reasons, it is necessary to take special care. The ailment can increase the risks of post-operative infections or generate a slower healing, in addition to heart, fluid, electrolyte or kidney problems, among other possibilities.

To make an adequate preparation for surgery, it is necessary that the medical team be duly informed about the patient's medical history, so that all the collections can be taken.

To talk about this topic we interview Dr. Mario Vega Carbó, an endocrinology specialist, he works as an endocrinologist at the Vega & Vado Office.

Doctor Mario,
1. How should a patient with diabetes prepare for surgery?

In the weeks before the operation it is important to strengthen the controls of the disease. This includes following a healthy and balanced diet, keeping glucose values within the objectives, taking medication in a timely manner, avoiding episodes of hypoglycemia and hyperglycemia, and preventing the development of ketoacidosis.

In addition, the doctor should be notified about all medications that are being taken. If you are using metformin, it may be suspended for 2 days before and 2 days after the intervention to reduce the risk of lactic acidosis.

2. What will the doctor control before the operation?

Before the surgery, the medical team must carry out a general control of the patient and provide all the necessary recommendations prior to the intervention. A glycemic check will be carried out to determine if it is suitable for carrying out the operation or not.

In these cases, it is recommended to continue surgery if glycosylated hemoglobin is less than 7.5% or is between 7.5 and 9%. If it is greater than 9, it is advisable to reprogram it until the results are improved.

3. What care should be taken during surgery?

Once in the hospital, it is recommended to check the patient's weight and perform a glycemic profile. As general anesthesia masks the symptoms and signs of hypoglycemia, frequent monitoring of its levels is necessary.

On the other hand, the increase in stress from the operation can generate a tendency to hyperglycemia and ketoacidosis, while the circulatory alterations associated with anesthesia and surgery can interfere with the absorption of insulin administered subcutaneously.

4. What will be the main objective during surgery regarding diabetes?

The main goal will be to avoid hypoglycemia, ketoacidosis and hyperglycemia. During the operation it is advisable to keep glucose controls between 100 and 180mg / dl. If the patient is fasting, it is necessary to manage insulin to avoid ketoacidosis.

5. How is insulin supplied during the operation?

The night before surgery, the patient should eat and receive his insulin treatment in the normal way. On the day of the operation, at the usual time when the person takes their dose, a drip of glucosated serum with electrolytes and a second route with an insulin infusion begins. The fact of using two separate flasks allows adjusting the infusion rate of insulin in order to maintain the blood glucose level between 100 and 180 mg / dl.

6. What should be done after the operation?

After the intervention, the patient or nurses should check frequently in blood sugar level. They may be altered as a result of post-surgical stress, eating problems, lack of activity or the use of medications.

To ensure controls, people with diabetes often have to stay in the hospital longer than those without this disease.

7. What are the signs to be alert to?

In addition to checking blood sugar levels frequently, you should be aware of symptoms of infection, such as fever or an incision that is red and hot to the touch, with more pain or suppuration. Pressure sores should be prevented, for which it is important to move constantly.

Chapter 57. Insulin Resistance: Metformin

Type 2 diabetes mellitus is a chronic disorder that prevents proper glucose metabolism, causing it to accumulate in the blood. This can be caused by an insulin resistance that eventually leads to a deficit in the production of this hormone in the pancreas.

To treat resistance it is necessary to modify the lifestyle, exercise regularly and control body weight. Also adopt a balanced diet, with lower consumption of saturated fats. If these changes are not enough, the doctor may recommend the use of drugs. Among them, the most used is Metformin.

To talk about this topic, we interview Mario Vega Carbó, an endocrinologist with more than 20 years of experience.

Doctor Mario,
1. How does Metformin work?

This drug lowers blood glucose levels by reducing and delaying the amount that is absorbed from food at the intestinal level. It also decreases the sugar produced by the liver and promotes its storage as glycogen, and increases the body's response to insulin, improving its use.

2. How should this medication be taken?

Metformin is marketed in liquid or tablets. It is usually taken 2 or 3 times a day, with or after meals. The initial dose is usually 500 mg, which is adjusted based on blood glucose levels. There are prolonged-release tablets that are taken once a day, with the evening meal.

3. What should be done if you forget to take a dose?

You should ingest it as soon as you remember. However, if it is almost time for the next dose, it is better to skip it and continue with the regular dosage. In no case should a double dose be taken to compensate for the one that was forgotten.

4. What side effects does Metformin have?

At the beginning of the treatment it is possible that the patient presents nausea, vomiting, diarrhea, flatulence, constipation, abdominal pain, swelling and loss of appetite, which disappear soon after. If diarrhea persists you should see your doctor to reduce the dose or stop your treatment.

When it is used for a long time, in some cases there is a reduction in the absorption of vitamin B12, increasing the risk of anemia.

In patients with severe renal impairment, it can generate lactic acidosis, a rare metabolic complication in which this acid accumulates in the blood when oxygen levels decrease in the cells. Some of its symptoms are respiratory distress, abdominal pain, muscle cramps, extreme tiredness, asthenia and hypothermia, which can eventually lead to a coma.

5. What are the most frequent errors while using this medicine?

Sometimes, people neglect diet and exercise because they think that with the intake of metformin the disease is already controlled. In other cases, its use is not temporarily suspended in special situations, such as surgery or radiological examinations with intravenous iodinated contrasts; the patient's renal function is not contemplated during treatment; or the dose is not adjusted over time based on the evolution of diabetes.

6. What other aspects should be taken into account while using Metformin?

Before starting the treatment it is important to inform the doctor about any other medication, vitamin or supplement that is being used, so that it evaluates whether the combination can be harmful.

You should also notify if you have other conditions, such as kidney or heart problems; if you are pregnant or planning to conceive in the short term, or if you are breastfeeding.

On the other hand, the use of oral contraceptives can worsen glycemic metabolism and make Metformin less effective, so it will be necessary to readjust the dose.

In addition, while using alcohol should be avoided, which can increase the risks of lactic acidosis and reduce blood sugar.

Finally, this medicine should be stored in a suitable place, at room temperature and out of the reach of children.

Chapter 58. Hypoglycemic drugs

In addition to Metformin, there are other drugs that are used in the treatment of type 2 diabetes, when lifestyle changes are not enough. They are known as hypoglycemic drugs and help lower blood glucose levels.

These antidiabetics are distinguished by their chemical structure and their mechanism of action. Among them are sulfonylureas, meglitinides, thiazolidinediones and alpha-glucosidase and dipeptidylpeptidase 4 inhibitors.

To talk about this topic, we interview Mario Vega Carbó, an endocrinologist with more than 20 years of experience.

Doctor Mario,
1. How do hypoglycemic drugs work?

These drugs can work in different ways. Some stimulate the pancreatic secretion of insulin, while others sensitize the peripheral tissues to the hormone, alter the gastrointestinal absorption of glucose or increase the presence of sugar in the urine.

They are generally used in combination with Metformin, or when it is not tolerated or contraindicated.

2. How do sulfonylureas help in diabetes control?

These oral medications, among which are gliclazide, glimepiride, glibenclamide and glipizide, stimulate insulin secretion in pancreatic beta cells (by this action they are called secretagogues). In the long term they increase the metabolic response to circulating insulin. In general they are taken once or twice a day, before meals.

3. What are its adverse effects?

These medications can cause hypoglycemia and an increase in body weight. They are not recommended for children or pregnant women, during breastfeeding, or for patients with type 1 diabetes, diabetic ketoacidosis or advanced liver and kidney failure. In case of hypoglycemia, if it is not resolved quickly, it can worsen quickly and cause epileptic seizures and brain damage.

4. How do thiazolidinediones or glitazones work?

These drugs act by increasing the sensitivity of muscle, fat and liver to insulin and decreasing peripheral resistance to this hormone. They can be used alone or in combination with sulfonylureas or with Metformin. Thiazolidinediones may be beneficial in the treatment of non-alcoholic fatty liver.

5. What care should be taken while taking these medications?

Cases of heart failure associated with the administration of thiazolidinediones have been reported, and are therefore not recommended in patients with heart disease. In the past some drugs caused acute liver failure. Although this problem no longer appears, periodic checks of liver function during use are advised. In addition, in many cases an increase in weight has been observed, due to fluid retention and increased adipose tissue mass.

6. How do alpha-glucosidase inhibitors work?

These medications, such as acarbose and miglitol, decrease the absorption of carbohydrates from the digestive tract, thus reducing sugar levels after meals. While they are less effective than the other drugs, they can be given in combination to improve treatment. Among its side effects are dyspepsia, flatulence and diarrhea.

7. Finally, how do dipeptidyl peptidase-4 inhibitors work?

These drugs, such as vildagliptin, sitagliptin, linagliptin and saxagliptin, are based on the action of incretin hormones, which help control the function of the pancreas. By inhibiting the enzyme DDP-4 this organ produces more insulin after meals.

Some of its side effects are nasal congestion, sore throat and headache, diarrhea, inflammation of the pancreas, rashes, swelling of the face and difficulty breathing.

Chapter 59. Use of insulin for the control of Diabetes

Insulin is the hormone produced by the pancreas, responsible for regulating sugar in the body and its use as a source of energy in the cells.

People with diabetes have a high blood glucose level because they do not produce enough insulin or because the body does not respond adequately to it. This can cause serious problems in the heart, eyes, kidneys, nerves and feet. A replacement therapy can help these patients maintain their stable values.

To learn more about this topic, we interview Mario Vega Carbó, an endocrinologist with more than 20 years of experience.

Doctor Mario,
1. Who needs to use insulin?

In those patients with type 1 diabetes the pancreas does not produce enough insulin, so they should take replacement hormone every day. In those with type 2 diabetes, there is usually an insulin resistance and the body does not use it properly. These people need to take it when other treatments and drugs cannot control blood sugar levels.

2. How does this therapy work?

This medicine replaces the insulin that the body does not produce naturally and works by helping to move blood sugar to the other tissues of the body, where it is used as a source of energy. In addition, it also prevents the liver from producing more glucose.

3. How many types of insulin are there?

There are different types. Among them are fast-acting insulin, which is taken before meals and starts working at 15 minutes and lasts 4 hours; the baseline, which begins to take effect at 2 hours and lasts from 12 to 18 hours; and the long-lasting one, which helps control glucose throughout the day. Depending on the case, these can be used individually or in combination.

4. How is insulin given?

Generally the therapy consists of the administration of three or more daily injections to maintain a normal blood sugar level. These are applied to the abdomen, upper arm, thighs or hips.

Another option is the use of an insulin pump, a device the size of a mobile phone that administers the hormone continuously for 24 hours. To do this, a tube connects the reservoir to a catheter, which is inserted under the skin of the abdomen.

It is also possible to use a disposable insulin pen, which is released under the skin using a needle; or a powder inhaler. The hormone cannot be administered orally because stomach acids destroy it.

5. How much insulin is given?

The dose and frequency of use depend on several factors, such as the patient's weight, the amount of food he consumes, his degree of physical activity, the level of blood sugar and whether or not he suffers from other health problems. Therefore, it is important that these people learn to measure glucose and to carry out periodic checks. Based on these results, the treatment will be adjusted according to the needs, to maintain an appropriate range.

6. What precautions should be taken into account during use?

Before starting the treatment it is important to inform the doctor about any other medication, vitamin or supplement that is being used, so that it evaluates whether the combination can be harmful.

It should also be notified if other conditions are suffered, such as nerve damage, heart failure, kidney or heart problems; if you are pregnant or planning to conceive in the short term; or if you are breastfeeding.

On the other hand, in certain situations it may be necessary to adjust the dose of insulin being taken. For example, before and after surgery, in times of stress or trips to other time zones, or when you are sick, you exercise a lot, drink alcohol or eat too much.

7. What side effects can this medicine cause?

In some cases, patients may have redness, swelling or irritation at the injection site; skin changes; weight gain; and constipation In severe cases, there may be difficulty breathing, blurred vision, irregular heartbeat, swelling in arms and legs, and muscle cramps.

8. What happens if a very high dose of insulin is used?

Insulin overdose can cause hypoglycemia, a condition in which blood sugar levels are below normal. If this is not resolved quickly, it can worsen quickly and cause epileptic seizures and brain damage.

To avoid this disorder, it is recommended to regularly measure glucose levels and maintain a fixed schedule for meals. Also follow the medical therapy indicated for the control of diabetes and take the medications at the time and at the indicated doses.

In addition, if you are going to practice physical activities, it is advisable to drink liquid and eat before, and always have glucose tablets or candies on hand.

9. What other aspects should be taken into account during treatment?

When administering the injections, the application on muscles, scars or moles should be avoided, and a different site should be used for each time, within the same area.

On the other hand, it is important for the patient to understand that insulin controls blood sugar, but does not cure diabetes. Therefore, it should continue to be used even when you feel well.

Finally, closed medication should always be kept in the refrigerator, out of the reach of children.

Chapter 60. Glucose monitoring and self-control

People with Diabetes should permanently monitor their sugar levels, in order to adequately control the disease.

In addition to the tests performed in hospitals, it is important that these patients learn to measure their own glucose and ketone values domestically. For this there are electronic devices known as glucometers, which analyze the amounts of these substances in blood and urine simply and instantly.

Based on these results, diabetes treatment can be adjusted according to the needs, in order to control the symptoms and avoid serious consequences.

To learn more about this topic, we interview Mario Vega Carbó, an endocrinology specialist, who works as an endocrinologist at the Vega & Vado Office.

Doctor Mario,
1. Who should monitor your glucose levels permanently?

These controls are recommended for all patients with diabetes, especially for those who use insulin or take pills to treat the disease.
In addition, they are also very important in cases of intensive therapies with this hormone and in situations of pregnancy and of very low or very high blood sugar levels.

2. What are the benefits of these measurements?

These controls are the best way to know if the treatment that is being followed against Diabetes is effective. In addition, they allow timely detection of acute complications related to the disease, such as Hypoglycemia, Hyperglycemia, Coma Hyperosmolar and Ketoacidosis.

On the other hand, keeping sugar levels within the desired ranges helps prevent the occurrence of serious problems in the heart, eyes, kidneys, nerves and feet. These measurements make it possible to establish a balance between the foods that are consumed, the exercises that are carried out and the drugs that are used to treat this condition, in addition to knowing how the body responds to each situation.

3. How is a self-monitoring done?

A portable electronic meter called a glucometer is used for it. After washing your hands, a puncture element is used to prick the fingertip and get a drop of blood. This is placed on a test strip covered with a chemical in the device, which marks the level of glucose on the screen.

In order for the doctor to make comparisons and analysis of the results, it is important to carry out the measurements at the same times each day and also record the food ingested, the dose of medication used and the exercise performed.

4. What values are considered normal?

The recommended glucose levels will depend on each patient, their age and their health status. Values between 70 and 100 milligrams per deciliter (mg / dL) are considered normal when the fasting measurement is performed; between 80 and 130 mg / dL before meals; and less than 170 mg / dL two hours after them.

5. How many daily checks are recommended?

The amount of measurements will depend on each patient based on the medical recommendation. In cases of people using insulin injections, 6 daily controls are usually advised. These are usually done before the 3 main meals (breakfast, lunch and dinner), and two hours after each of them, the last before bedtime.

For those who use long-acting insulin, two monitoring per day is usually recommended, one in the morning and one at night. Meanwhile, patients with type 2 diabetes who do not use insulin and who treat the disease with diet and exercise in general do not require daily measurements.

In situations of stress, illness or changes in the dose of medications, more frequent controls are required.

6. What is postprandial glycemia?

It is the level of blood sugar after eating. Usually, after meals it rises during the first two hours and the production of insulin in the body grows.

7. What values are expected after meals?

The glucose level should not exceed 170 mg / dL after more than 90 minutes after eating food. In addition, these values should return to normal at 3 hours of intake.

8. What are continuous glucose monitors?

They are devices that measure glucose frequently, through a sensor placed under the skin. They reflect sugar levels at all times and have an alarm that is activated when the values are too high or too low. They are usually recommended for patients with type 1 diabetes who use insulin.

9. What care should be taken during these measurements?

To ensure the effectiveness of these controls it is important to verify that the glucometer and the rest of the elements used are clean and that they are at room temperature. It is also necessary to ensure that the test strips are not expired or damaged, that the meter is well calibrated and that the size of the blood drop is indicated.

10. How are urine glucose controls?

These measurements are similar to blood. In these cases, the color at which the test strip changes indicates the glucose level. However, urine controls are not as accurate as blood controls, so they are not highly recommended unless there is no other option.

This monitoring is used to detect ketones, acids that appear when there is not enough insulin in the body. Their presence is an indication that the body is using fats as an energy source instead of sugar, something that usually occurs more frequently in patients with type 1 diabetes.

11. What is the glycosylated hemoglobin or HbA1c test?

It is a test that measures the average blood glucose level attached to hemoglobin, the part of the red blood cells that carries oxygen, during the last three months. It is used to detect diabetes or prediabetes in adults, or to monitor the progression of the disease and the results of its treatment. Diabetics are recommended to perform this test at least twice a year.

12. How is this study conducted and what are the expected values?

For this analysis, a blood sample is drawn from a vein in an arm using a needle. The results are given in percentages and are generally normal below 5.7%, indicate prediabetes between 5.7 and 6.4%, and diabetes if they are greater than that value. For people who already have the disease, it is recommended to keep this value below 6.5%.

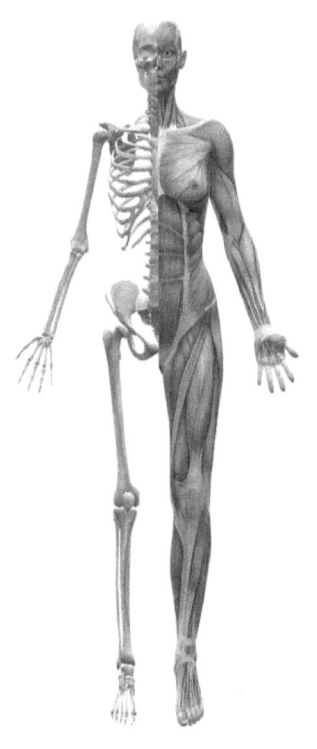

SECTION II ENDOCRINOLOGY

The second section of this book of interviews goes a little deeper into issues related to the clinical Endocrinology discipline. In each of its parts and chapters we invite the reader to identify which are the main glands of the endocrine system, how they work and what situations derive from their diseases.

We begin by talking about the thyroid, a gland that functions as "a great initiating machine for all metabolic processes in the body." We will clarify your doubts about diseases such as hypothyroidism, hyperthyroidism, its complications, medications for its treatment, and we will talk about other less known diseases, such as sick euthyroid syndrome, to more serious conditions such as thyroid cancer and methods for diagnosis and treatment.

Similarly, the thyroid gland participates in the regulation and metabolism of calcium, which is the second part of this section. You will understand how calcium is used in the body in different cellular processes, which hormones control your blood levels, and the diseases that result from their alterations. We will study the parathyroid gland, and the processes of regulating your parathyroid hormone.

The third part of this second section deals with the adrenal glands, a pair of glands in close relationship with the kidneys, which are true endocrine regulators, since their hormones control the processes related to carbohydrate metabolism, levels of electrolytes (sodium, potassium) and are a source of production of sex hormones (androgens). We will discuss some pathologies given by their hypo or hyperfunction, factors that alter this function and its management.

In the fourth part of this section we talk about the controlling center of all the endocrine organs of the body, the pituitary gland or pituitary gland. It is located in the skull, being responsible for releasing hormones that are stimulants of the action of the rest of the body's endocrine glands, also involved the process of regulating said hormonal secretion. We will clarify doubts about diseases that compromise the function of the pituitary gland, symptoms, diagnosis and treatment.

Then deepen your knowledge in *Endocrinology*.

Part IV Thyroid

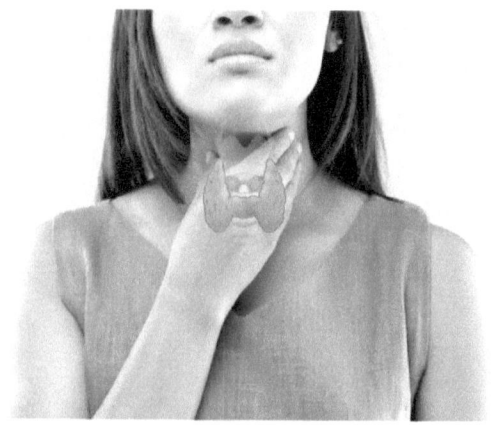

Chapter 61. Ectopic Thyroid

Ectopic Thyroid is a rare congenital anomaly, in which the gland is not in its normal location. This occurs due to a defective displacement of the organ from the blind hole to its final pretracheal position. In most cases, the most frequent location of thyroid tissue is at the base of the tongue and sublingual.

This disorder can be asymptomatic or present with different complications, such as hypothyroidism. Its clinical incidence is estimated in 1 case per 200 thousand people, being more common in women.

To talk about this issue we interview Dr. Mario Vega Carbó, an endocrinology specialist, who currently works as an endocrinologist at the Vega & Vado Office.

Doctor Mario,
1. How is the Ectopic Thyroid generated?

This gland appears as an epithelial proliferation on the floor of the pharynx and subsequently migrates until it reaches its pretracheal location in the seventh week of gestation. During this process it remains attached to the base of the tongue through a conduit that then disappears.

When alterations occur in the course of this displacement, the thyroid develops in another location. If the descent does not start, the gland remains in its original position at the base of the tongue. If it can move, it can be lodged in the sublingual, submandibular, prelaryngeal or tracheal region, and even appear in areas away from the neck.

It is believed that this anomaly is due to the alteration in the function of various genes that regulate thyroid development.

2. What are your main symptoms?

In many cases, the Ectopic Thyroid is asymptomatic. In others it may present difficulty or inability to swallow, dysphonia, choking and breathing problems, sensation of a foreign body in the mouth or pharynx, cough and blood expectoration.

In babies there is usually a decrease in activity and an increase in sleep, as well as difficulty in feeding and constipation.

3. How is the Ectopic Thyroid detected?

In view of its symptoms, a physical examination and neck palpation, analysis of hormonal levels, scintigraphy and radiological tests are usually performed to more accurately determine the size of ectopic thyroid tissue and differentiate it from other causes of cervical mass.

4. What is your treatment?

In cases of lingual thyroid without symptoms and small in size, conservative behavior with regular controls and thyroid function tests is recommended. If the gland has a moderate size, a treatment based on suppression with T3 and T4 is usually carried out so that its size decreases gradually.

If the signs get worse, there is severe obstruction, suspicion of malignancy, ulceration or bleeding, surgery may be necessary.

5. What other complications can this ailment bring?

Thyroid hormone is essential for brain development and growth. In cases where the Ectopic Thyroid results in Congenital Hypothyroidism, if the patient is not treated in time, he may suffer intellectual disabilities and a maturational delay. As for carcinomas derived from ectopic thyroid tissue, they are usually rare.

Chapter 62. Goiter

Goiter is a swelling in the neck that is caused by an abnormal enlargement of the thyroid gland. It is usually not painful, but it can cause coughing and difficulty swallowing and breathing.

The most common cause of this condition is the lack of iodine in the diet, although it can also appear as a result of excessive or insufficient production of certain hormones or thyroid nodules. Most of these packages are non-cancerous.

The thyroid gland is responsible for controlling the metabolism and its task is essential for normal growth and development in childhood, and for the functioning of the brain throughout life.

To learn more about this topic, we interview Mario Vega Carbó, an endocrinologist with more than 20 years of experience.

Doctor Mario,
1. What are the symptoms of goiter?

Its most common sign is a visible lump at the base of the neck. In addition, the swollen thyroid can put pressure on the trachea and esophagus and cause coughing, hoarseness, dryness and difficulty swallowing and breathing. However, in some cases the goiter has no symptoms.

2. Who are more likely to have it?

Goiter can affect anyone, be congenital or appear over time. Women, especially pregnant women, those over 40 and those with a family history of autoimmune diseases have a higher risk of suffering from it.

Also people with Graves disease, hypothyroidism or thyroiditis, those who consume certain medications such as lithium, smokers and those who received radiation in the neck or chest.

3. How is this disease detected?

To confirm the diagnosis, physical exams and blood tests are usually performed to control the levels of hormones produced by the thyroid and pituitary gland. A neck ultrasound and a thyroid scan and biopsy may be necessary.

4. What is your treatment?

The therapy will depend on the size of the goiter and its symptoms. If it is small and does not cause problems, periodic checks are usually only required. If the cause is the lack of iodine, a diet rich in this mineral will be recommended, along with potassium iodide supplements.

If the problem is Hypothyroidism, a replacement of the thyroid hormone with Levothyroxine will be performed, while if it is hyperthyroidism, its effects will be blocked with propylthiouracil or methimazole.

For inflammation of the gland, aspirin or a corticosteroid can be taken. In severe cases, surgery may be necessary to remove the organ or its reduction with the intake of radioactive iodine. If that happens, the patient should take hormone replacement pills for life.

5. What other aspects are recommended to consider?

For people with goiter it is advisable to eat foods rich in iodine, such as fish, shrimp and shellfish. Also avoid some vegetables, such as cauliflower, cabbage, broccoli and cabbage, which make it difficult to operate this mineral. In many countries iodine is added to salt.

Chapter 63. Ultrasound or ultrasound of the thyroid

Ultrasound or ultrasound of the thyroid is an imaging test that is performed in order to observe in detail this gland, responsible for producing hormones that control metabolism, cardiovascular balance, energy consumption and growth.

This is a study that uses high frequency sound waves that allow you to see internal organs and structures of the body in real time. Unlike x-rays, this test does not expose to radiation.

Among other possibilities, ultrasound of the thyroid makes it possible to see if the gland is enlarged or swollen, or if it has nodules and even cancer. In addition, it allows guiding the needle in case of biopsy.

To learn more about this test, we consulted Dr. Mario Vega Carbó, an endocrinology specialist in charge of the Vega & Vado Office.

Doctor Mario,
1. When is it necessary to perform an ultrasound of the thyroid?

If the patient shows symptoms of abnormal functioning of the gland or if it has a swelling or strange growth, the doctor may want to check its structure and size and confirm if there are nodules.

2. How is pre-exam preparation?

To perform an ultrasound, no previous preparation or fasting is necessary. The patient should wear comfortable and loose clothes, take off necklaces and chains, and lie on a stretcher.

3. How is ultrasound performed?

A water-based conductive gel is applied to the patient, which allows the adaptation of the ultrasound transducer. This is a small portable device, which is connected to a computer by means of a cable. The transducer slides on the skin to send high-frequency acoustic waves and obtain real-time images on a monitor. Usually the exam for between 15 and 30 minutes, and is completely painless.

4. What can be seen in the study?

The ultrasound allows you to observe the shape and internal structure of the thyroid, and check if it is enlarged or has a smaller volume; see if there are nodules and what are their sizes, location and characteristics, to determine whether they are benign or malignant.

In the case of Doppler, a type of ultrasound that also shows blood flow, vascularization of the gland can be observed, which helps in the diagnosis of thyroiditis or Graves-Basedow disease. The results obtained in the study are fundamental to determine the steps to follow in the treatment.

5. What other uses does this test have?

Ultrasound also makes it possible to detect tumors in the parathyroid glands, located behind the thyroid and very important for regulating calcium levels in the body. In addition, it is very useful to carry out controls after surgical interventions in the area, to assess the function of the vocal cords and to observe lymph nodes and other tumors and cysts that may appear in the neck.

On the other hand, it is also used as a guide to perform an aspiration thyroid biopsy. In that case, the ultrasound allows the needle to be directed into the cyst or hematoma in order to remove a small amount of tissue, drain it, analyze its contents or infiltrate a medication. This procedure makes it possible to differentiate with greater certainty whether the thyroid lesion is benign or malignant.

Chapter 64. Fine needle biopsy for the study of thyroid nodules

Most of the nodules that appear in the thyroid, 90 - 95%, are benign in nature. However, there are several types of cancer that can affect it. When it is necessary to obtain a sample of your cells to detect or rule out any disease, it is possible to perform a fine water biopsy.

During this procedure, it is inserted into the gland to remove fluid and tissues, which are sent to the laboratory for analysis.

In order to learn more about this topic, we interview Mario Vega Carbó, an endocrinology specialist with more than 20 years of experience.

Doctor Mario,
1. How is this study done?

This biopsy is very simple and can be carried out with or without anesthesia. Once the sample is removed, pressure is applied to the area to stop any bleeding and then covered with a bandage. In cases where it is not possible to feel the area, an ultrasound or scanner is used to guide the needle into the cyst or hematoma. Usually the exam for 15-30 minutes.

2. How does ultrasound work?

A water-based conductive gel is applied to the patient, which allows the adaptation of the ultrasound transducer. This is a small portable device, which is connected to a computer by means of a cable. The transducer slides on the skin to send high-frequency acoustic waves and obtain real-time images on a monitor.

3. How is the preparation for this exam?

This type of study does not require much prior preparation. You should only inform the doctor about all the medications you are taking, if you suffer from any type of allergy or disease, or if you are pregnant.

In case of taking anticoagulant remedies, such as aspirin and ibuprofen, it is possible that the patient should suspend them temporarily for a few days before the intervention.

4. What are the benefits of this procedure?

The fine needle biopsy allows us to differentiate with greater certainty whether the thyroid lesion is benign or malignant. It is a less invasive examination than the surgical one, it almost does not leave a scar and does not involve exposure to ionizing radiation.

5. What abnormalities can be found in the biopsy?

The results may show some type of thyroid disease, such as goiter or thyroiditis, benign tumors or cancer.

6. What side effects does it have?

In some cases you may feel a slight discomfort in the neck or have a small bruise that disappears in a day or two. Generally the patient can resume his activities without problems after the procedure and the bandage that is placed is removed in a few hours.

7. Does the fine needle biopsy have any risk?

The procedure is very safe and the risks are very low. In some very few cases the patient may have bleeding at the site of the examination, infection or damage to any of the structures adjacent to the thyroid.

Chapter 65. Thyroid Cancer

Thyroid Cancer is one that occurs in the thyroid gland responsible for the production of hormones that influence metabolism, growth and most of the body's functions, such as heart rate and blood pressure.

Located on the neck, just below the Adam's nut, this organ is shaped like a butterfly, with two lobes joined by a central area. Most of the nodules that appear in it, between 90 - 95%, are benign in nature. However, there are several types of cancer that can affect it. The most common and least dangerous is Papillary Carcinoma, which usually occurs in women of reproductive age and spreads slowly. Others are Anaplastic Carcinoma, the most harmful but rare; Follicular Tumor, which is very likely to reappear; and Medullary Carcinoma, which affects non-thyroid cells found in the gland and tends to run in families.

In order to learn more about this topic, we interview Mario Vega Carbó, an endocrinology specialist with more than 20 years of experience.

Doctor Mario,
1. What are the symptoms of Thyroid Cancer?

Its signs may vary depending on the type of cancer, but they usually have a lump or swelling in the neck, cough, difficulty swallowing, enlargement of the thyroid gland, changes in the voice with increased hoarseness, sore throat, breathing problems and swollen lymph nodes.

2. Who are more likely to have it?

Thyroid Cancer can appear at any age, although it is more common in adults and women. People who have received radiation in the neck or head area, and those with a family history are more likely to have it.

3. How is it produced?

Thyroid Cancer originates when the cells located there undergo genetic changes that allow them to grow and multiply rapidly. In addition, this mutation causes them to lose the ability to die, as normal cells would. Its accumulation in the gland forms a tumor, which can invade nearby tissues and spread throughout the body.

4. How is thyroid cancer detected?

Faced with its symptoms, a physical examination is usually done to look for lumps in the gland and swollen lymph nodes in the neck. To confirm the diagnosis, studies of calcitonin in the blood, laryngoscopy, biopsy and ultrasound of the thyroid, computed tomography of the neck and tests of thyroid function are carried out.

5. What is your treatment?

Therapy depends on the type of Thyroid Cancer. Usually a surgery is performed in which the entire gland is removed. If they have spread, it may also be necessary to remove lymph nodes from the neck. After treatment, the patient should take thyroid hormone pills throughout his life.

This process can be accompanied by external radiotherapy or with iodine, which comes in the form of capsules or drinking liquid. It can cause side effects such as nausea, dry mouth and eyes, fatigue and changes in taste and smell.

If the cancer does not respond to surgery or radiotherapy, it can be tested with chemotherapy or with targeted therapy, with substances that attack cancer cells without harming normal ones.

6. What is the forecast?

The treatment of most types of thyroid cancer is usually effective if it is diagnosed in a timely manner.

7. What other complications can this disease bring?

This condition can cause injury to the larynx, damage to the vocal cords and hoarseness after surgery, low calcium levels due to accidental removal of the parathyroid glands and spread of cancer to the lung, bones or other parts of the body.

8. What other aspects are recommended to take into account to face this disease?

Due to the stress and concern that this disease can cause, psychological support and participation in therapeutic groups with people suffering from the same disease is recommended.

Chapter 66. Thyroid surgery and its complications

Thyroid surgery is the most common endocrine operation. It is done to treat different gland problems, such as cancer, goiter or hyperthyroidism.

If only one part is removed during surgery, it is possible that the thyroid can continue to function normally. On the other hand, if the removal is total, the patient should take hormone replacement medications for life. Thyroidectomy is usually a safe procedure. However, as with any surgery, complications may arise.

To learn more about this topic, we consulted Dr. Mario Vega Carbó, an endocrinology specialist, who currently works at the Vega & Vado Office.

Doctor Mario,
1. What are the most frequent reasons for thyroid surgery?

Cancer is the most common cause for thyroidectomy. Also goiter, a swelling in the neck that is caused by an abnormal enlargement of the gland and can cause breathing or swallowing difficulties.

Other possible reasons are hyperthyroidism, a disease in which the thyroid produces too much thyroxine hormone; and the appearance of certain suspicious nodules that present a risk of being malignant.

2. What is this intervention?

There are several ways to carry out a thyroidectomy. In the conventional method a cut is made in the center of the neck to have direct access to the gland. In the transoral this incision is avoided by making it inside the mouth. In the endoscopic small cuts are made in the neck through which a small video camera is inserted that guides the doctor during the intervention. Another option is to perform surgery from the armpit.

3. What complications may occur during the operation?

The thyroid is highly vascularized which can cause bleeding and risk of infection. In addition, bleeding may cause airway obstruction.

On the other hand, during surgery an involuntary lesion of the parathyroid glands, which are located behind the thyroid, can occur. This can lead to hypoparathyroidism, a disorder in which little parathyroid hormone is produced, responsible for controlling the use and elimination of calcium, phosphate and Vitamin D from the body.

In turn, after a thyroidectomy some people have neck pain or a hoarse or weak voice, as a result of an injury to the nerves of the vocal cords and larynx.

Finally, in severe cases of untreated hyperthyroidism a sudden aggravation of its symptoms can occur and cause what is known as Thyroid Storm.

4. Why can voice changes occur after the operation?

When a thyroidectomy is performed there are risks of damage to the recurrent laryngeal nerve, which passes through the internal and posterior part of the gland. Therefore, some patients may present hoarseness or weak voice. These symptoms are temporary and are due to the tube to maintain pulmonary ventilation that is inserted into the trachea during the operation or to a nerve irritation caused by surgery

Usually in 2 or 3 weeks these signs disappear, without the need for treatment. In a few cases, traumatic intubation, excessive stretching of the nerve or accidental cutting can cause a definite alteration of the voice and breathing.

5. What damage can cause skin surgery?

The effects on the skin are those of the incision that needs to be made to practice the intervention. When a cut is made in the neck it is inevitable that after the operation a scar will remain.

In the first weeks in the wound there may be some tightness and some pain and even numbness around it. These signs are normal and transient. On the other hand, infections and bruises on the skin are very unlikely.

6. What is Thyroid Storm?

Thyroid Storm is the acute increase in the symptoms of hyperthyroidism, which endangers the functioning of the organs and the patient's life. It is a rare crisis that can be triggered by an infection or surgery, causing high fever, diarrhea, tachycardia, shock and death.

It usually occurs in patients in whom thyroid hyperactivity is poorly controlled or even undiagnosed.

Chapter 67. Hypothyroidism or Hypoactive Thyroid

Hypothyroidism is a disease in which the thyroid does not produce enough thyroid hormone. This gland is one of the most important in the body and its activity influences metabolism and most of the bodily functions, such as heart rate and blood pressure.

That there are usual levels of this hormone in the body is essential for normal growth and development in childhood, and for the functioning of the brain throughout life. If not treated correctly, hypothyroidism can cause numerous health problems, such as obesity, joint pain, infertility or heart disease.

To talk about this topic, we interview Dr. Mario Vega Carbó, an endocrinology specialist, who works as an endocrinologist at the Vega & Vado Office.

Doctor Mario,
1. What is the cause of hypothyroidism?

The most common cause is Hashimoto's Disease or Chronic Thyroiditis. It is caused by a reaction of the immune system, in which antibodies directed against the thyroid lead to inflammation of the gland. It is not known for sure why this occurs, but it is believed to be related to a virus, a bacterium or a genetic failure. The chronic damage caused by this condition usually causes a decrease in the levels of thyroid hormone in the blood.

In addition, Hypothyroidism can also be caused by viral or respiratory infections, pregnancy, certain medications such as lithium, some types of chemotherapy, congenital diseases and Sheehan Syndrome.

Other reasons are treatments with radioactive iodine or drugs against hyperthyroidism, radiotherapy, or a tumor or surgery of the thyroid or pituitary gland.

2. Who has more risks of having it?

Hypothyroidism can occur in anyone of any age. However, it is more common in women of middle age and over 60 years. Those who have autoimmune or family diseases with a history of thyroid problems, those who treated against hyperthyroidism and those exposed to high levels of radiation are more likely to suffer from it. Also women who were pregnant or gave birth in the last 6 months.

3. What are your main symptoms?

The disease usually develops slowly and initially shows no signs. Over time, the patient may have constipation, difficulty concentrating, pale dry skin, swelling in the front of the throat, fatigue, brittle hair and nails, irregular menstruation, increased sensitivity to cold, weight gain, depression, pain in the joints and muscle weakness.

If left untreated, in more severe cases there may be a decrease in the sense of taste and smell, hoarseness, thickening of the skin, slow heart rate and swelling of the face, hands and feet.

4. How is this disease detected?

When your symptoms occur, a physical exam and various studies are usually done to measure the levels of thyroid hormone, thyroid stimulating hormone, cholesterol and glucose, and an antibody test. Other specialized tests of the gland may also be necessary.

5. What is your treatment?

The therapy involves replenishing the thyroid hormone that is missing in the body with Levothyroxine, which should generally be taken for life. This oral medication restores adequate levels of the hormone and reverses the signs and symptoms of the disease. Periodic controls are essential during treatment, since at the appropriate dose this drug has no side effects. If ingested more than necessary, the patient may have an accelerated pulse, tremor, weight loss, tiredness and hyperactivity.

6. What other complications can hypothyroidism bring?

If not treated properly, it can cause infections, goitre, heart problems, peripheral neuropathy, depression, reduced libido, infertility and miscarriage. Also myxedema, the most severe form of hypothyroidism, which causes a medical emergency that must be treated in the hospital. Its symptoms are low temperature, decreased breathing, low blood pressure and blood glucose, lethargy and loss of consciousness.

On the other hand, babies of women with untreated hypothyroidism can be born with congenital defects.

Chapter 68. Medications for Hypothyroidism: Levothyroxine and Lyothyronine

Hypothyroidism is a disease in which the thyroid does not produce enough thyroid hormone. The usual levels of it is essential for normal growth and development in childhood, and for the functioning of the brain throughout life.

The treatment for this medical condition consists in replenishing the hormone that is missing in the body, for which Levothyroxine and Lyothyronine are used, which generally must be taken for life.

To learn more about this topic, we interview Mario Vega Carbó, an endocrinologist with more than 20 years of experience.

Doctor Mario,
1. How do levothyroxine and lithothyronine work?

These medications replace the thyroid hormone that the body normally produces. They come in tablets and capsules, and in general they are taken once a day, on an empty stomach, half an hour before breakfast. It is usually started with a low dose, which is gradually increasing.

In the case of babies, they should be crushed and administered mixed with water or breast milk, using a dropper or syringe.

2. How do they differ from each other?

Usually in the treatment of hypothyroidism only Levothyroxine is used. However, in some cases where symptoms persist, combined therapy with lithiotylin may be more effective. Liothyronine has a faster onset of action and a shorter half-life in relation to Levothyroxine.

3. What should be done if you forget to take a dose of these medications?

You should ingest it as soon as you remember. However, if it is almost time for the next dose, it is better to skip it and continue with the regular dosage. In no case should a double dose be taken to compensate for the one that was forgotten.

4. What side effects do these drugs have?

When they are administered in the appropriate dose they do not usually present side effects, so periodic controls are important to adjust the dose. Sometimes, patients may gain or lose weight, feel a headache or suffer from vomiting, diarrhea, changes in appetite and menstrual cycle, fever, heat sensitivity and leg cramps.

In more severe cases there may be difficulty breathing, rash, redness, and swelling of the hands, feet, ankles or lower legs.

5. What happens if a larger than adequate dose is given?

If ingested more than necessary, the patient may have an accelerated pulse, chest pain, irritability, shortness of breath, tiredness, hyperactivity and loss of consciousness. When taken in large amounts with amphetamines and methamphetamines, it can cause serious, life-threatening problems.

6. What other aspects should be taken into account during use?

Before starting the treatment it is important to inform the doctor about any other medication, vitamin or supplement that is being used, so that it evaluates whether the combination can be harmful.

You should also notify if you have other conditions, such as kidney or heart problems; if you are pregnant or planning to conceive in the short term, or if you are breastfeeding. Levothyroxine and liothyronine should not be used in treatments for obesity or to cause weight loss.

On the other hand, some foods and beverages, especially those that contain soy and dietary fiber, can interfere with the absorption of these medications. It is important that the patient understands that these drugs control Hypothyroidism, but do not cure it. Therefore, they should continue to be used even when the patient feels well.

Finally, these medications should be stored in a suitable place, at room temperature and out of reach of children.

Chapter 69. Mixedematous Coma

Mixedematous Coma is a serious complication of hypothyroidism that puts the patient's life at risk. It is a rare disorder in which the lack of thyroid hormone production is poorly controlled or even undiagnosed.

Among its main symptoms are intense cold intolerance and drowsiness, followed by deep lethargy and loss of consciousness. Mixedematous Coma should be treated urgently.

To talk about this issue we interview Dr. Mario Vega Carbó, an endocrinology specialist who works as an endocrinologist at the Vega & Vado Office.

Doctor Mario,
1. What causes Mixedematous Coma?

This condition occurs in patients with poorly controlled hypothyroidism for years. When this disease is not treated, a situation of severe stress, trauma, a heart attack, surgery, an infection, cold exposure, hip fracture, gastrointestinal bleeding or the use of anesthetics, sedatives or narcotics, can generate a sudden worsening of your symptoms and cause a crisis.

2. Who has more risks of suffering it?

This disorder is more common in elderly women and occurs more frequently in the winter months, since exposure to cold is a precipitating factor.

3. What are your main symptoms?

Its most common signs include severe cold intolerance, respiratory failure, hypothermia, constipation, fatigue, joint pain, slow heart rate, dry skin, alopecia, hoarse voice and swelling of the face, hands and feet.

On the other hand, the mental state usually progresses from the alteration of consciousness to disorientation, deep lethargy and finally coma, which can be accompanied by convulsions.

4. How is Mixedematous Coma detected?

Signs such as involuntary lowering of body temperature are taken into account for diagnosis; the low level of glycemia and sodium and the increase in creatine phosphokinase and thyroid stimulating hormone; the absence of sufficient oxygen in the tissues to maintain bodily functions; slow heart rate and alterations in the state of consciousness. Urine and respiratory system are also tested for infections.

5. What is your treatment?

The therapy must be early and multidisciplinary. It will include the gradual warming of the patient, the correction of blood glucose alterations, the monitoring of cardiovascular function and the mechanical ventilation and adequate hydration. In addition, hypothyroidism will be controlled with high doses of Levothyroxine, orally or intravenously, and broad-spectrum glucocorticoids and antibiotics will be administered to fight infections. Also, arterial hypotension, hydroelectrolytic disorders and triggers of the crisis will be treated.

6. What are the expected results?

The evolution will depend on age, associated diseases and, fundamentally, the control of hypothermia. In all cases the early diagnosis is vital, because the delay in treatment worsens the prognosis.

Chronic Thyroiditis or Hashimoto's Disease is a disorder caused by a reaction of the immune system against the thyroid gland. It causes a decrease in thyroid function, which results in hypothyroidism.

This medical condition mainly affects middle-aged women, although it can also occur in men and boys. Hashimoto's disease develops slowly and may take a long time to be detected. Your hormone replacement treatment usually gives good results.

To talk about this topic, we interviewed Dr. Mario Vega Carbó, an endocrinology specialist in charge of the Vega & Vado Office in Managua, Nicaragua.

Doctor Mario,

1. What causes Chronic Thyroiditis?

Hashimoto's disease is caused by a reaction of the immune system, in which antibodies directed against the thyroid lead to inflammation of the gland. It is not known with certainty why this occurs, but it is believed to be related to a virus, a bacterium or a genetic failure.

The chronic damage caused by this condition usually causes a decrease in the levels of thyroid hormone in the blood. In a few cases, the disease may be related to other endocrine disorders, such as adrenal insufficiency and type 1 diabetes.

2. Who has more risks of having it?

Chronic thyroiditis can occur in anyone of any age. However, it is more common in middle-aged women. Those who suffer from immune or family diseases with a history of thyroid problems and those exposed to high levels of radiation are more likely to suffer from it.

215

3. What are your main symptoms?

The patient usually has constipation, difficulty concentrating, pale and dry skin, swelling in the front of the throat, fatigue, hair loss, brittle nails, irregular menstruation, greater sensitivity to cold, increased tongue size and weight , depression, joint pain and muscle weakness.

4. How is this disease detected?

When your symptoms occur, a physical exam and various studies are usually done to measure the levels of thyroid hormone, thyroid stimulating hormone, cholesterol and glucose, and an antibody test. Other specialized tests of the gland may also be necessary.

5. What is your treatment?

If you have hypothyroidism, it is treated with Levothyroxine, a pill that contains thyroid hormone. In this therapy it is necessary to carry out periodic controls to adjust the dose and the medicine should probably be taken for life. If there is no hormonal deficiency and the thyroid is functioning normally, only its evolution should be monitored.

6. What happens if a higher dose of hormones is given to the appropriate one?

If ingested more than necessary, the patient may have an accelerated pulse, weight loss, tiredness and hyperactivity. That is why periodic checks are essential for its administration correctly, since in the proper dose it has no side effects.

7. What other complications can Chronic Thyroiditis bring?

Hashimoto's disease can occur along with other autoimmune disorders, such as adrenal insufficiency and type 1 diabetes. If left untreated it can also cause goiter, heart problems, depression, reduced libido and myxedema. In addition, in rare cases you may develop lymphoma or thyroid cancer. On the other hand, babies of women with untreated hypothyroidism can be born with congenital defects.

Chapter 71. Subacute thyroiditis and viral infections

Subacute thyroiditis is an inflammation of the thyroid gland that usually occurs after a viral infection. It is a rare disease that occurs shortly after having suffered an infectious picture of the upper respiratory tract, such as mumps (mumps), flu or a common cold. Its symptoms include fever and neck pain.

In the first weeks about half of the patients register an excessive production of the thyroid hormone (hyperthyroidism) that is later normalized. This ailment mainly attacks middle-aged women and usually disappears within a few months.

To learn more about this topic, we interview Mario Vega Carbó, an endocrinologist with more than 20 years of experience.

Doctor Mario,
1. What are the symptoms of subacute thyroiditis?

Usually the patient has fever and pain in the front of the neck, although this discomfort can spread to the jaw and ears. That is why many times their signs are confused with a dental problem, pharyngitis or otitis. In these cases the gland usually increases in size asymmetrically and is swollen and sensitive to touch. In addition, pain may increase when swallowed or when the head is turned. Other frequent symptoms are hoarseness, fatigue and a feeling of weakness.

At the beginning of the disease there are also signs associated with hyperthyroidism, such as anxiety, nervousness, difficulty concentrating, diarrhea, vomiting, increased appetite, sweating, palpitations, hair and weight loss, and sleeping problems.

2. How is this disease detected?

When your symptoms occur, a physical exam and different studies are usually done to measure thyroid hormone levels. To confirm the diagnosis, specialized tests with ultrasound and scintigraphy, including radioactive iodine uptake and fine needle aspiration biopsy, may be necessary.

3. What is your treatment?

The therapy will seek to reduce pain and inflammation, and treat hyperthyroidism if it occurs. The discomfort caused by Subacute Thyroiditis can be resolved with nonsteroidal anti-inflammatory drugs, such as ibuprofen, or corticosteroids, such as prednisone.

In addition, to resolve the symptoms of hyperthyroidism, beta-blockers may also be prescribed, which help improve heart rhythm disorders, tremors and anxiety.

If the thyroid becomes hypoactive during the recovery phase, replacement thyroid hormones may be necessary.

4. What can you expect from this therapy?

The treatment is effective and Subacute Thyroiditis usually heals spontaneously in a few months. However, in some cases the disease may reappear and, over time, may cause permanent hypothyroidism.

Chapter 72. Euthyroid Sick Syndrome

Euthyroid Sick Syndrome is a disorder in which the results of thyroid tests are abnormal, although the gland works correctly. This usually occurs when the patient has another serious illness, is malnourished or underwent surgery, which causes some hormones not to act regularly.

The thyroid is one of the most important glands in the body and its activity influences metabolism and most of the body's functions, such as heart rate and blood pressure.

To talk about this issue we interview Dr. Mario Vega Carbó, an endocrinology specialist who is currently in charge of the Vega & Vado Office.

Doctor Mario,
1. What is Euthyroid Sick Syndrome?

It is a little known pathology that appears in hospitalized patients, in which the serum values of thyroid hormones are altered, without there being a disease in the gland, but another systemic ailment.

2. What diseases can cause these alterations?

Certain gastrointestinal, pulmonary, cardiovascular, inflammatory and metabolic disorders can cause Euthyroid Sick Syndrome. Also, chronic renal failure, acute myocardial infarction, severe malnutrition, fasting, burns, severe trauma, diabetic ketoacidosis, nervous anorexia, surgical intervention, cirrhosis, sepsis, cancer or transplant of bone marrow

3. Why are the alterations in the results of thyroid tests?

The variations may be due to changes in the production of thyroid hormones, in the hypothalamic-pituitary-thyroid axis or in the peripheral metabolism of hormones. It can also occur by a combination of these three factors.

4. What are the most frequent altered results that appear on exams?

The variations that generally appear are low levels of triiodothyronine (T3), increased inverse T3 and reduced thyroxine (T4). In addition, thyroid stimulating hormone (THS) and free T4 may also be affected.

5. How is this syndrome detected?

Against their symptoms, the objective is to define if the patient has Hypothyroidism or Euthyroid Sick Syndrome. For this, a physical examination and different studies are carried out to measure hormonal levels. The safest test is that of the thyroid stimulating hormone, which in Hypothyroidism is very high, while in the syndrome it is usually low, normal or slightly elevated.

Similarly, serum cortisol levels tend to increase in the syndrome and be low or normal in hypothyroidism.

Some medications that affect thyroid hormones, such as iodine-rich contrast media, amiodarone, dopamine and corticosteroids, may make it difficult to interpret the results.

6. What is your treatment?

Since it is not a problem in the thyroid gland, no specific treatment or replacement of hormones is necessary. The therapy will focus on the underlying disease and, when it is resolved, the laboratory results will return to normal.

Chapter 73. Hyperthyroidism or overactive thyroid

Hyperthyroidism is a condition in which the thyroid produces too much thyroid hormone. This gland is one of the most important in the body and its activity influences metabolism, growth and most body functions, such as heart rate and blood pressure.

The most common reason for excessive thyroid secretion is Graves' disease, a condition in which the immune system produces antibodies that attack and damage it. Other causes may be an inflammation of the gland due to viral infections, some medications or postpartum thyroiditis; an overactive adenoma; tumors; the intake of large amounts of synthetic thyroid hormone; and exaggerated iodine consumption.

Hyperthyroidism can speed up the body's metabolism, which causes involuntary weight loss, arrhythmia and tachycardia.

To talk about this topic, we interviewed Dr. Mario Vega Carbó, an endocrinology specialist, with more than 20 years of experience.

Doctor Mario,
1. What are the most common symptoms of hyperthyroidism?

Its most common signs are anxiety, nervousness, fatigue, difficulty concentrating, diarrhea, fine and fragile hair, hand tremor, heat intolerance, increased appetite, sweating, menstrual irregularities, palpitations, sleeping problems and weight loss. Other symptoms include swelling or abnormal growth of the thyroid, breast development in men, high blood pressure, eye irritation, nausea, vomiting, hot skin and redness, nail changes, depression and skin rashes.

2. How is this disease detected?

When your symptoms occur, a physical exam and different studies are usually done to measure the levels of thyroid hormones, cholesterol and glucose. Specialized tests of the gland, with ultrasound and scintigraphy, or radioactive iodine uptake may also be necessary.

3. Who are more likely to have it?

This condition is more common in women, in people with other thyroid problems and in those over 60. It also occurs more frequently in those who have a family history of Graves' disease.

4. What is your treatment?

Therapy will depend on the cause of hyperthyroidism and the severity of its symptoms. It is usually treated with antithyroid medications, such as propylthiouracil or methimazole, that decrease or block the effects of the hormone. Both drugs cause serious liver damage, so they should be taken with caution and medical care.

In more severe cases, surgery may be necessary to remove the gland or reduce it with the intake of radioactive iodine. If that happens, the patient should take hormone replacement pills for life. Drugs may be prescribed to alleviate the symptoms of hyperthyroidism, such as beta-blockers, which help improve heart rhythm disorders, tremors and anxiety.

5. What can you expect from this therapy?

Patients usually respond well and improve with treatment. Some of its causes may even disappear without any therapy. However, hyperthyroidism caused by Graves' disease can get worse over time and affect the patient's quality of life.

6. What other complications can this condition bring?

Stress or infection can cause a sudden worsening of the symptoms of hyperthyroidism and generate fever, a change in consciousness and severe abdominal pain, which requires urgent medical attention. This medical condition can cause heart problems and osteoporosis.

In some rare cases, it can also affect your eyes and cause them to swell and dry. In addition, surgery to throw it away from the thyroid can cause injury to the larynx, damage to the vocal cords, hoarseness and low calcium levels due to damage or accidental removal of the parathyroid glands.

7. What other recommendations should these patients consider?

People with hyperthyroidism should control the intake of iodine, which may be present in food, vitamin supplements and in cough syrups, since its consumption can worsen the symptoms. It is also recommended that they avoid tobacco, which is associated with the development of eye problems in patients with Graves' disease.

On the other hand, exercising on a regular basis can help you maintain bone density and the cardiovascular system, and the practice of relaxation techniques relieves stress, which is an important risk factor in this condition.

Chapter 74. Thyroid Orbitopathy

Thyroid Orbitopathy is a disease of autoimmune origin that affects the functioning of the thyroid gland and the organs related to sight, together or in isolation. These patients usually present with hyperthyroidism and a series of changes that afflict the eyelids, the orbit and the muscles that move the eyes, causing their swelling. This causes them to leave the cavity and cause the appearance of bulging eyes.

On the other hand, Thyroid Orbitopathy can also cause strabismus, irritation, problems closing the eyes, tearing, gritty sensation, double vision and damage to the optic nerves.

To learn more about this topic, we interview Mario Vega Carbó, an endocrinologist, with more than 20 years of experience.

Doctor Mario,
1. What causes thyroid orbitopathy?

Usually this condition is caused by a reaction of the immune system, which generates antibodies that attack and damage the thyroid. This causes the gland to produce excess hormones, leading to hyperthyroidism.

On the other hand, these same antibodies can affect the organs related to vision, causing their swelling.

2. Who is affected by this condition?

Thyroid Orbitopathy is more common in women smokers between 40 and 60 years old, and usually affects both eyes.

3. What are your main symptoms?

This condition usually occurs months or years after thyroid disease. However, it can rarely precede it. Its initial signs are pressure around the eyeball, irritation, strabismus, tearing, difficulty closing the eyes and feeling gritty.

On the other hand, if the muscles or tissues are very swollen, they can compress the optic nerve and cause vision loss. Over time, the patient may have sequelae such as bulging eyes, eyelid bags and double vision.

4. How is thyroid orbitopathy treated?

The therapy depends on the severity of the disease and the symptoms presented. In mild cases, the administration of artificial tears, cold compresses and the use of sunglasses are usually sufficient to relieve their signs.

During the active phase of the condition, corticosteroids may be prescribed intravenously or radiotherapy may be used. If the condition is serious and there are risks for vision, a surgical procedure is performed that removes part of the bones surrounding the eyeball, to decompress the orbit. If it causes severe aesthetic problems, rehabilitation or eyelid surgery can be performed.

5. What are the expected results of this therapy?

In general, surgical treatments are usually safe and effective. In a few cases, inflammation, bleeding and infections that are treated with antibiotics may occur.

Chapter 75. Thyroid Storm or Thyrotoxic Crisis

Thyroid Storm is known as the acute increase in symptoms of hyperthyroidism, which endangers the functioning of the organs and the patient's life. It is a rare crisis, but one that has a high mortality rate, so it must be controlled urgently.

This sudden worsening is usually triggered by a stress situation, an infection, surgery or labor, and can cause high fever, diarrhea, tachycardia, shock and death. It usually occurs in patients in whom thyroid hyperactivity is poorly controlled or even undiagnosed.

To talk about this topic, we interview Dr. Mario Vega Carbó, an endocrinology specialist, who works as an endocrinologist at the Vega & Vado Office.

Doctor Mario,
1. When does a Thyroid Storm occur?

Hyperthyroidism is a condition in which the thyroid produces too much thyroid hormone. This gland is one of the most important in the body and its activity influences metabolism, growth and most body functions, such as heart rate and blood pressure.

When this disease is not treated, a serious stress situation, such as trauma, heart attack, surgery, labor or infection, can cause a sudden worsening of your symptoms and cause a crisis.

In a few cases, this can also be caused by the inadequate supply of iodine or thyroid hormone, in treatments for Graves' disease or obesity.

2. What are your main symptoms?

The most common signs are agitation, reduced level of consciousness, confusion, delirium, diarrhea, fever, acceleration of heart rhythm, hypertension, yellow appearance of eyes and skin, restlessness, tremor, sweating, nausea, vomiting and abdominal pain.

3. How is a Thyroid Storm detected?

There are no specific diagnostic tests for this condition, so its detection is based on clinical observations related to its symptoms. For this, blood pressure, heart rate and thyroid hormone levels are measured; renal and cardiac functions are checked and infections are sought. Ultrasound of the thyroid and other studies may also be done.

4. What is your treatment?

The management of Thyroid Storm involves the reduction of fever and the supply of oxygen and fluids in case of difficulty breathing and dehydration. It seeks to reduce the levels of thyroid hormone in the blood, either by supplying high doses of iodine or with antithyroid medications, such as methimazole or propylthiouracil.

In addition, the application of intravenous beta-blockers may be necessary to lower heart rate, blood pressure, tremor and anxiety. In case of infection, antibiotics are also given.

5. What complications can this disorder bring?

Heart failure and pulmonary edema can develop rapidly, cause shock and lead to death.

6. How is Thyroid Storm prevented?

The best way to prevent it is by treating and controlling hyperthyroidism. Exercising regularly can help maintain bone density and the cardiovascular system, and the practice of relaxation techniques relieves stress, which is an important risk factor in this condition.

Chapter 76. Treatments for hyperthyroidism: radioiodine and antithyroid

Hyperthyroidism is a condition in which the thyroid produces too much thyroid hormone. This condition is usually treated with antithyroid medications, such as propylthiouracil or methimazole, that decrease or block its effects.

In more severe cases, surgery may be necessary to remove the gland or reduce it with the intake of radioactive iodine. If that happens, the patient should take hormone replacement pills for life.

To learn more about this topic, we interview Mario Vega Carbó, an endocrinologist with more than 20 years of experience.

Doctor Mario,
1. How do antithyroid medications work?

These drugs inhibit the synthesis, release, peripheral conversion and effects on the organs of thyroid hormones. Both propylthiouracil and methimazole come as tablets and are taken 3 times a day, every 8 hours, with food.

2. What side effects do they have?

In some cases there may be skin rashes, itching, abnormal hair loss, vomiting, joint pain, drowsiness, dizziness and a decrease in the number of leukocytes and platelets.

In more serious situations, there may be headache, fever, bleeding, abdominal pain and yellowing of the eyes or skin. Propylthiouracil can cause serious liver damage. Therefore, it is only recommended for use in patients who cannot receive other treatments, such as surgery or radioactive iodine.

For its part, methimazole should not be used during pregnancy or during the period of breastfeeding, as it can cause birth defects. In these cases, propylthiouracil can be used during the first months of conception.

3. What should be done if you forget to take a dose of these medications?

You should ingest it as soon as you remember. However, if it is almost time for the next dose, it is better to skip it and continue with the regular dosage. In no case should a double dose be taken to compensate for the one that was forgotten.

4. What other aspects should be taken into account during the use of antithyroid drugs?

Before starting the treatment it is important to inform the doctor about any other medication, vitamin or supplement that is being used, so that it evaluates whether the combination can be harmful. You must notify if you have other conditions, such as kidney or heart problems, or any disease that affects the blood; if you are pregnant or planning to conceive in the short term, or if you are breastfeeding.

Finally, these medications should be stored in a suitable place, at room temperature and out of the reach of children.

5. What is radioactive iodine therapy used for?

Radioactive iodine is given as pills or liquid to reduce or kill thyroid cells, in order to control some diseases. In the case of hyperthyroidism, this treatment kills the overactive cells or decreases the size of the gland, which stops the hormonal production.

For cancer, after surgery to remove the thyroid, iodine destroys the remaining cancer cells and those that have spread in other parts of the body. After these therapies, patients may have to take hormone replacement pills for life.

6. What side effects does this therapy have?

In addition to the possibility of hypothyroidism, if its use is abused, the patient is exposed to a very low level of radiation that may be harmful. That is why it is not recommended for pregnant women or those who are breastfeeding.

In a few cases, patients may have low sperm count and infertility for up to 2 years in men and irregular periods for up to one year in women.

On the other hand, after treatment there may be swelling and tenderness in the neck and salivary glands, dry mouth and eyes, gastritis and changes in the sense of taste. In addition, very high doses may decrease saliva production or injure the colon or bone marrow.

7. What care should be taken after this treatment?

The patient should avoid possible contact with other people, especially children and pregnant women, for at least four days. That includes sleeping in a separate bed. For at least 6 months, you should also avoid conceiving or becoming pregnant.

On the other hand, every time you go to the bathroom, it is recommended to discharge twice or more to run the water. It is also advisable to bathe and wash your hands frequently, use disposable cutlery or wash them separately from others, and do not cook food for others.

Chapter 77. Radioactive iodine post thyroiditis

Post-radioactive iodine thyroiditis is an inflammation in the thyroid that appears after treatment with radioactive iodine, usually to combat cases of hyperthyroidism.

The thyroid is one of the most important glands in the body and its activity influences metabolism, growth and most body functions, such as heart rate and blood pressure. When it for some reason produces excess hormones, it must be treated. One of the therapies used is the reduction of the gland through the intake of radioactive iodine. In a few cases, the effects of mild radiation can cause an inflammation in the thyroid, known as post-radioactive iodine thyroiditis.

To learn more about this topic, we interview Mario Vega Carbó, an endocrinologist with more than 20 years of experience.

Doctor Mario,
1. In what cases does this disorder occur?

Post-radioactive iodine thyroiditis is a rare phenomenon that occurs in less than 1 percent of patients to whom this treatment is applied. Usually its symptoms appear within two weeks of its realization and it is characterized by an increase in the size of the gland, neck pain and fever.

2. Who is more at risk of suffering it?

This condition is more common in women and there are more risks when the dose of radioactive iodine administered is considerably greater than 15 mCi.

3. What is your treatment?

If thyroiditis is mild, it does not require treatment. If it is moderate, pain and inflammation can be resolved with nonsteroidal anti-inflammatory drugs, such as ibuprofen. In severe cases, it is treated with steroids.

Occasionally, as a result of this disease, patients register an excessive production of thyroid hormone, which is then normalized. Beta-blockers may be prescribed to treat the symptoms of hyperthyroidism.

On the other hand, if the thyroid becomes hypoactive during the recovery phase, replacement thyroid hormones may be needed.

4. What can you expect from this therapy?

The treatment is usually effective and thyroiditis usually disappears shortly.

5. What other aspects should be taken into account?

In patients receiving radioactive iodine treatment, the possibility of thyrotoxicosis after application should always be analyzed. This can cause heart problems such as atrial fibrillation, supraventricular tachycardia and ventricular arrhythmias.

Chapter 78. Nuclear Medicine for Thyroid

Nuclear Medicine is a specialty of medicine that is used for the diagnosis and treatment of diseases. It uses a carrier drug and a radioactive isotope that are applied inside the body, usually intravenously or orally. From there they emit signals, which are detected by a special camera, known as a gamma camera.

This device is responsible for storing information digitally, which is then processed into images. Unlike those obtained in radiology, these show how the organs and tissues explored work and reveal alterations thereof at a molecular level. Usually, Nuclear Medicine exams are not invasive and lack serious side effects.

To learn more about this topic, we interview Dr. Mario Vega Carbó, an endocrinology specialist, in charge of the Vega & Vado Office.

Doctor Mario,
1. In which cases is Nuclear Medicine used to treat thyroid?

Usually this specialty is used to perform a scintigraphy, in which the anatomy of the gland is analyzed and evaluated, and surgical remains, ectopic thyroid tissue, cysts or nodules are sought.
In cases of severe disease, radioactive iodine treatment is also used to destroy hyperactive or cancerous cells.

2. What is the preparation for these studies?

The patient is usually asked not to eat food after midnight the day before the exam. Also, if you are taking any thyroid drug, you should stop at least three days before the test. The person should advise if they are taking any medicine that contains iodine or if they are having diarrhea, as they may interfere with the results.

In turn, before beginning the study, jewelry, dentures and other metals should be removed.

3. How is thyroid scintigraphy performed?

For this procedure a pill containing a small amount of radioactive iodine is administered. Then they wait between 4 and 6 hours for this chemical to accumulate in the thyroid and the first scan is performed. To do this, the camera is placed on the neck, so that it takes pictures of the gland from different angles. During that process, the patient must remain completely still.

After 24 hours, another measurement may be necessary. Later, radioactive iodine is expelled from the body through urine.

4. What results does this test offer?

Among other possibilities, the scan allows to see if there are nodules, goiter or thyroid cancer and find the cause of hyperthyroidism. If the gland is enlarged or shifted to the side, it may be a sign of a tumor.

If you accumulated too much iodine, it may be due to an overactive thyroid. Instead, he did little, there may be inflammation. If the nodules are dark, it means that they have absorbed a lot of iodine, that they are very active and the possible cause of excessive hormone production.

5. What is the treatment with radioactive iodine?

This Nuclear Medicine therapy allows to treat hyperthyroidism and thyroid cancer. It involves the intake of a small dose of radioactive iodine, through capsules or liquid, which accumulates in the gland and destroys its cells.

Hyperthyroidism occurs when the thyroid produces an excess of hormones. Radioactive iodine treats this condition by killing hyperactive cells or decreasing the size of the gland, which stops production. In the case of cancer, after surgery to remove the thyroid, iodine destroys the remaining cancer cells and those that have spread in other parts of the body.

After these therapies, patients may have to take hormone replacement pills for life.

6. What side effects does Nuclear Medicine have?

This technique is not invasive, except for intravenous injections, and is usually painless and has no major side effects. However, if its use is abused, the patient is exposed to a very low level of radiation that might be harmful. That is why it is not recommended for pregnant women or those who are breastfeeding.

In a few cases, patients may also experience swelling and tenderness in the neck and salivary glands, dry mouth and eyes, and changes in the sense of taste.

7. What care should be taken after this treatment?

The patient should avoid possible contacts with other people, especially children and pregnant women, for at least four days. That includes sleeping in a separate bed. On the other hand, every time you go to the bathroom, it is recommended to discharge twice or more to run the water. It is also advisable to bathe and wash your hands frequently, use disposable cutlery or wash them separately from others, and do not cook food for others.

For at least 6 months, you should also avoid conceiving or becoming pregnant.

Part V. Calcium Metabolism

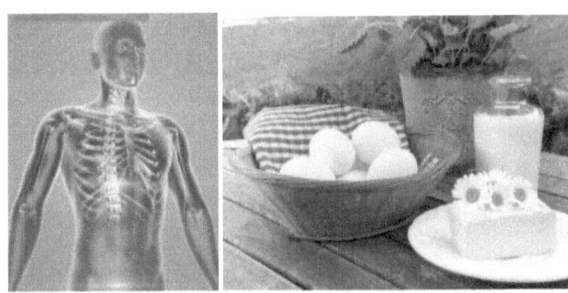

Chapter 79. Hypocalcaemia

Hypocalcaemia is a disorder in which blood calcium levels are low. This mineral plays an important structural role in the body by being part of the teeth and bones, and contributing to its development and maintenance.

In addition, it participates in blood coagulation, nerve impulse transmission, muscle contraction and relaxation, stimulation of hormonal secretion and heart rate, among other tasks. A prolonged deficit of calcium levels can lead to bone malformation or make them brittle and with a tendency to fracture.

To learn more about this topic, we interview Mario Vega Carbó, an endocrinology specialist, who works as an endocrinologist at the Vega & Vado Office.

Doctor Mario,
1. What causes hypocalcaemia?

Hypocalcaemia can be due to different factors, such as a diet low in calcium, blood disorders or vitamin D and magnesium deficiency, which are essential for fixation in the bone system. Other possible causes are alcoholism; chronic renal failure; problems in the parathyroid hormone and intestine; certain medications such as diuretics; chemotherapy; inflammation of the pancreas; the syndrome of hungry bones and the consumption of coffee or tea.

2. What are your main symptoms?

Some frequent signs are muscle spasms, especially in the hands, feet and face; the cramps; the contractures; the tingling sensation; numbness and problems of arthritis in the fingers.

238

In addition, the patient may present excessive tiredness, sweating, palpitations, irregular contractions, shortness of breath, irritability, vomiting, fever, nausea, diarrhea, anxiety attacks and depression.

3. How is this disorder detected?

Against his symptoms, a blood count is usually performed to control blood calcium levels. When the values are below 8.5 mg / dl, the patient is considered to have hypocalcaemia. In addition, albumin, creatinine, magnesium and phosphorus levels are also controlled. On the other hand, to complete the diagnosis, an electrocardiogram, x-rays and ultrasound may be necessary.

4. What is your treatment?

Therapy depends on what causes hypocalcaemia. However, as a first step, it is generally sought to add more calcium, magnesium, phosphorus and vitamin D to the diet.

Calcium-rich foods include dairy products, such as milk, cheese and yogurt; green leafy vegetables, such as broccoli; soft-bone fish, such as canned sardines and salmon; cereals; almonds; Brazil nuts and fruit juices.

If necessary, calcium or vitamin D supplements or infusions may be prescribed. In severe cases, the mineral may be administered intravenously. If Hypocalcaemia is a consequence of another disease, it must be treated.

5. What other recommendations can be given to these patients?

People with hypocalcaemia are advised to maintain healthy lifestyle habits, such as a balanced diet and daily exercise, with control to avoid bumps and falls. It is advisable to maintain an adequate body weight and avoid tobacco and excessive alcohol consumption.

Chapter 80. Hypocalcaemic Crisis

Hypocalcaemia is a disorder in which blood calcium levels are below 8.5 mg / dl. Some frequent signs of this condition are muscle spasms, especially in the hands, feet and face; the cramps; the contractures; the tingling sensation; numbness and problems of arthritis in the fingers.

In addition, the patient may present excessive tiredness, sweating, palpitations, irregular contractions, shortness of breath, irritability, vomiting, fever, nausea, diarrhea, anxiety attacks and depression.

In many cases, hypocalcemia can generate a serious situation that requires urgent therapeutic measures.

To learn more about this topic, we interview Mario Vega Carbó, an endocrinology specialist, who is in charge of the Vega & Vado Office.

Doctor Mario,
1. What are the symptoms of a hypocalcemic crisis?

In severe cases, the patient may present with muscle spasms, laryngospasm, impaired renal function, hypotension, heart failure, arrhythmias and fainting, seizures and decreased state of consciousness.

Hypercalcemic crises, in general, are caused by large tumors in the parathyroid glands, which produce higher plasma concentrations of calcium and parathyroid hormone. They may also be due to renal failure, inflammation of the pancreas, administration of phosphates or excess tissue damage.

2. How are these crises treated?

Severe hypocalcemia, below 7 mg / dL, requires immediate treatment with calcium and vitamin D intravenously. Usually 100-200 mg of elemental calcium is applied in the form of calcium gluconate, followed by a continuous infusion of 0.5-1.5 mg / kg / h. Perfusion should be slow to avoid cardiovascular complications.

Another option is to use calcium chloride, although this is used less than gluconate because it is more irritating locally. This therapy should be maintained until the patient is able to receive oral calcium.

As for vitamin D substitutes, calcitriol, a medicine that acts in a few hours, can be used.

3. What contraindications does calcium gluconate have?

This medicine should not be used in cases of severe renal disease or in patients undergoing digitalis. Among other side effects, calcium gluconate can cause itching, hot flashes, vertigo and tissue necrosis.

On the other hand, when applied too quickly or in very high doses, it can cause hypercalcemia. This increases the risks of hypotension, bradycardia, arrhythmia, syncope and cardiac arrest.

4. What other aspects should be taken into account during a hypocalcemic crisis?

In these cases seizures and spasms of the larynx should also be prevented, and heart rhythm controlled. It is common for patients with hypocalcemia to also have hypomagnesemia, especially if they are alcoholics or suffer from severe malnutrition or malabsorption.

Therefore, during a crisis it is also important to treat low levels of magnesium in the blood, as this causes resistance to parathyroid hormone and reduces its secretion. The usual dose is 2 g of 10% magnesium sulfate, followed by an infusion of 1 g / 100 ml / h.

Finally, if there is also hyperphosphatemia, an increase in the inorganic phosphate content of the blood, its values are corrected by hemodialysis in end-stage renal failure, or by administering phosphate-fixing antacids.

Chapter 81. Supplementation: calcium, vitamin D and magnesium

Calcium, vitamin D and magnesium are indispensable for the human body. They help form teeth and bones, and contribute to their development and maintenance. In addition, they participate in blood coagulation, nerve impulse transmission, muscle contraction and relaxation, stimulation of hormonal secretion and heart rate, among other tasks.

A prolonged deficit of these substances can lead to bone malformation or make them brittle and with a tendency to fracture.

To learn more about this topic, we interviewed Cuban doctor Mario Vega Carbó, a specialist in clinical endocrinology.

Doctor Mario,
1. What is hypocalcaemia and what are its causes?

Hypocalcaemia is a disorder in which blood calcium levels are low. It may be due to different factors, such as a diet poor in this mineral, blood disorders or vitamin D and magnesium deficits, which are essential for fixation in the bone system.

Other possible reasons are alcoholism; chronic renal failure; problems in the parathyroid hormone and intestine; certain medications such as diuretics; chemotherapy; inflammation of the pancreas; the syndrome of hungry bones and the consumption of coffee or tea. On average, adults should consume between 1,000 and 1,200 mg of calcium per day.

2. What is your treatment?

The therapy will depend on what causes hypocalcaemia. However, as a first step, it is generally sought to add more calcium, magnesium, phosphorus and vitamin D to the diet.

Calcium-rich foods include dairy products, such as milk, cheese and yogurt; green leafy vegetables, such as broccoli; soft-bone fish, such as canned sardines and salmon; cereals; almonds; Brazil nuts and fruit juices.

If necessary, calcium or vitamin D supplements or infusions may be prescribed. In severe cases, the mineral may be administered intravenously.

3. Who should evaluate taking calcium supplements?

People who follow a vegan diet, those who consume large amounts of protein or sodium, those who receive long-term treatment with corticosteroids and those who have lactose intolerance, osteoporosis or some digestive or intestinal disease that decreases calcium absorption may need to consume supplements of this mineral.

4. How are calcium supplements taken?

These are sold in tablets, capsules, liquids or powders, and are generally better absorbed if they are ingested in small doses (less than 500 mg) distributed in meals.

However, it is important to keep in mind that these supplements can change the way the body absorbs certain medications, such as those used to control blood pressure, synthetic thyroid hormones, antibiotics and iron pills. Depending on the drugs used, the doctor will recommend whether it is better to take them with or between meals.

5. Do these supplements present any risk or side effects?

Usually they are very well tolerated. On rare occasions the patient may present with flatulence, constipation and swelling. If taken in large quantities, they can cause hypercalcaemia and generate an increased risk of bone fractures, high blood pressure, heart problems, kidney stones or a serious kidney ailment.

On the other hand, although the studies are inconclusive, there could be a relationship between these supplements and the increased likelihood of prostate cancer.

6. What is the role of vitamin D?

This substance is essential for the normal formation of bones and teeth, for the absorption of calcium and phosphorus at the intestinal level, and for the functioning of the nervous, muscular and immune system.

When the proper amount of vitamin D is not received, or when the body has trouble using it, this can cause loss of bone density, osteoporosis, osteomalacia and rickets.

7. How is vitamin D obtained?

This substance can be obtained in two ways: by exposure to sunlight or by eating foods that contain it, such as milk, eggs, fatty fish, cereals, meats, bread and orange juice.

8. Why do some people have problems absorbing this substance?

This could be a consequence of different conditions such as Celiac disease; intestinal, heart or immune diseases; some types of cancer; renal problems; rheumatoid arthritis; and tuberculosis. In addition, surgeries that remove the stomach or intestine can cause problems absorbing vitamin D

9. Who may need vitamin D supplements?

People with dark skin, those who live in geographical areas with little exposure to sunlight, those who remain indoors and those who use very powerful sunscreen may need to consume supplements of this substance. Also those who have lactose intolerance, those who do not eat or drink dairy products, vegetarians and those who consume certain anticonvulsant and antiretroviral drugs.

The same goes for those who suffer from cancer, kidney failure and liver diseases.

10. Can eating too much vitamin D be harmful?

Yes, the excess of this substance can also be harmful and damage the kidneys and raise calcium levels in the blood. This can cause heart rhythm problems, nausea, vomiting, lack of appetite, constipation and weight loss. Usually the excess of vitamin D is due to the exaggerated consumption of supplements of this substance.

11. What is the function of magnesium?

This mineral is involved in the maintenance of healthy teeth, heart and bones, participates in energy metabolism and the activation of enzymes that release glucose, helps in the production of energy and protein, and acts in nerve transmission, among other important functions of the organism.

12. What foods is it present in?

It can be obtained from vegetables, green vegetables, nuts, legumes, cereals, white corn, fruits such as bananas or apricots, soy products, chocolate, fish, shellfish, whole grains and milk, among other foods.

13. Who can have a magnesium deficit?

Although it is not usual, alcoholics, newly operated people, those with diabetes, and those who suffered burns or the removal of much of the intestine may have a significant magnesium deficit. Its most common symptoms are excessive excitability, muscle weakness and drowsiness.

Anyway, the use of supplements of this mineral is only recommended for very special cases and it is always better to obtain it naturally.

14. What side effects can magnesium supplements cause?

The body generally removes excess magnesium. However, its indiscriminate use can cause diarrhea, nervous disturbance and muscle contraction and kidney failure.

Chapter 82. Rickets and lack of vitamin D

Rickets is a childhood disorder, which causes softening and weakness in the bones of children. This is usually due to the prolonged lack of vitamin D, which is responsible for promoting adequate levels of calcium and phosphorus in the body. This usually causes stunted growth, arched legs, thickened wrists and ankles, and pain in the spine, pelvis and legs.

Its treatment consists of the addition of vitamin D or calcium supplements to the diet, medications and, in some cases, corrective surgery.

To learn more about this topic, we interview Mario Vega Carbó, an endocrinology specialist, who works as an endocrinologist at the Vega & Vado Office.

Doctor Mario,
1. What is the cause of Rickets?

Vitamin D is essential for the normal formation of bones and teeth and for the absorption of calcium and phosphorus at the intestinal level. When the proper amount of this substance is not received, or when the body has trouble using it, this can cause Rickets.

2. How is vitamin D obtained?

This substance can be obtained in two ways: by exposure to sunlight or by eating foods that contain it, such as milk, eggs, fatty fish, cereals, meats, bread and orange juice.

3. Why do some people have problems absorbing this substance?

This could be a consequence of different conditions such as Celiac disease; intestinal, heart or immune diseases; some types of cancer; renal problems; rheumatoid arthritis; and tuberculosis.

4. Who are more likely to suffer Rickets?

People with dark skin, premature babies and children of mothers with vitamin D deficiency during pregnancy are at greater risk of suffering it.

Also children living in geographical areas with little exposure to sunlight, those who remain indoors and those who consume certain anticonvulsant and antiretroviral drugs.

On the other hand, children with lactose intolerance, babies fed exclusively with breast milk and those with a family history are also more likely to develop it.

5. What complications can this disease bring?

If left untreated Rickets can cause growth problems, abnormal curvature of the spine, skeletal deformities, dental abnormalities and seizures. It can also generate cramps, pain, bone fractures without cause and a decrease in muscle tone.

6. How is Rickets detected?

To confirm their symptoms, physical and blood tests, bone x-rays and arterial blood gas tests are usually performed, among other studies.

7. What is your treatment?

Therapy for Rickets aims to remedy the causes that cause it and relieve its symptoms. In most cases, adding calcium, phosphorus and vitamin D to the diet solves the problem. Children with gastrointestinal disorders or other diseases may need prescription supplements.

On the other hand, some skeletal deformities may require corrective surgery, while others may be resolved with the use of orthopedic devices.

8. Can eating too much vitamin D be harmful?

Yes, the excess of this substance can also be harmful and damage the kidneys and raise calcium levels in the blood. This can cause heart rhythm problems, nausea, vomiting, lack of appetite, constipation and weight loss. Usually the excess of vitamin D is due to the exaggerated consumption of supplements of this substance.

Chapter 83. Bone Densitometry and the diagnosis of Osteoporosis

Bone Densitometry is a medical study that measures the density of a person's bones. It is usually used for the diagnosis of Osteoporosis, to assess the chances of suffering fractures and to analyze whether a treatment for this disease is being effective.

This is a painless test that allows you to estimate how many grams of calcium and other bone minerals are in the bone. The test usually lasts between 10 and 30 minutes, and exposes the patient to a very small amount of radiation.

To learn more about this study, we consulted Dr. Mario Vega Carbó, an endocrinology specialist, in charge of the Vega & Vado Office.

Doctor Mario,
1. What is Bone Densitometry?

This is a test also known as dual energy X-ray absorptiometry (DXA), which measures bone bone density. To do this, it uses a very small dose of ionizing radiation to produce images of the inside of the body. The study is simple, fast and non-invasive.

2. In which cases is this study used?

Bone Densitometry is recommended for patients who have lost height, have fractured a bone, have used steroid medications for a long time, received an organ or bone marrow transplant, or have suffered a decrease in their hormonal levels. Also in those with dorsal and lower limb pain, hunched posture or any sign related to Osteoporosis.

In addition, it is advised for post menopausal women who do not ingest estrogen, and for people with a history of smoking, rheumatoid arthritis, type 1 diabetes, liver or kidney disease, hyperthyroidism or hyperparathyroidism.

3. How is the preparation for a bone densitometry?

These exams do not require any special preparation and you do not need to be fasting. It is only recommended to wear loose and comfortable clothes and avoid taking calcium supplements for at least 24 hours before conducting the study.

In case of pregnancy, if you have performed a recent barium test or received an injection of contrast material for a CT scan or radioisotopia, you should inform the doctor.

Before starting, the patient should remove all metal objects from the pockets, such as keys, wallets or coins, in addition to jewelry, dentures and metal lenses.

4. In what part of the body are the tests performed?

Bone Density tests are usually performed on the bones that are more likely to break due to Osteoporosis. They are the lumbar vertebrae located in the lower part of the spine, the femur next to the hip joint and the bones of the forearm.

5. What results are expected?

Bone Densitometry allows you to estimate how many grams of calcium and other bone minerals are in the bones. The higher the mineral content, the greater the density and strength thereof, and the lower the chances of suffering fractures.

The study offers two numbers as a result: the T-score, which compares bone density with the average of a young and healthy adult of the same sex, and the Z-score, which it does with other people of the same age group, size and gender.

Although this test allows to know if there is a low bone density, it does not provide information on what is the cause, so in these cases more complete exams will be necessary.

6. Is radiation exposure during Bone Densitometry dangerous?

No. The exposure is very low, even less than that emitted during a chest x-ray.

7. Are Densitometry and Scintigraphy the same?

No, the studies are different. Bone scintigraphy requires a previous injection and is generally used to detect fractures, cancer, infections and other bone abnormalities.

Chapter 84. Osteoporosis and bone weakness

Osteoporosis is a disease that thins and weakens the bones, causing them to become brittle and break easily. This decrease in bone mass density especially affects the hip, spine and wrist. While anyone can suffer it, it is more common in women, from 50 years.

Alcoholism, certain medications, kidney failure and inflammatory, rheumatic, liver and endocrine diseases can cause osteoporosis. In some cases, bone loss and thin bones are hereditary.

To learn more about this topic, we consulted Dr. Mario Vega Carbó, an endocrinology specialist with more than 20 years of clinical experience.

Doctor Mario,
1. When does osteoporosis occur?

Bones are living tissues that break and renew constantly. Osteoporosis occurs when the formation of new bones is not enough to replace the one that was removed.

2. How is this condition detected?

Osteoporosis is a silent disease, that is, it has no symptoms until the damage is significant and a fracture occurs, for example. When advanced, it can cause back and lower limb pain, loss of height, hunched posture and fragile bones.

To control the health of bone tissue, it is recommended to perform a mineral density test to see and analyze what state it is in and to prevent any complications.

3. What aspects increase the risk of fractures?

The possibility of fracturing increases if not enough calcium and vitamin D are consumed or if they are not absorbed correctly by the body. The risks also grow as the years go by and with alcohol consumption, smoking, lack of exercise and body weight, malnutrition, certain medications such as prednisone and cortisone and eating disorders.

4. What is the relationship of this medical condition with hormones?

Osteoporosis is usually more frequent in people with higher or lower hormone levels than normal. For example, the decrease in estrogen in menopausal women and testosterone in men over the years increases the risk of suffering from it.

The same goes for hormonal problems related to the thyroid, pituitary, parathyroid and adrenal glands.

5. What other diseases can influence the development of Osteoporosis?

Conditions such as celiac disease, lupus, cancer, multiple myeloma, rheumatoid arthritis and intestinal, kidney, liver, endocrine, rheumatic and inflammatory diseases can increase the risk of suffering from it.

6. What is the treatment?

As a first step to treat osteoporosis it is recommended to maintain healthy lifestyle habits, such as a balanced diet rich in calcium and daily exercise, with control to avoid bumps and falls. In addition, it is advised to avoid tobacco and excessive alcohol consumption.

On the other hand, some people may need calcium and vitamin D supplements, and medications to strengthen bones. Among the latter are bisphosphonates, estrogen and estrogen receptor modulators, which prevent bone loss. On the other hand, teriparatide stimulates the formation of new tissue.

If there is an endocrine, liver or other problem that causes Osteoporosis, it should also be treated. Hormone replacement therapy may be necessary if the levels are too high or low.

7. What can be done to keep bones healthy?

As I said, the ideal is to eat a diet rich in calcium and vitamin D, exercise daily, maintain an adequate body weight and not smoke. In older people, it is important to avoid falls, which are the main cause of fractures.

Hip and spine fractures are especially important since they require surgical intervention, hospital admission and affect the patient's quality of life.

Chapter 85. Hypoparathyroidism, calcium and vitamin D

Hypoparathyroidism is a disorder in which the parathyroid glands produce little parathyroid hormone, responsible for controlling the use and elimination of calcium, phosphate and Vitamin D from the body. When this occurs, blood calcium levels drop and phosphorus levels rise. In children, this medical condition can cause poor growth, abnormal teeth and slow mental development. In adults, bone malformation and tendency to fracture.

To learn more about this topic, we interview Mario Vega Carbó, a specialist in clinical endocrinology.

Doctor Mario,
1. What causes hypoparathyroidism?

This is usually due to an involuntary injury to the parathyroid glands during thyroid or neck surgery. In addition, it can also be caused by radiation treatment, very low level of magnesium in the blood or an autoimmune reaction.

On the other hand, in some cases babies are born directly without the parathyroid glands. This is known as Di George Syndrome and is a chromosomal disorder that causes poor development in several of the body's systems.

2. What are your main symptoms?

This disorder usually develops slowly and, in many cases, has no signs or they are very mild. As the condition progresses there may be abdominal pain, brittle nails, cataracts, calcium deposits in some tissues, dry hair and skin, muscle cramps and spasms, tingling or burning sensation, fatigue and painful menstruation. Also impaired renal function, arrhythmias and fainting, depression, anxiety, seizures and decreased state of consciousness.

3. How is this disease detected?

Faced with its symptoms, physical, urine and blood tests are performed to check the levels of parathyroid hormone, calcium, phosphorus and magnesium. On the other hand, to complete the diagnosis, an electrocardiogram may be necessary to check the heart rate and a CT scan to see if there are calcium deposits in the brain.

4. What is your treatment?

The therapy will seek to reduce the signs of hypoparathyroidism and restore the balance of calcium and minerals in the body. In general, the administration of calcium and vitamin D supplements will be necessary, which in many cases will have to be taken for life. For this, periodic controls should be carried out to regulate the dose. In addition, a diet rich in calcium and low in phosphorus is recommended.

Among foods with calcium are dairy products, such as milk, cheese and yogurt; green leafy vegetables, such as broccoli; soft-bone fish, such as canned sardines and salmon; almonds; Brazil nuts and fruit juices. In turn, fizzy drinks, meats, hard cheeses and whole grains should be avoided. In severe cases, calcium and vitamin D may be given intravenously. Seizures, spasms of the larynx should also be prevented and the rhythm of the heart will be controlled.

5. What other complications can this disease bring?

If left untreated in time, Hypoparathyroidism can cause poor growth in children, abnormal teeth, cataracts and brain calcifications that are irreversible. In addition, excessive treatment with calcium and vitamin D can lead to hypercalcemia and kidney failure.

On the other hand, this condition increases the risks of Addison's disease, pernicious anemia and Parkinson's disease.

Chapter 86. Hyperparathyroidism: causes, symptoms and consequences

Hyperparathyroidism is a disorder in which the parathyroid glands produce too much parathyroid hormone, responsible for controlling the use and elimination of calcium, phosphate and Vitamin D from the body.

This disease is more common in people over 60, but it can also manifest itself in young adults. Its appearance in childhood is very unusual and women are more likely to suffer from it than men.

In most cases it is unknown what is the underlying cause that causes it. However, it is known that receiving ionizing radiation in the head, chronic use of lithium and some genetic syndromes increase the risk of suffering from it.

Similarly, renal or calcium insufficiency in the diet, conditions that make it difficult to break down phosphate, problems absorbing nutrients from food and vitamin D disorders can also generate it.

To learn more about this topic, we interviewed Cuban doctor Mario Vega Carbó, a specialist in clinical endocrinology.

Doctor Mario,
1. What are the parathyroid glands?

These are four glands that are about the size of a grain of rice and are found in the neck. Its main function is to produce parathyroid hormone, which together with Vitamin D are responsible for controlling the amount of calcium in the body, especially in the bones and blood.

The calcium and phosphorus that circulate throughout the body help in the transmission of signals in nerve cells, participate in muscle contraction and affect various systems. Therefore its regulation is very important.

2. What are the causes of Hyperparathyroidism?

Excessive production of parathyroid hormone may be due to a growth of some of the parathyroid glands and, to a much lesser extent, to a cancerous tumor in them. Hyperparathyroidism can also result from a severe deficiency of calcium or vitamin D, or chronic renal failure.

3. What are the main symptoms of this disease?

Usually their symptoms are related to damage to organs or tissues caused by an elevated level of calcium in the blood, or by their loss in the bones. These may include bone or abdominal pain, depression, lack of memory, fatigue and physical weakness, fragile bones that fracture easily (osteoporosis), kidney stones, nausea, vomiting, loss of appetite, excessive urine and frequent urination.

4. How is Hyperparathyroidism confirmed?

In case of presenting its signs, blood tests are performed to verify parathyroid hormone, calcium and phosphorus levels; and urine to confirm the diagnosis. In addition, by means of radiographs and a study of bone mineral density, the state of the bones can be established and possible fractures found.

On the other hand, through tests on the kidneys and urinary tract it is possible to know if there are calcium deposits or an obstruction, and it is also necessary to analyze the neck for tumors or changes in the parathyroid glands.

5. What is the treatment of Hyperparathyroidism?

The therapy will depend on the cause that is causing this ailment. If calcium levels are too high, surgery may be necessary to remove the parathyroid gland that produces the excess hormone. If the problem is in the kidney, the patient may need dialysis or a transplant.

On the other hand, some medications such as mimetic calcium mimic the calcium that circulates in the blood and can cause the parathyroid glands to release less hormone. In milder cases, some habit changes can help improve the disorder, such as exercising more, following a proper diet, not smoking, and drinking more fluid to prevent kidney stones.

On the other hand, women who have reached menopause and show signs of osteoporosis, may need a hormone replacement treatment with the application of estrogens, to help retain calcium in the bones.

6. What disorders can this disease bring?

If uncontrolled, hyperparathyroidism can cause an increased risk of bone fractures, high blood pressure, heart disease, kidney stones or a serious kidney ailment. On the other hand, surgery of the parathyroid glands can damage the nerves that control the vocal cords.

Chapter 87. Parathyroid Surgery

Parathyroids are four glands located around the thyroid, which secrete parathyroid hormone. This substance is responsible, along with vitamin D, to balance calcium, magnesium and phosphorus in the body, maintaining a balance of its levels in the blood and bones.

These minerals that circulate throughout the body help in the transmission of signals in nerve cells, participate in muscle contraction and affect various systems. Therefore its regulation is very important. Parathyroidectomy or parathyroid surgery is done to remove the gland or a tumor from it.

To learn more about this topic, we interviewed Cuban doctor Mario Vega Carbó, a specialist in clinical endocrinology.

Doctor Mario,
1. In which cases is thyroid surgery performed?

This intervention is usually performed in cases of hyperparathyroidism, a disorder in which parathyroids produce too much parathyroid hormone. When this condition is due to a growth of one of the glands or a cancerous tumor in them, an excision surgery is usually performed.

2. What is this procedure?

There are several ways to perform a parathyroidectomy. In traditional surgery a small amount of radioactive marker is injected, so that the affected glands stand out. Then, using a probe, they are located and a cut is made in the neck by which the removal is carried out.

In video-assisted surgery, two small shorts are made in the neck, one to introduce the camera that allows you to see the area and the other for the instruments with which the affected glands are removed.

261

Meanwhile, the endoscopic intervention is similar. In this case, small cuts are made in the front of the neck and another in the upper part of the sternum, through which the endoscope is inserted, a thin tube with a light and a camera at its end. This reduces visible scarring, pain and recovery time. In rare situations where the four glands need to be removed, part of one of them can be transplanted into the forearm to ensure that the calcium level remains at a healthy level.

3. How is the preparation for this surgery?

Before the operation it is important to inform the doctor about all the medications that are being taken, if any type of allergy or illness is suffered, or if you are pregnant. On the other hand, since parathyroids are very small, it may be necessary to perform a CT scan or ultrasound before surgery so that the surgeon can find the glands more easily.

In case of taking anticoagulant remedies, such as aspirin and ibuprofen, the patient may have to suspend them temporarily before the intervention.

4. What complications can occur during parathyroidectomy?

During surgery, an involuntary injury to the thyroid gland may occur or the need to remove part of it. This can lead to hypothyroidism, a disorder in which little thyroid hormone is produced. On the other hand, the operation can also cause hypoparathyroidism and cause blood calcium levels to fall and phosphorus levels to rise. This is usually handled with calcium supplements.

In turn, after a parathyroidectomy some people have neck pain or a hoarse or weak voice, as a result of an injury to the nerves of the vocal cords and larynx. In addition, as in any surgery, there may be abnormal reactions to medications, breathing problems, blood clots or infections.

5. What care should the patient follow after the intervention?

After surgery, the area where the incision was made should be kept clean and dry. During the first weeks there may be swelling and redness, which will gradually disappear. In addition, the patient may have to drink fluids and eat soft foods for a day.

On the other hand, blood calcium may be lower than normal and you may need to take tablets for a while. Among the symptoms of hypocalcaemia there may be tingling of the lips and the tips of the fingers and toes. After the intervention, periodic checks will be necessary to measure the levels of the different minerals in the body to detect deficiencies.

6. How are the scars after the operation?

Small lateral incisions can be closed with plastic surgery and remain virtually invisible in a few months. The central scars are more noticeable but can also go almost unnoticed a year after the operation.

Chapter 88. Hypercalcemia and excess calcium

Hypercalcemia is a condition in which blood calcium levels are above normal. Among other disorders, this can weaken the bones, form kidney stones and interfere with the functioning of the heart and brain.

Usually, this medical condition occurs when the parathyroid glands produce too much parathyroid hormone, responsible for controlling the use and elimination of calcium, phosphate and Vitamin D from the body. This is known as hyperparathyroidism. Although it can occur in people of any sex and age, Hypercalcemia is more common in women over 50 years.

To learn more about this topic, we interviewed the Cuban doctor Mario Vega Carbó, an endocrinology specialist with more than 20 years of experience.

Doctor Mario,
1. What are parathyroids and what causes hyperparathyroidism?

Parathyroids are four glands found in the neck. Its main function is to produce parathyroid hormone, which together with Vitamin D are responsible for controlling the amount of calcium in the body, especially in the bones and blood.

The excessive production of this hormone may be due to a growth of some of the parathyroid glands and, to a much lesser extent, to a small non-cancerous tumor in them. It can also be a consequence of a severe deficiency of calcium or vitamin D, or chronic renal failure.

2. In addition to Hyperparathyroidism, what can cause Hypercalcemia?

This may also be due to severe dehydration; certain types of cancer, such as breast and lung cancer; excess vitamin D and calcium in the diet; and to remain prostrate for many days. On the other hand, hyperthyroidism; kidney problems; certain medications, such as lithium and diuretics; some infectious and inflammatory diseases, such as tuberculosis and sarcoidosis; and some hereditary factors can also cause it.

3. What are your main symptoms?

If Hypercalcemia is mild, it usually has no sign. In more severe cases, there may be bone or abdominal pain, depression, lack of memory, disorientation, fatigue and physical weakness, spasms, fragile bones that fracture easily (osteoporosis), kidney stones, nausea, vomiting, constipation, loss of appetite , excessive urination and frequent urination. In addition, it can rarely cause palpitations and fainting.

4. How is this disease detected?

In case of presenting its signs, blood tests are performed to check the levels of parathyroid hormone, calcium and vitamin D; and urine to confirm the diagnosis. In addition, by means of radiographs and a study of bone mineral density, the state of the bones can be established and possible fractures found.

On the other hand, through tests on the kidneys and urinary tract it is possible to know if there are calcium deposits or an obstruction, and it is also necessary to analyze the neck for tumors or changes in the parathyroid glands

5. What is the treatment of hypercalcemia?

The therapy depends on the cause that is causing this disorder. If elevated calcium levels are due to Hyperparathyroidism, surgery may be necessary to remove the parathyroid gland. If the problem is in the kidneys, the patient may need dialysis or a transplant.

On the other hand, some medications such as mimetic calcium mimic the calcium that circulates in the blood and can cause the parathyroid glands to release less hormone. In addition, calcitonin, bisphosphonates and prednisone can also help control Hypercalcemia.

On the other hand, women who have reached menopause and show signs of osteoporosis, may need a hormone replacement treatment with the application of estrogens, to improve calcium retention in the bones.

6. What other complications can Hypercalcemia cause?

If left unchecked, this disorder can cause an increased risk of bone fractures, high blood pressure, heart problems, kidney stones or a serious kidney ailment. Also pancreatitis, peptic ulcer disease, bone cysts, dehydration, osteoporosis, depression, dementia and difficulty concentrating and thinking.

Chapter 89. Renal lithiasis: causes, consequences and treatment of the famous "stones" in the kidneys

Renal lithiasis, also known as "stones" in the kidneys, is a condition caused by the presence of urinary tract stones. It is one of the most painful diseases that exists and is estimated to affect about 15 percent of men and 8 percent of women.

Its most frequent symptoms are severe pain in the lower back, blood or the elimination of sand in the urine, sweating, nausea and vomiting.

However, in many cases it does not present specific signals and is usually detected by chance on radiographs or ultrasound examinations that are performed for other reasons.

To learn more about this medical condition, we speak with Mario Vega Carbó, an endocrinology specialist who currently works as an endocrinologist at the Vega & Vado Office.

Doctor Mario,
1. How are "stones" formed in the kidneys?

Renal lithiasis originates when the urine has a high concentration of mineral salts that are not diluted correctly. The most frequent calculations, between 75 and 80 percent, are formed by calcium oxalate, while the remaining 20-25 percent correspond to uric acid, magnesium ammonium phosphate and cystine.

2. What consequences do these calculations have? Can they cause death?

Its effects vary according to the size and movement that they have inside the ducts. Many times the stones are very small and are expelled naturally without causing pain or producing any effect. Others, on the other hand, are very painful and should be treated with serum to prevent urine from accumulating and causing an infection.

It is difficult for lithiasis to lead to death but there have been cases of dialysis patients who have suffered severe complications in renal function as a result of it.

3. Who suffers from this disease and how often?

The maximum incidence occurs between 15 and 44 years of age and occurs more in men than in women, although the difference is slight. There is also an important genetic component that makes the children of people who have suffered this ailment more likely to suffer from it.

On the other hand, patients who have had kidney stones tend to relapse throughout their lives, most likely as the years go by.

4. What can be done to prevent renal lithiasis?

The most important thing is to always keep the body well hydrated. In that sense, it is advisable to drink at least 2.5 liters of water per day. On the other hand, it is also recommended to lead a healthy life and do sports, since obesity and sedentary lifestyle increase the possibility of generating stones.

As for the diet, it is important to avoid salt and sodium, sugars, alcohol and excess meat and animal proteins.

5. What happens when the stones are not expelled naturally?

In recent years there have been significant advances in treatments and today it is possible to remove the stones using increasingly less invasive techniques, such as lithotripsy and endoscopic surgery. In the first case, it is a procedure that uses shock waves to break the stones into small pieces, which are then expelled through the urine.

As for the endoscopic extraction, the calculation is divided mechanically or through laser and then its remains are removed.

6. What recommendations would you give to a patient who suffered from renal lithiasis?

I would advise you not to stop medication or preventive care, such as constant hydration, healthy living, good nutrition, exercise, because, as I mentioned earlier, studies show that the majority of patients who had this problem regenerate Stones over time.

Chapter 90. Bone Paget Disease

Paget's Disease, also known as Deforming Osteitis, is a condition that interferes with the process of gradual renewal of bone tissue. Over time, this causes the bones to become brittle and deformed. It usually affects the pelvis, skull, spine, arms, clavicles and legs.

It is the second most common bone condition, behind Osteoporosis, and the risk of getting it increases with age. Among other complications it can cause fractures, hearing loss and compression of the nerves of the spine.

To learn more about this topic, we interview Mario Vega Carbó, an endocrinologist with more than 20 years of experience.

Doctor Mario,
1. What causes Paget's Disease of Bone?

Although its exact origin is unknown, it is believed that it could be related to a viral infection, such as measles or rubella. On the other hand, there is also a genetic component, since it is very common for several members of the same family to suffer, and environmental, because it is more frequent in Europe and Oceania.

2. What are your symptoms?

In most cases this disease has no signs and is usually detected when an x-ray is taken or blood tests are performed for another cause. Some people may feel bone pain, joint stiffness, hearing loss, decreased height, tingling and fragile bones that fracture easily. In addition, in severe cases there may be an arching of the legs, an enlargement of the head and other deformations.

3. Who are more likely to have it?

People over 40, men, those who live in Europe and Oceania and those who have a family history with this disease have more risks.

4. What is your treatment?

In some cases where the disease has no symptoms, no treatment is necessary. On the contrary, if there is pain, noticeable bone changes or deformities, it will be necessary. Certain medications, such as bisphosphonates and the hormone calcitonin, help prevent further bone formation and breakdown. On the other hand, paracetamol and non-steroidal anti-inflammatories serve to relieve pain. In addition, some deformities, damaged joints and fractures may require orthopedic surgery. In general, the results of the therapy are positive.

5. What complications can this disease bring?

People who suffer from this disorder have a higher risk of suffering from neurological, cardiovascular and orthopedic problems. Abnormal bone growth can affect certain nerves, such as the auditory when the condition occurs in the skull. Complications may also include osteoarthritis, fissures, fractures, hypercalcemia and heart failure, paraplegia and narrowing of the spine. In a few cases, it can lead to bone cancer, known as osteosarcoma.

6. What other recommendations should be taken into account?

People with Paget's disease are advised to follow a diet rich in calcium and vitamin D, exercise daily, maintain an adequate body weight and not smoke. In older people, it is important to avoid falls, which are the main cause of fractures. In some cases it may be necessary to use a cane or a walker.

Chapter 91. Osteomalacia and bone softening

Osteomalacia is a disorder that causes a marked softening of the bones. This is usually due to the prolonged lack of vitamin D, which is responsible for promoting adequate levels of calcium and phosphorus in the body. This can cause arched legs during growth, bone pain and more chances of bone fractures, especially those of the ribs, spine and legs. In children, this condition is called Rickets.

To learn more about this topic, we interview Mario Vega Carbó, a specialist in endocrinology, nutrition and family medicine, who works as an endocrinologist at the Santa Fe Medical Center and the Vega & Vado Office.

Doctor Mario,
1. What is the cause of Osteomalacia?

Vitamin D is essential for the normal formation of bones and teeth and for the absorption of calcium and phosphorus at the intestinal level. When the proper amount of this substance is not received, or when the body has trouble using it, this can cause osteomalacia.

For example, surgeries that remove the stomach or intestine can cause problems to absorb vitamin D. Celiac disease, some kidney and liver problems, rheumatoid arthritis, tuberculosis and certain medications to treat seizures.

2. How is vitamin D obtained?

This substance can be obtained in two ways: by exposure to sunlight or by eating foods that contain it, such as milk, eggs, fatty fish, cereals, meats, bread, yogurt and orange juice.

3. Who are more likely to have Osteomalacia?

People with dark skin, those who live in geographical areas with little exposure to sunlight, those who remain indoors and those who use very powerful sunscreen have a higher risk of suffering it. Also those who have lactose intolerance, those who do not eat or drink dairy products, vegetarians and those who consume certain anticonvulsant and antiretroviral drugs. The same goes for those who suffer from cancer, kidney failure and liver diseases.

4. What are your main symptoms?

People with osteomalacia usually suffer fractures without a certain cause, muscle weakness, tingling of arms and legs, and hand and foot cramps. Also bone pain, especially in the back, pelvis, hips, legs and ribs.

5. How is osteomalacia detected?

To confirm your symptoms, physical and blood tests are usually done to check levels of vitamin D, creatinine, calcium, phosphate, electrolytes, alkaline phosphatase and parathyroid hormone. X-rays may also be necessary to detect possible fractures and bone loss, and a biopsy to see if there is a softening of the bones.

6. What is your treatment?

The therapy will aim to remedy the causes that cause it and relieve its symptoms. Generally, it will seek to add calcium, phosphorus and vitamin D to the diet and, if necessary, oral supplements will be administered. On the other hand, kidney or liver diseases that affect metabolism should be treated.

Part VI Kidney glands

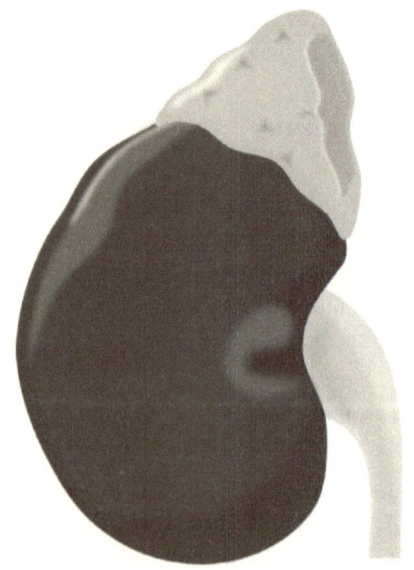

Chapter 92. Lipotimias and Fainting

Lipotimia is known as sudden loss of consciousness due to a decrease in cerebral blood flow. This includes syncope, seizures and some epileptic seizures.

During the syncope a temporary faint occurs, with spontaneous recovery and without subsequent sequelae. While it can be alarming, it generally has no major consequences. In many cases there are no premonitory signs and the loss of consciousness is sudden. In others there may be nausea, feeling faint, blurred vision, pale skin and coldness.

To learn more about this topic, we interview Mario Vega Carbó, an endocrinologist with more than 20 years of experience.

Doctor Mario,
1. What causes a lipotimia?

It is caused by a decrease in the blood flow of the brain. This could be due to fatigue; fatigue; lack of food; a sudden impression, joy or emotion; the anxiety; the fear; fever; dehydration or excess heat.

Other possible causes are blood draws, low blood pressure, severe pain, shortness of breath, phobias and alcohol or drug use. In more abrupt cases, it can be a consequence of a heart problem, such as arrhythmias.

2. What are your main symptoms?

In some cases there are no previous signs. In others there may be a feeling of weakness, paleness, cold sweating, blurred vision, weak pulse, shallow breathing, nausea and sudden fall.

In epileptic seizures, they may be preceded by abnormal numbness and shaking of some parts of the body, visual hallucinations and changes in behavior.

3. What complications can a lipotimia bring?

Fainting itself usually has no consequences. The inconveniences may arise from the area in which they occur, for example due to the blow to the ground or other objects, or because they occur while the person is driving or climbing a ladder.

4. What to deal with fainting?

Before a lipotimia it is important to lay the person in a cool place with the legs up, to facilitate the return of blood to the brain. You should also loosen your clothes, ask him to cough several times and take a deep breath, taking a breath through his nose and expelling it through his mouth.

When you have recovered, you should get up slowly, if possible with the help of another person, and check if you have any bumps or injuries.

If the person does not regain consciousness, it should be placed in a ventilated place and on the side, to avoid drowning in case of vomiting. If it is cold, a blanket can be placed on it so that it does not cool. If the fainting lasts more than five minutes, it is advisable to ask for medical help.

5. Can lipotimia be prevented?

So that it does not occur it is important to always stay well hydrated, especially on hot days. Also avoid closed places and strong emotions.

6. What other care should be taken into account?

Pregnant women and those over 50 should pay special attention to fainting, as it can be a symptom of a more serious problem. In the case of a person with Diabetes, the cause may be a sudden drop in glucose, so you have to give some sugary soda or a spoonful of honey or sugar.

If there are seizures, it can be an epileptic seizure, a disorder in which the activity of nerve cells in the brain is interrupted. In front of her, the person should be placed on the floor with a pillow on her head to avoid being hit. You should also take off your glasses, loosen your clothes and move away any sharp elements or with which you can collide. In no case do you have to put objects in your mouth or hold it tightly to avoid its movements. When the crisis passes, you have to let it rest on its side to recover.

Chapter 93. Addison's disease and adrenal insufficiency

Addison's disease is a condition that occurs when the adrenal glands do not produce enough hormones. It is a rare disorder that can affect anyone of any age and, if left untreated, can lead to death. Usually its cause is a problem with the immune system.

The adrenal glands are located above the kidneys and are responsible for producing hormones, such as cortisol and aldosterone, which are essential for life. Among other essential functions, these allow normal growth and regulate metabolism, energy levels, blood pressure and stress response.

To learn more about this topic, we interview Mario Vega Carbó, an endocrinology specialist who currently works as an endocrinologist at the Vega & Vado Clinic.

Doctor Mario,
1. What causes this medical condition?

Addison's disease is usually due to a problem with the immune system, which mistakenly attacks its own tissues and damages the adrenal glands. When this occurs, it is called Primary Adrenal Insufficiency. Other possible causes are some infections such as tuberculosis or HIV, cancer or hemorrhage within the glands.

On the other hand, the pituitary gland produces a hormone called adrenocorticotropin, which stimulates the adrenal cortex to generate its hormones. When it undergoes a tumor, inflammation or surgery, it stops producing hormones, which also ends up affecting the work of the adrenal glands. This is known as Secondary Adrenal Insufficiency.

2. Who has more risks of suffering from Addison's disease?

People with certain diseases, such as chronic thyroiditis, hyperthyroidism, Graves' disease, herpetiformis dermatitis, hypoparathyroidism, hypopituitarism, myasthenia gravis, pernicious anemia, testicular dysfunction, type 1 diabetes, vitiligo and genetic defects are more likely to suffer from it.

3. What are your main symptoms?

The disease usually progresses slowly so that initially there are no signs. As it progresses, in cases of Primary Adrenal Insufficiency there may be chronic diarrhea, nausea, vomiting, darkening in some areas of the skin, dehydration, abdominal and muscular pain, dizziness when standing, low blood pressure, weakness, extreme fatigue , craving for salt, irritability, depression, fainting and weight loss with reduced appetite.

The signs of Secondary Adrenal Insufficiency are similar, although they are more likely to have low blood sugar and not have hyperpigmentation, severe dehydration and low blood pressure.

4. How is this disease detected?

To make a diagnosis, it is necessary to carry out physical examinations and analyze the medical history and the medications that the patient is taking. Blood, saliva and urine studies are usually done to measure hormone levels and antibodies related to the disease, and diagnostic imaging tests to detect abnormalities in the pituitary gland and adrenal glands.

5. What is your treatment?

The therapy usually involves a replacement of hormones that are not being produced, with corticosteroids (hydrocortisone, prednisone, fludrocortisone acetate) and mineralocorticoids. Usually these medications should be taken for life.

In addition, the patient must undergo regular checks to adjust the dose and, in cases of infection, injury, surgery or stress, it may be necessary to increase the dose.

6. What other complications can Addison's disease bring?

People with Addison's disease are at risk of having an adrenal crisis, as a result of very low blood cortisol levels. This causes diarrhea, vomiting, dehydration and a drop in sugar in the body that require immediate attention.

In addition, people with this medical condition usually suffer from associated autoimmune diseases, such as diabetes, chronic thyroiditis, hypoparathyroidism, testicular insufficiency, pernicious anemia and hyperthyroidism.

7. What other aspects should be taken into account during this disease?

It is important that these patients wear a bracelet or special card that indicates their condition, to alert others in emergency situations. There you must state the medication and the dose they use.

It is also recommended that they have extra drugs in the workplace, travel bag or purse, since not taking the medication even for a single day can be dangerous. In addition, they are advised to carry out regular check-ups and carry a kit with an emergency hydrocortisone injection. It must be applied immediately in cases of an adrenal crisis.

Chapter 94. The Adrenal Crisis or Acute Adrenal Insufficiency

The Adrenal Crisis is an acute deficit of the hormones produced by the adrenal glands, which produces a critical situation that requires urgent treatment. It usually occurs when there is insufficiency of cortisol, the hormone responsible for adjusting energy levels, blood pressure, vascular function, glucose concentrations, the immune system and the stress response, among other essential aspects for the body's health.

People with Addison's disease, Congenital Adrenal Hyperplasia and other disorders of the thyroid glands can suffer a crisis of this type if they are not treated properly, if they stop taking the medications abruptly or if they face stressful situations. When this occurs, blood pressure and blood sugar levels drop, while potassium levels rise, and can even cause death.

To learn more about this topic, we interview Mario Vega Carbó, an endocrinology specialist with more than 20 years of experience.

Doctor Mario,
1. How does an adrenal crisis occur?

This situation occurs when there is a sharp reduction in the levels of hormones produced by the adrenal glands in the body. This usually occurs when people with Addison's disease, Congenital Adrenal Hyperplasia and other similar disorders suddenly stop hormone replacement therapy with corticosteroids.

It can also be the result of massive bilateral hemorrhage or sudden damage to the adrenal glands, or when the aforementioned diseases are not well treated. In these cases, an infection, a dehydration, a trauma, a stress situation or surgery can trigger the crisis.

2. What are your main symptoms?

People with Acute Adrenal Insufficiency usually present with fever, tachycardia, dehydration, extremely low blood pressure, respiratory distress, sugar fall, abdominal pain, diarrhea, nausea, vomiting, loss of appetite, dizziness, fatigue, severe weakness, confusion and reduction of conscience level. Symptoms manifest rapidly and progressively and require immediate attention.

3. What is your treatment?

The therapy must be administered quickly and consists of replenishing the volume of fluid in the blood and administering hydrocortisone intravenously to stabilize the patient. Alterations of ions, such as sodium and potassium, and blood pressure should also be corrected. Once the emergency is resolved, the causes that caused the crisis should be treated.

4. What disorders can cause an Adrenal Crisis?

If not treated quickly, it can cause a shock in which the body does not receive sufficient blood flow and cause death.

5. What other aspects should be taken into account during an Acute Adrenal Insufficiency?

It is important that patients with adrenal problems wear a bracelet or special card that indicates their condition, to alert others in emergency situations. There you must state the medication and the dose they use. In addition, they are advised to carry out regular check-ups and carry a kit with an emergency hydrocortisone injection. It must be applied immediately in cases of an adrenal crisis.

In cases of illness, before facing surgery or if they are very stressed, patients with Addison's disease are generally advised to increase the dose of the glucocorticoid medication temporarily.

Chapter 95. Cortisol Replacement: Glucocorticoids

Cortisol is a steroid hormone produced by the adrenal glands, which fulfills essential functions within the body. Among other tasks, it adjusts energy levels and is responsible for increasing the level of blood sugar; the metabolism of fats, proteins and carbohydrates; and the stress response.

Several synthetic forms of cortisol, known as corticosteroids or glucocorticoids, are used to treat a wide variety of different diseases.

To learn more about this topic, we interviewed Cuban doctor Mario Vega Carbó, a specialist in clinical endocrinology.

Doctor Mario,
1. What are glucocorticoids and what are they used for?

Glucocorticoids are medications that mimic the effects of hormones that the body naturally produces in the adrenal glands and are characterized by their anti-inflammatory, antiallergic and immunosuppressive power. In endocrinology they are used to replace cortisol deficiency in hormone replacement therapies, to treat Addison's disease and other cases of adrenal insufficiency.

Due to its wide scope, they are also used for the control of various ailments, such as arthritis, asthma, lupus, multiple sclerosis, allergies and other skin conditions and some types of cancer. In addition, they are also used to prevent rejection of organs in transplant recipients.

However, being very potent drugs that can cause serious side effects, they are usually indicated for short periods of time.

2. What are the most commonly used glucocorticoids?

Among them are beclomethasone, budesonide, cortisone, deflazacort, dexamethasone, hydrocortisone, Methylprednisolone, prednisone, prednisolone and triamcinolone. Due to its short action, low cost and low incidence of adverse effects, prednisone is the most prescribed glucocorticoid. However, for cases of adrenal insufficiency, cortisone or hydrocortisone acetate is preferred, using prednisone only when these are not available.

On the other hand, for perioperative and acute adrenal crisis, the use of injectable hydrocortisone is recommended according to the patient's need.

3. How are these medications given?

They come in different presentations. There are tablets, capsules and syrups that are ingested orally and are generally used to treat inflammations and pains associated with chronic ailments, such as rheumatoid arthritis and lupus.

In cases of cortisol hormone replacement, in the treatment of Addison's disease and other adrenal insufficiencies, a tablet is usually given at 7 or 8 in the morning, and half a tablet at 5 in the afternoon. However, some patients may require higher doses or frequencies, depending on blood pressure and potassium levels, which should be in normal ranges.

On the other hand, there are also nasal inhalers and sprays, which are used for asthma and nasal allergies, and topical creams and ointments that help cure skin diseases.

Meanwhile, glucocorticoid injections are used to treat muscle and joint pain, and in cases of perioperative and adrenal crises, as I mentioned earlier.

4. What side effects can these drugs cause?

Oral glucocorticoids, by affecting the entire body and not just the area for which they are taken, are the ones that can cause the most side effects. These may include fluid retention, hypertension, mood swings, glaucoma, memory and behavioral problems, confusion, weight gain, cataracts, hyperglycemia, osteoporosis, increased risk of infections, nausea, muscle weakness, psychotic crises, thin skin and slower wound healing.

On the other hand, in children it can cause growth problems. Inhaled, meanwhile, can cause hoarseness and fungal infection in the mouth, while the topics can generate thin skin, red skin lesions and acne.

In turn, injectables can cause hyperglycemia, facial redness, insomnia, severe pain and thinning and loss of skin color near the injection site.

5. How can these side effects be limited?

The supply of a single dose, even high, does not usually generate toxic problems. On the other hand, treatments of less than one week usually do not cause damage.

In prolonged treatments of more than two weeks, to reduce side effects, lower concentrations or intermittent doses can be tested, and other presentations can be chosen instead of oral ones.In these cases it is also recommended to take calcium and vitamin D supplements to avoid osteoporosis. In addition, periodic checks are advised to assess possible risks.

On the other hand, when interrupting its supply, this should be done gradually and not suddenly because it can cause severe adrenal insufficiency.

6. What are mineralocorticoids?

Mineralocorticoids are other hormones secreted by the adrenal glands. The most important is aldosterone, which helps maintain the right amount of sodium in the body, by regulating its elimination through urine, sweat glands and intestines. In addition, it participates in the secretion of potassium and in the increase of blood pressure.

7. What are synthetic mineralocorticoids used for?

These drugs, such as fludrocortisone, are used for the treatment of hormone replacement in cases of adrenal insufficiency or in congenital adrenal syndrome. They help control the amount of sodium and fluids in the body, preventing large amounts from being lost in the urine. In addition, they are also used to increase blood pressure.

8. How is fludrocortisone given?

This medicine comes as a tablet to take by mouth.

9. What side effects can it cause?

Its use can cause stomach upset, vomiting, headache, dizziness, insomnia, agitation, anxiety, acne, increased hair growth and menstrual irregularities. In severe cases there may be skin rashes, vision problems and swelling of the face, legs or ankles. It can also cause depression and increased suicidal thoughts.

10. What other aspects should be taken into account while using these medications?

In cases of adrenal insufficiency, it is important that these patients wear a wristband or identification card that indicates their condition, to alert others in emergency situations. There you must state the medication and the dose they use.

It is also recommended that they have extra drugs in the workplace, travel bag or purse, since not taking the medication even for a single day can be dangerous. In addition, they are advised to perform regular checkups to avoid a crisis.

Chapter 96. Autoimmune Polyglandular Syndrome

Autoimmune Polyglandular Syndromes are a series of disorders in which two or more diseases of the endocrine system occur, associated with other pathologies of autoimmune etiology.

The most common endocrine ailments that appear within these groups are Diabetes Mellitus, Adrenal Insufficiency, Hyperthyroidism, Hypothyroidism, Hypoparathyroidism, Alopecia, Vitiligo and rheumatic diseases. Meanwhile, autoimmune conditions are usually of a cutaneous nature.

The association between the different disorders shows recurring patterns. This has allowed Autoimmune Polyglandular Syndromes to be classified into types I, II and III.

To learn more about this topic, we interview Mario Vega Carbó, an endocrinologist with more than 20 years of experience.

Doctor Mario,
1. What is Autoimmune Polyglandular Syndrome type I?

This disorder usually appears in childhood and usually has hypoparathyroidism along with mucocutaneous candidiasis in the mouth. This fungal infection is usually chronic and resistant to conventional therapy. Near adolescence, kidney failure is added to the diagnosis.

This syndrome is hereditary and is caused by the mutation of a single autoimmune gene located on chromosome 21. Among other symptoms, it can cause abnormalities in the teeth, chronic diarrhea and problems in the bones, joints, skin, nails, nails. ovaries, testicles, eyes and other internal organs.

Other endocrine ailments that may manifest are hypogonadism and hypothyroidism. Rarely also Diabetes. On the other hand, more than half of women under 30 with this disease also develop Primary Ovarian Insufficiency.

2. How is Autoimmune Polyglandular Syndrome type II?

It begins in adulthood and is characterized by the presence of adrenal insufficiency along with an autoimmune thyroid disease. Type 1 Diabetes may also appear. It is not known for sure what causes it, but it is believed to be related to a combination of genetic and environmental factors.

This syndrome is more common in women than in men. Other endocrine problems such as Primary Hypogonadism, Myasthenia Gravis and Celiac Disease can also be added to it.

3. What is Autoimmune Polyglandular Syndrome type III?

This type is characterized by an autoimmune thyroiditis combined with another condition, which can be type 1 diabetes, pernicious anemia, vitiligo, myasthenia gravis or alopecia, among other possibilities.

It usually affects women during middle age. Its cause is unknown, but it is estimated to be caused by an autoimmune disease derived from environmental and genetic factors. In many cases, more than one member of the same family suffers from it.

4. How are these syndromes treated?

Therapy for Autoimmune Polyglandular Syndromes is based on addressing each of the endocrine conditions that appear. Generally, hormone replacement is the mainstay of treatment.

In type I, medications are also used to treat candidiasis. In this infection, recurrences in the digestive tract should be monitored, since it can cause cancer of the epithelium.

Chapter 97. Vitiligo Loss of skin color

Vitiligo is a degenerative skin disease, which is characterized by depigmentation of skin areas. This loss of color generates white patches of different sizes and shapes, which can affect any part of the body. It is not contagious and its consequences are mainly aesthetic, since the texture of the skin does not change.

Although it has a strong inherited component, it usually appears associated with other autoimmune diseases, such as celiac disease, diabetes, rheumatoid arthritis or pernicious anemia. About 2% of the population suffers from Vitiligo, which often has a psychological and social impact on the patient.

To learn more about this topic, we interviewed Cuban doctor Mario Vega Carbó, a specialist in clinical endocrinology.

Doctor Mario,
1. What causes Vitiligo?

This condition appears when the cells responsible for pigmentation, known as melanocytes, die or suspend melanin production. While the exact cause is unknown, this is believed to occur due to an immune problem, where the cells of this system destroy the melanocytes by mistake.

This can also happen as a result of sunburn, stress or exposure to industrial chemicals.

2. Who are more likely to have it?

Vitiligo can appear at any age and there is a greater propensity in people with a family history. It affects both men and women equally.

On the other hand, people who suffer hormonal changes (pregnancy, menopause, stress), or who suffer from diabetes, Addison or thyroid disease and pernicious anemia are also more likely to suffer from it.

3. What are your symptoms?

Vitiligo is characterized by the appearance of areas of a different color in the body. Dark skinned people usually have pink spots, while those with light skin are white. These patches usually appear on the face, hands, feet, knees and elbows. They can also occur in the back, torso, genitals, arms and legs, although less frequently.

In some cases it affects the inside of the mouth and nose, eyes and hair, which turns white or gray on the scalp, eyelashes, eyebrows or beard prematurely.

4. What is your treatment?

Vitiligo is difficult to treat and takes time to show concrete results. The use of phototherapy and lasers could help repigment the skin. On the other hand, certain medications with corticosteroids, creams or immunosuppressive ointments or topical drugs such as methoxalene may favor the production of melanin.

In some cases, a skin graft can be performed from an area that is not affected to another that is. In addition, natural remedies such as evening primrose oil, ginkgo biloba and aloe vera can improve the appearance of Vitiligo

For extreme situations in which the disease has spread to most of the body, depigmentation of the unaffected areas can be performed. This color removal will be permanent and the person will be extremely sensitive to sunlight.

5. What can you expect from this therapy?

In many cases the treatment manages to restore the color of the affected skin. However, it does not prevent the continuous loss of pigmentation or completely prevent its spread to other parts of the body.

On the other hand, certain special makeups can hide your symptoms.

6. What other aspects should consider those who suffer from this disease?

Depigmented skin has no natural protection and is more exposed to the effects of UV rays. To avoid serious burns, it is recommended to use sunscreen or sunscreen with a factor above 30, wide-brimmed hats and clothing that covers the entire body. It is also important to avoid stress, which in many cases increases the symptoms of Vitiligo, and tattoos not related to treatment.

7. What other complications can this disease cause?

People with Vitiligo are more likely to suffer sunburn and skin cancer, and eye and ear problems. On the other hand, those who suffer from this faction tend to suffer from lack of self-esteem, shame and depression due to the change in appearance, so it is advisable to accompany the treatment with psychological and family support.

Chapter 98. Secondary Hypertension. Diseases that cause it

Secondary hypertension is high blood pressure caused by other diseases, such as those affecting the kidneys, arteries, heart and endocrine system. It differs from primary school, which is the most common, and is related to hereditary issues, poor diet, lack of exercise and obesity.

Blood pressure is the force exerted by the blood that circulates against the walls of the arteries. When it increases, hypertension occurs, which is a condition suffered by a third of the adult population. If left untreated, it can cause serious complications, such as heart attack, stroke and kidney and visual damage.

To learn more about this topic, we interview Mario Vega Carbó, an endocrinologist with more than 20 years of experience.

Doctor Mario,
1. What are the symptoms of high blood pressure?

Usually this condition has no symptoms and is detected through measurements. In very severe cases there may be headache and chest pain, nausea, vomiting, nasal bleeding, sweating, blurred vision and confusion.

2. What causes Secondary Hypertension?

There are many conditions that can cause it, especially those related to the kidneys, arteries, heart and endocrine system. The most common are Diabetes, cysts in the kidneys, Cushing's syndrome, tumors in the adrenal glands, thyroid problems, hyperparathyroidism, aortic narrowing and sleep apnea.

In addition, Secondary Hypertension may appear due to obesity, pregnancy or the consumption of various medications, supplements and illegal drugs.

3. Who are more likely to have it?

Older people, obese people, those suffering from stress, those who drink alcohol excessively, smokers and those with a family history are more likely to suffer from high blood pressure

4. What other disorders can cause secondary hypertension?

If left unchecked, it can cause hardening and thickening of the arteries and cause a heart attack or stroke. It can also generate an aneurysm, metabolic disorders, heart failure or weakened, thickened or broken blood vessels in the kidneys or eyes.

5. How is it diagnosed?

The only way to detect it is through its measurement. Many people can have it for years without knowing it. When the patient is not obese, he has no family history and high blood pressure appears suddenly, possibly it is a secondary hypertension.

In that case, blood and urine tests, kidney ultrasound, electrocardiogram and other studies are performed to detect the condition that is causing it.

6. What is the treatment of Secondary Hypertension?

First of all the disease that causes it should be treated. Once this is resolved or controlled, Secondary Hypertension can normalize. On the other hand, there are specific medications to maintain low blood pressure, such as thiazide diuretics, beta blockers and angiotensin converting enzyme inhibitors. Usually, a combination of drugs is used for treatment.

7. What other recommendations are provided for these cases?

As with Primary Hypertension, leading a healthy life, exercising, drinking plenty of fluids and eating well can help with treatment.

Within foods, a diet rich in fruits, vegetables, whole grains and dairy products is recommended, and avoid salt, saturated fats and total fats. Potassium, present in potatoes, spinach and bananas, helps control the pressure. It is also advised to maintain a healthy weight, correct vitamin deficiencies, avoid alcohol and quit smoking.

Finally, to control stress, you can practice muscle relaxation techniques, such as yoga or meditation.

Chapter 99. Benign and Malignant Adrenal Incidentaloma

An Adrenal Incidentaloma is an unexpected tumor that appears in one or both adrenal glands. It is an increasingly common condition, which can be benign or malignant (cancerous).

The adrenal glands are located above the kidneys and are responsible for producing hormones, such as cortisol and aldosterone, which are essential for life. Among other essential functions, these allow normal growth and regulate metabolism, energy levels, blood pressure and stress response.

Adrenal Incidentaloma can manifest itself at any age, although it is more common in children under 5 years and adults over 50. On the other hand, diabetic, obese and hypertensive people are more likely to suffer from it.

To learn more about this topic, we interview Mario Vega Carbó, an endocrinologist with more than 20 years of experience.

Doctor Mario,
1. Why is this condition "booming"?

At present, the number of incidents discovered casually during ultrasound, computed tomography, magnetic resonance imaging and scintigraphy have increased. This is due on the one hand to the greater development and resolution that the imaging tests have achieved and also to the progressive aging of the population, which makes the pathologies increase.

2. What causes an Adrenal Incidentaloma?

Some cause the adrenal glands to produce too much hormones and generate what is called an active functional tumor. This can be caused by various conditions such as Cushing's Syndrome, Hyperaldosteronism, Congenital Adrenal Hyperplasia or a Pheochromocytoma.

On the other hand, when the indicentaloma does not cause excessive hormone production, it is called a non-functional tumor. In these cases it can be an adenoma, a cancer or a cyst inside or outside the glands.

3. How is it diagnosed?

As I said, these types of tumors are usually detected by chance during an imaging test to investigate another disorder. Once found, they usually analyze the patient's medical history and perform physical exams and blood and urine tests to measure hormone levels and identify their causes.

4. What are your symptoms?

Symptoms vary depending on whether the tumor is functional or not. If there is an excess of hormones, the patient may have weight loss, obesity in the middle and upper body, purple streaks, thin and fragile skin, acne, muscle weakness, high blood pressure and increased blood sugar.

On the other hand, in women it can generate hirsutism (excessive development of body hair) and irregular or non-existent menstrual periods, and in men decreased libido and fertility, and erectile diffusion. In addition, patients may suffer from depression, anxiety, irritability, sweating and sleep disorders.

5. What is the treatment for Adrenal Incidentaloma?

About 85% of these tumors are not functional and may not require treatment. Only your periodic check. In some cases, radiation therapy, chemotherapy or surgery will be necessary to remove the tumor or one or both adrenal glands. Also treatment to normalize hormonal levels.

Cancer in the adrenal glands is very rare and its treatment can be used to delay its progression. Although it is usually very aggressive, if detected in time there is a possibility of cure.

6. What other aspects are recommended to consider?

In the case of a malignant tumor, it is recommended to seek psychological support and participation in therapeutic groups with people who are suffering from this same disease, to treat the anxiety, anguish and stress that the disease can cause.

Chapter 100. Hypercortisolism or Cushing's Syndrome

Cushing's syndrome is a disorder caused by prolonged exposure to excess cortisol, produced by the adrenal glands that are located in the upper part of the kidneys.

This hormone is responsible for adjusting energy levels, blood pressure, vascular function, glucose concentrations, the immune system and the response to stress, among other functions essential to the health of the body. The cause of this condition may be due to a benign tumor in the pituitary gland or chronic use of glucocorticoids and other medications to treat inflammatory diseases, such as asthma and rheumatoid arthritis. In addition, it can be caused by abnormalities in the adrenal glands.

Also known as Hypercortisolism, Cushing's Syndrome is a rare condition, which occurs in less than 40 people per million inhabitants.

To learn more about this topic, we interview Mario Vega Carbó, an endocrinology specialist with more than 20 years of experience.

Doctor Mario,
1. What are the symptoms of this condition?

The usual signs of Cushing Syndrome are obesity in the middle and upper body, generating a kind of fat hump between the shoulders, and the rounded and red face. Other symptoms are thin arms and legs, purple streaks, thin, fragile skin, slow recovery of cuts and easy bruising.

2. How is it diagnosed?

In general it can be difficult to detect Hypercortisolism, because its symptoms are similar to other diseases, such as obesity and metabolic syndromes.

To make a diagnosis, it is necessary to carry out physical examinations and analyze the medical history and the medications that the patient is taking. In addition, blood, saliva and urine studies are usually performed to measure hormone levels, and diagnostic imaging tests to detect abnormalities in the pituitary gland and adrenal glands. It is also advisable to measure the thickness of the skin fold.

3. What is the treatment for Hypercortisolism?

The therapy will depend on what is causing the excess cortisol in the body. For example, if the reason is a tumor, surgery, radiotherapy and other treatments may be necessary. On the other hand, if the problem is caused by a medication, the dose can be lowered or changed to a similar one that does not produce these symptoms.

On the other hand, there are different drugs to control the excessive production of cortisol, among which are ketoconazole, mitotane, methirapone, pasireotide and mifepristone.

4. Do these medications have side effects?

Yes, these drugs can cause fatigue, nausea, vomiting, diarrhea, headaches and abdominal pain, muscle aches, high blood pressure, low potassium and swelling. Side effects are quite frequent.

5. What other health problems can this ailment cause?

Cushing's syndrome can lead to a decrease in bone mass, high blood pressure, increased blood sugar, excessive urination, frequent infections, vertebral fractures, acne and obesity.

On the other hand, in women it can generate hirsutism (excessive development of body hair) and irregular or non-existent menstrual periods, and in men decreased libido and fertility, and erectile diffusion.

In addition, patients with this medical condition may suffer from depression, anxiety, irritability, insomnia, cognitive difficulties, hallucinations and paranoid symptoms.

6. What influence do corticosteroid medications have?

In many cases, hypercortisolism may be due to taking oral corticosteroids in high doses for a prolonged period of time.

These medications, such as prednisone, have the same effect on the body as cortisol and are used to treat inflammatory conditions such as rheumatoid arthritis, lupus and asthma, or to prevent the body from rejecting an organ transplant. In general, steroids that are inhaled or that come in creams are less likely to cause Cushing's Syndrome than those given orally.

7. Is Cushing Syndrome hereditary?

Very rarely people inherit a tendency to suffer tumors in their endocrine glands, which affects cortisol levels and causes Hypercortisolism.

8. What are the usual results of your treatment?

In general, if cortisol production is normalized in the body, the prognosis is good. However, in some cases patients may have more tendency to obesity, osteoporosis and depression than the normal population.

Chapter 101. Pheochromocytoma and increased blood pressure

Pheochromocytoma is a tumor in the adrenal glands, which is usually non-cancerous (benign). It stimulates the exaggerated secretion of epinephrine and norepinephrine, two hormones that control heart rate, metabolism and blood pressure.

If left untreated, it can cause serious damage to other body systems, especially the cardiovascular system, the brain and the kidneys. Removal of the pheochromocytoma by surgery usually causes blood pressure levels to return to normal.

To learn more about this topic, we interview Mario Vega Carbó, an endocrinologist, nutritionist and master in satisfactory longevity with more than 20 years of experience.

Doctor Mario,
1. What causes a pheochromocytoma?

The causes for which this tumor appears are not known, but in general it develops in the center of one or both adrenal glands, in cells called pheochromocytes. These release certain hormones, such as epinephrine and norepinephrine, that help control many body functions, such as heart rate, blood pressure and blood sugar.

The appearance of a pheochromocytoma causes an irregular and excessive release of these hormones, which generates an increase in blood pressure.

2. Who has more risks of suffering it?

Pheochromocytoma can occur at any age, but it is more common in people between 20 and 50 years old. In a few cases, the condition appears in several family members.

Those who have inherited disorders such as multiple endocrine neoplasia type II, von Hippel-Lindau disease, neurofibromatosis 1 and paraganglioma syndromes have a higher risk of developing these tumors.

3. What are your main symptoms?

In addition to an increase in blood pressure, the person may experience headache, severe sweating, heart palpitations, tremor, shortness of breath and extreme paleness. Generally these signs occur in the form of episodes when the tumor releases hormones and can last a few minutes or extend for longer.

They can also be triggered by situations of anxiety or stress, physical exertion or the consumption of certain foods, medications or stimulants. As the pheochromocytoma grows, the attacks increase in frequency, duration and severity.

4. How is pheochromocytoma detected?

For diagnosis, physical, blood and urine tests, and various imaging tests are usually performed. These may include computed tomography, scintigraphy and magnetic resonance imaging of the abdomen; adrenal biopsy; and analysis of catecholamines, glucose and plasma methanephrine.

In addition, a genetic analysis may also be necessary to determine if the tumor is related to an inherited disorder.

In many cases the pheochromocytoma is found by chance during studies that are carried out for other reasons.

5. What is your treatment?

The most common therapy is the removal of pheochromocytoma by surgery. Before performing it, it is necessary to stabilize the patient's blood pressure and pulse with medications. After the intervention, the levels of the hormones norepinephrine and epinephrine generally return to normal.

Other treatment options include radiotherapy, chemotherapy and targeted therapy, where substances are used to identify and attack cancer cells, without harming healthy ones.

6. What other complications can pheochromocytoma generate?

If left untreated, the high blood pressure caused by this tumor can damage several organs and cause heart disease, stroke, kidney failure, breathing difficulties and damage to the ocular nerves.

On the other hand, in rare cases the pheochromocytoma is malignant and the cancer cells spread to other parts of the body causing metastasis.

Chapter 102. Primary Hyperaldosteronism and Blood Pressure

Primary hyperaldosteronism is a hormonal disorder in which the adrenal glands produce an excessive amount of aldosterone in the blood. It is due to a non-cancerous (benign) tumor in the glands.

Aldosterone is a hormone that helps maintain the right amount of sodium and potassium in the body, by regulating its elimination in the urine, sweat glands and intestines.

Primary Hyperaldosteronism causes a loss of potassium and an excess of sodium, which generates a fluid retention that increases blood volume and blood pressure.

To learn more about this condition, we consulted Dr. Mario Vega Carbó, an endocrinology specialist, who currently works at the Vega & Vado Office.

Doctor Mario,
1. What are the causes of primary hyperaldosteronism?

This is usually due to a non-cancerous (benign) tumor in the adrenal glands, known as Conn syndrome. It can also be the result of hyperactivity of both glands and, rarely, a cancerous lump or hereditary aldosteronism.

2. What are your main symptoms?

Its most common signs are high blood pressure, low potassium level, fatigue, headache, numbness and muscle weakness.

3. Who has more risks of suffering it?

Primary hyperaldosteronism is more common in people 30 to 50 years of age. Those with a family history of high blood pressure, the obese, those who lead a sedentary lifestyle, smokers and those who consume a lot of alcohol are more likely to suffer from it.

4. How is this disorder detected?

A physical examination, a CT scan of the abdomen, ultrasound in the kidneys are usually performed, and the levels of aldosterone, renin, sodium and potassium in the blood and urine are measured. Aldosterone measurements may include studies of saline infusion and fludrocortisone suppression.

In some cases, adrenal vein sampling may also be necessary to verify which of the two glands is producing too much aldosterone.

5. What is your treatment?

Therapy for Primary Hyperaldosteronism includes medications, lifestyle changes and surgery. The first option is to treat the medical condition with drugs and with a healthy diet. Medications that block the action of aldosterone, such as spironolactone, may be prescribed, while diuretics help improve fluid accumulation in the body.

In some cases, removal of the tumor or gland can control the symptoms. If the blood pressure continues, it will be necessary to take some drug to remedy it.

6. What other aspects should be taken into account?

Blood pressure medications are more effective when accompanied with a healthy lifestyle. This includes controlling weight and eating a well-balanced diet low in sodium, avoiding condiments and eliminating salt, and adding more fruits, vegetables, lean proteins and whole grains.

Also do physical activity for at least 30 minutes most days, and avoid smoking and consuming alcohol and excessive caffeine.

7. What complications can cause Primary Hyperaldosteronism?

This medical condition generates a very high blood pressure, which can damage many organs, especially the kidneys, eyes, heart and brain. Some of the possible complications are heart attack, stroke, kidney failure and premature death.

On the other hand, low sodium levels can cause weakness, arrhythmias, muscle cramps and excess thirst and urination. In addition, prolonged use of medications to control Primary Hyperaldosteronism can cause erection and gynecomastia problems in men.

Chapter 103. Carcinoid Syndrome

A series of symptoms associated with tumors that bear the same name and that affect the small intestine, colon, appendix, rectum and lungs is called Carcinoid Syndrome. This is a rare and usually slow-growing condition.

Carcinoid tumors secrete a large amount of the hormone serotonin and other substances, which causes blood vessels to dilate and the syndrome appears. Its symptoms usually manifest only in the final stages of the disease. The most common are diarrhea and redness of the skin.

To learn more about this topic, we interview Mario Vega Carbó, an endocrinologist with more than 20 years of experience.

Doctor Mario,
1. How is this condition diagnosed?

In most cases, carcinoid tumors are detected when studies are done for other reasons, such as during abdominal surgery.

To confirm the diagnosis, blood and urine tests, computed tomography and magnetic resonance imaging of the chest and abdomen, ultrasound and scintigraphy are performed. Only a small percentage of carcinoid tumors secrete the chemicals that cause the syndrome, so it occurs in very few cases (between 5 and 8%). When this occurs, it is usually because the disease has spread to the liver or lung.

2. What are the main signs of the syndrome?

Its most common symptom is the dilation of small blood vessels on the surface of the skin, mainly on the face, neck and upper chest. This redness may appear for no reason or occur due to stress, physical activity or alcohol consumption. It can be brief or last for hours, usually accompanied by palpitations.

307

Other signs include difficulty breathing, diarrhea, facial injuries, abdominal cramps, nausea, vomiting and heart problems, such as tachycardia or high or low blood pressure.

3. How is this condition treated?

The treatment for Carcinoid Syndrome is the same as for cancer, along with certain specific medications to control your symptoms. Usually, the first thing that is done is surgery to remove the tumor.

This can be accompanied by drugs that block the secretion of hormones produced by cancer cells, which helps reduce their signs and strengthen the immune system. Therapy may also include chemotherapy and the removal of cancer cells in the liver with cold or heat.

On the other hand, in advanced cases in which the tumor cannot be surgically removed, octreotide or lanreotide injections are applied to treat it and to decrease the symptoms of the syndrome.

4. What is the expectation of this therapy?

The prognosis depends on where the tumor is and its degree of progress. If it is diagnosed early, treatment is usually effective.

In cases of patients presenting with Carcinoid Syndrome, the tumor is usually advanced and has spread to the liver, which reduces the survival rate.

5. What other complications can this disease bring?

This condition can lead to increased falls and injuries as a result of low blood pressure, obstruction and gastrointestinal bleeding, and thickening of the heart valves, which causes heart disease. The latter can lead to fatigue and difficulty breathing during physical activity.

On the other hand, exposure to certain triggers, such as anesthesia used during surgery, can cause a carcinoid crisis. This is characterized by severe episodes of redness, low blood pressure that causes hypotension and difficulty breathing. It can be deadly.

6. What other care should these patients take?

People with Carcinoid Syndrome should avoid alcohol, hearty foods and foods rich in tyramine (mature cheese, nuts, chicken liver, chocolate, red wine and certain fish), as they can trigger their symptoms. The same goes for some medications, such as Prozac, which can increase serotonin levels.

It is also convenient to try to avoid stressful situations, rest well and take a vitamin supplement to counteract the effects of diarrhea.

Finally, it is recommended that they lead a healthy lifestyle and, if necessary, seek psychological support to better cope with the disease.

Chapter 104. Multiple Endocrine Neoplasia

Multiple Endocrine Neoplasia encompasses a series of rare inherited disorders, in which several endocrine glands grow excessively or have benign or malignant tumors. They are caused by genetic mutations, which usually affect the entire family group. Your symptoms, which vary depending on the affected glands, can occur at any age.

In general, Multiple Endocrine Neoplasia produces an overproduction of hormones that must be treated. There are three classes: type 1, type 2A and type 2B.

To learn more about this topic, we interview Mario Vega Carbó, an endocrinologist with more than 20 years of experience.

Doctor Mario,
1. What is Multiple Endocrine Neoplasia type 1?

This class is characterized by the presence of tumors or by the hyperactivity of two or more glands, among which are usually the pancreas, parathyroids and pituitary gland. Tumors are usually benign and cause excessive secretion of hormones. When it occurs in parathyroids, it can raise blood calcium levels and cause kidney stones.

When it appears in the pancreas it causes an excess of gastrin and can generate an overproduction of stomach acid and form peptic ulcers.

Meanwhile, if it develops in the pituitary gland, it can cause an increase in prolactin or growth hormone and cause menstrual abnormalities, galactorrhea, lack of libya, acromegaly and erectile dysfunction.

2. How is Multiple Endocrine Neoplasia type 2A?

This class is characterized by the presence of tumors or by the hyperactivity of two or more glands, which usually include the thyroid, parathyroid and adrenal glands. In most cases, thyroid medullary carcinoma develops and the appearance of pheochromocytomas that cause hypertension is also common.

In some patients, obstructions in the large intestine and a pruritic skin disease known as cutaneous amyloid lichen are observed.

3. What is Multiple Endocrine Neoplasia type 2B?

This class is characterized by the appearance of medullary thyroid cancer, parathyroid hyperplasia, adenomas, pheochromocytomas and nerve cell tumors in the mucous membranes or other places. On some occasions, patients who have this disease do not have a family history with this condition, but it is the result of a new genetic mutation.

Due to benign tumors in the mucous membranes, the lips and eyelids may appear thick. Neuromas can also appear on the tongue, the inside of the mouth and the eyes.

These patients often have a slender body, with thin arms and legs. Alterations in the spine and abnormalities in the bones of the skull are also common.

4. How is Multiple Endocrine Neoplasia diagnosed?

Genetic tests are usually performed and hormonal levels are measured through blood and urine tests. In some cases, imaging studies may also be necessary to determine the location of the tumors.

5. What is your treatment?

The neoplasm itself has no cure, so the therapy aims to resolve the changes that are generated in each of the affected glands individually. In case of tumors, they can be removed by surgery. On the other hand, hormonal imbalances are treated with medications.

If the neoplasm is type 2A or 2B, preventive removal of the thyroid gland is often performed to prevent the appearance of a thyroid medullary carcinoma, which can be fatal. After surgery, thyroid hormone should be taken for life.

6. What other complications can this disease bring?

Complications depend largely on which glands are affected. In many cases the tumors may continue to reappear. That is why regular checks are essential.

Chapter 105. Benign and Malignant Neuroendocrine Tumors

Neuroendocrine tumors are abnormal lumps that originate from neuroendocrine cells, responsible for producing hormones. They are rare and usually occur in the lungs, appendix, small intestine, rectum and pancreas. They can also appear in the thyroid, parathyroid, adrenal and pituitary glands, and other organs such as the kidney, bladder and prostate.

Neuroendocrine tumors are usually slow growing, although they can also develop aggressively and spread to other parts of the body.

To learn more about this condition, we consulted Dr. Mario Vega Carbó, an endocrinology specialist, who currently works at the Vega & Vado Office.

Doctor Mario,
1. What are the main symptoms of Neuroendocrine Tumors?

Many people have no signs and the disease can go unnoticed for years or be detected casually. When there are symptoms, they vary depending on the location of the tumor. The most common are reddening of the skin, diarrhea, sweating, abdominal pain and variation in blood glucose levels. Usually signs appear when the tumor generates an exaggerated elaboration of certain hormones.

2. What are the most frequent Neuroendocrine Tumors?

These include carcinoid tumors, medullary thyroid cancer, pheochromocytomas, insulinomas, neuroendocrine carcinoma of the skin, adrenal gland cancer, small cell lung cancer and large cell carcinoid tumor.

3. Who has more risks of suffering them?

Neuroendocrine tumors occur in both men and women, most often around 50 years. Although they are not usually associated with an inherited genetic mutation, in a few cases they appear alongside other family syndromes, such as Multiple Endocrine Neoplasia type 1.

In addition, people with Diabetes Mellitus or stomach diseases and smokers have more risks of suffering from them.

4. What is your treatment?

The therapy will depend on the type of tumor, its location, if it affects hormone production and if it has spread to other parts of the body. Some treatments may include surgery, radiation therapy, chemotherapy and targeted therapy. Also the use of certain medications to prevent the growth and spread of the tumor or to block the secretion of hormones produced by cancer cells. This helps reduce their signs and strengthen the immune system.

For people with cancer that has spread to the liver, transplantation may be an option.

5. What other care should these patients take?

These tumors can be slow growing and can cause metabolic and nutritional problems related to hormone overproduction, metastasis or treatment side effects. That is why regular checks are important.

It is also convenient that these patients try to avoid stressful situations, for which the practice of relaxation techniques such as yoga or meditation is advised. In addition, it is recommended that they lead a healthy life; may they rest well; that perform light physical activity, such as gymnastics, Pilates or daily walks; and that they take a vitamin supplement to counteract the effects of diarrhea, if any.

6. What other aspects should be taken into account during the illness?

In the case of a malignant tumor, it is recommended to seek psychological support and participation in therapeutic groups with people who are suffering from the same disease, to treat the anxiety, anguish and stress that can cause.

Part VII Hypothalamus and Pituitary

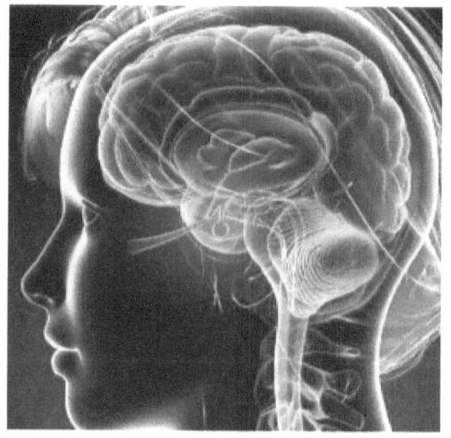

Chapter 106. Syndrome of Inappropriate Antidiuretic Hormone Secretion

The Syndrome of Inappropriate Antidiuretic Hormone Secretion (SSIHA) is a disorder in which the body produces too much of this substance.

The antidiuretic hormone is generated in the hypothalamus and helps the kidneys conserve water by concentrating urine and reducing its volume. The SSIHA causes the body to retain excess fluid and lower the level of sodium in the blood, affecting the normal functioning of the organs.

To learn more about this topic, we interviewed the Cuban doctor Mario Vega Carbó, an endocrinology specialist with more than 20 years of experience.

Doctor Mario,
1. What causes the Syndrome of Inappropriate Antidiuretic Hormone Secretion?

This disorder can be caused by the consumption of certain medications for diabetes, blood pressure, heart, seizures, depression and cancer. It can also be the result of hormonal treatment, inherited causes, surgery with general anesthesia, certain brain disorders or a lung disease, in the spinal cord, hypothalamus or pituitary gland.

2. What are your main symptoms?

Patients with SSIHA usually present with fatigue, muscle and headaches, dark urine, decreased appetite, increased thirst, diarrhea, nausea, vomiting, irritability, seizures, confusion and memory problems.

3. How is this disease detected?

A physical exam and blood and urine tests are usually done to measure the levels of sodium and other chemicals and the functioning of the organs. In some cases, chest radiography, CT scan of the head and fluid challenge tests are also performed to check retention and elimination levels in the urine.

4. What is the treatment of the syndrome of inappropriate secretion of antidiuretic hormone?

In general, the first thing that is done is to limit fluid intake to prevent its accumulation in the body. Then, to relieve symptoms, saline solutions are usually given intravenously, to increase the percentage of sodium in the blood.

If the excessive production of the antidiuretic hormone is caused by a tumor, it can be removed by surgery. If the cause is a certain drug, the dose can be adjusted or replaced by another. Some medications such as demeclocycline, lithium, conivaptan and tolvaptan also help lower levels of this hormone.

5. What other complications can SSIHA bring?

When the sodium level drops rapidly in severe form, it can cause brain herniation, a decrease in mental lucidity, hallucinations or coma.

6. What other aspects should be taken into account during the illness?

In some cases it may be necessary to follow a special diet with more salt and high protein content, such as beans, nuts, eggs, chicken and fish.

Chapter 107. Polyuria or excessive urination

Polyuria is the abnormal production of large amounts of urine, which causes an excessive need to go to the bathroom. A healthy adult urinates an average of 700 milliliters and 2.5 liters per day, depending on how much fluid he drank and the total amount of water in the body. When it exceeds 3 liters in 24 hours, it is very possible that you suffer from this ailment.

Polyuria should be distinguished from polaquiuria, which is the need for frequent urination, while maintaining normal volumes. Often these two symptoms appear together. Most people urinate about 4 to 7 times per day.

Many patients discover that they suffer from this disorder when they have to get up in the bathroom at night, which is known as nocturia. This can also happen if you drink a lot of fluid near bedtime.

Polyuria is a fairly common symptom and may be due to different factors. To learn more about this condition, we consult Dr. Mario Vega Carbó, an endocrinology specialist, in charge of the Vega & Vado Office.

Doctor Mario,
1. What are the most frequent causes of Polyuria?

Two of the most common reasons are diabetes insipidus, a condition whereby the kidneys are unable to avoid fluid removal, and diabetes mellitus, in which blood sugar or glucose levels increase as a result of a deficit in the production of insulin in the pancreas. Another frequent cause is to drink large amounts of water during the day.

On the other hand, among the less common reasons are renal or heart failure, certain medications such as diuretics and lithium, high or low calcium levels, alcohol or caffeine intake, sickle cell anemia and Sjögren's syndrome, a system disorder immunological characterized by dry eyes and mouth.

2. Are the causes the same in the case of Polish?

No. The increased frequency of going to the bathroom is usually due to cystitis (inflammation of the bladder), involuntary urination, prostate growth or urinary tract stones. Pain or burning when urinating, fever and lumbar or flank discomfort may indicate an infection.

On the other hand, if there is difficulty in starting urination, a weak stream of urine and dripping at the end may mean a prostate lesion.

3. Returning to Polyuria, how is this ailment diagnosed?

Before going to the doctor, it is important that the patient controls his daily urine levels, recording the frequency with which he needs to go to the bathroom, the amount he produces each time and the total amount of fluid he drinks. Together with these data, to make a diagnosis, it will be necessary to know the person's medical history and perform physical exams, urine and blood sugar tests, and osmolarity and water deprivation tests, among other studies.

In women, the examination usually requires a gynecological examination and sampling of cervical and vaginal fluid to detect sexually transmitted diseases. In men, the penis is examined for the presence of secretion and a rectal examination is performed to assess the prostate.

4. What other issues should be taken into account during exams?

Among other important points, we must watch for signs of obesity or malnutrition, which may reflect the presence of some type of cancer or eating disorders. During the head and neck examination, the presence of dry eyes or mouth (Sjögren's syndrome) must be analyzed and the skin checked for hyperpigmented or hypopigmented lesions, ulcers or subcutaneous nodules that indicate sarcoidosis.

On the other hand, it is important to find out if Polyuria appeared abruptly and if the patient has night sweats, coughs, weight loss, if he has a history of smoking and if he suffers from psychiatric disorders.

5. What is the treatment of Polyuria?

Therapy depends on what is the cause of the problem. For example, if it is due to diabetes Insipidus, it can be controlled with desmopressin, a synthetic medication that favors fluid retention and prevents dehydration. In the case of diabetes mellitus it will be necessary to apply an insulin substitute or oral antidiabetics, and follow a special diet.

On the other hand, excess urine can be reduced by decreasing the consumption of coffee or alcohol, and, in the case of being treated with diuretics, adjusting the dose.

6. What special care must be taken into account?

If a person with Polyuria has weakness in the legs, they should go to the hospital immediately, as they may have a spinal cord disorder. On the other hand, if you have fever and low back pain, you should urgently consult a doctor, because it can be an infection in the kidneys.

7. Are the elderly more likely to suffer from this disorder?

Yes. Older men tend to urinate more frequently due to an increase in the prostate and, in the case of women, the same occurs due to various factors, such as weakness of the pelvic floor after delivery and the loss of estrogen after menopause.

Chapter 108. Care and treatment of diabetes insipidus

Diabetes Insipidus (DI) is a condition in which the kidneys are unable to avoid fluid removal, as a result of a deficiency of the hormone vasopressin, secreted by the pituitary gland, or by an insensitivity of the kidneys to respond to this hormone.

Most of the body's water is reabsorbed and only a small portion is discarded. When this condition occurs, retention capacity is lost and large amounts of diluted urine are produced.

ID is a rare condition, which can affect people of any age and sex. It is caused by genetic or kidney diseases, infections, surgeries, tumors or other diseases that damage the hypothalamus or pituitary gland. Its main symptoms are urination and excessive thirst, the need to drink a large amount of fluids, urinary incontinence and confusion due to dehydration and a higher than normal level of sodium.

In the cases of young children, there may also be growth arrest, lack of weight gain or loss, constipation and recurrent fever.

To talk about this topic, we interview Mario Vega Carbó, an endocrinologist with more than 20 years of experience.

Doctor Mario,
1. How is diabetes insipidus detected?

Once its signs are presented, it is necessary to carry out a series of tests to confirm the diagnosis. In general, studies of osmolarity and sodium in the blood, urinalysis, magnetic resonance imaging and tests of water deprivation and provocation with desmopressin are usually performed.

2. What are normal urination levels?

Normally, a healthy adult urinates an average of 2 liters per day. A person with ID, if he drinks a lot of liquid, can exceed 15 liters, depending on the severity of the disease.

3. What is the treatment of diabetes insipidus?

First of all, the cause that causes this condition should be treated, either an abnormality in the pituitary gland or in the hypothalamus. DI can be controlled with desmopressin, a synthetic medication that favors fluid retention and prevents dehydration. It is given as a nasal spray, tablets, wafers under the tongue or injections, and should be used only when necessary.

In most people, vasopressin deficiency is not complete, and the amount of hormone the body produces varies from day to day. In milder cases, you only need to drink more water to ensure proper hydration.

On the other hand, when the kidneys do not respond adequately to the hormone, a low-salt diet is recommended to help reduce the amount of urine they produce.

4. What happens if a person consumes more desmopressin than necessary?

This can cause fluid retention and low levels of sodium and salts in the blood, which is very dangerous, even leading to seizures. The symptoms of excessive water retention in the body are weight gain, swollen legs, elevated blood pressure figures and headache.

5. Is diabetes insipidus the same as diabetes mellitus?

No. In Diabetes Mellitus, which is more common, blood sugar or glucose levels increase, as a result of a deficit in the production of insulin in the pancreas. The causes and treatments are different. What both diseases have in common is that there is a lot of thirst and a lot of fluid is urinated.

6. What complications can ID bring?

Improper fluid intake can cause dehydration and an electrolyte imbalance. This can lead to low blood pressure, fever, high concentration of sodium in the blood, headache, rapid heart rate, fatigue, nausea, muscle cramps and other serious problems.

7. What other care should people with ID take?

It is recommended that these patients wear a bracelet or special card that indicates their condition, to alert others in emergency situations. Also, always have a bottle of water and a supply of your medicine on hand, and transfer it with them wherever they go.

On the other hand, alcohol intake usually decreases vasopressin secretion, so it is recommended to avoid it.

Chapter 109. Hypopituitarism

Hypopituitarism, or Multiple Pituitary Hormone Deficiency (DHHM), is a condition in which the pituitary does not produce the normal amount of some or all of its hormones. This alteration may be present from birth or subsequently generated as a result of tumors or other problems.

The first sign of this condition is usually related to the decrease in bone development speed and short stature, due to a deficiency of growth hormone. Other common symptoms are abdominal and headache, loss of appetite, lack of sexual desire, dizziness or fainting, tiredness, excessive urination and thirst, infertility, loss of body hair, weight changes, cold sensitivity, anemia, low blood pressure and decrease in blood sugar levels.

These signs may occur gradually and vary depending on the amount of missing hormones and the severity of the condition.

To learn more about this topic, we interviewed Cuban doctor Mario Vega Carbó, a specialist in clinical endocrinology.

Doctor Mario,
1. What is the pituitary gland?

The pituitary gland is an internal secretion gland located at the base of the skull, behind the nose and between the ears. It is responsible for controlling the activity of other glands and regulating certain functions of the body, such as growth and sexual activity. The hormones it produces are essential to maintain the health, development and regulation of metabolism.

2. What are the causes of hypopituitarism?

DHHM may be due to inherited disorders, but it is usually acquired and is usually the result of a pituitary tumor. It can also be caused by head trauma; a stroke; a tumor, an inflammation or an infection in the brain; surgery or radiotherapy in the head area; or metabolic, hypothalamus or immune system diseases.

On the other hand, certain medications, such as prednisone and dexamethasone, can cause an inhibition in the normal functioning of this gland.

3. How is DHHM detected?

When your symptoms occur, some tests are necessary to confirm your diagnosis. These may include a CT scan of the brain, an MRI of the pituitary gland and tests to control the levels of different hormones in the body.

4. What is your treatment?

To replenish hormones that are not produced by the pituitary gland correctly, the patient will need a lifelong hormonal therapy. This may include corticosteroids (cortisol), Levothyroxine, growth hormone, sex hormones, thyroid hormone and desmopressin, among other medications.

If pituitary insufficiency is caused by a tumor, it may be necessary to treat it with radiotherapy or remove it with surgery.

5. How are these hormones given?

Depending on the type of hormone, some can be administered orally through pills and others by injections, skin patches or creams.

6. What can you expect from this therapy?

Usually this condition is permanent, so you should follow a treatment for life. Anyway, with a suitable therapy and periodic controls to adjust the doses you can lead a normal life.

7. Can teenagers with hypopituitarism have habitual sexual development?

Yes, when there is a deficiency of sex hormones, the appropriate use of testosterone in men and estrogen in women allows for a normal onset and progression of puberty and full sexual development. This treatment should continue during adulthood to ensure genital function and trouble-free sexual behavior.

8. What other care should people with DHHM take into account?

It is recommended that these patients wear a bracelet or special card that indicates their condition, to alert others in emergency situations or accidents on public roads. This is important especially in people with cortisol and growth hormone deficiencies, due to the high risk of severe hypoglycemia or arterial hypotension in stressful situations.

Chapter 110. Sheehan syndrome and severe bleeding during childbirth

Sheehan syndrome is a medical condition that occurs when a woman has severe bleeding or blood pressure that is too low during childbirth. When this occurs, the pituitary tissue can die and cause the gland to not function properly, which means that it does not produce normal amounts of one or more hormones. This condition is a rare type of hypopituitarism.

The pituitary gland is responsible for controlling the activity of other glands and regulating certain functions of the body, such as growth, breast milk production and sexual activity. The hormones it generates are essential to maintain the health, development and regulation of metabolism, so a failure in its production can cause various disorders.

To learn more about this topic, we interviewed the Cuban doctor Mario Vega Carbó, an endocrinology specialist, with more than 20 years of experience.

Doctor Mario,
1. What conditions can increase the risk of bleeding during childbirth?

Multiple pregnancies (twins or triplets) and problems in the placenta may increase the risks. Anyway, it is a very rare condition that occurs in 1 every 10,000 births and proper medical attention further reduces the chances of bleeding in these cases.

2. What are the symptoms of Sheehan syndrome?

Among its most common signs are the inability to breastfeed, fatigue, absence of menstrual periods, loss of pubic and axillary hair, hypoglycemia, lack of appetite, cold intolerance, reduction of breasts and low blood pressure.

Some women may also suffer from a decrease in mental function, weight gain and difficulty staying alert as a result of poor thyroid activity. Many times these symptoms manifest themselves after childbirth, and months and even years can pass.

3. How is this condition detected?

Since its symptoms coincide with those of other diseases, it can be difficult to diagnose. For this it is necessary to carry out some studies, which may include a CT scan of the brain, an MRI of the pituitary gland and blood tests to control the levels of different hormones in the body.

4. What is your treatment?

To replace the hormones that are not produced by the pituitary gland correctly, the patient will need hormonal therapy. In the case of estrogen and progesterone, they should be applied at least until the normal age of menopause. On the other hand, thyroid and adrenal hormones will have to be taken for life.

In the face of situations of serious illness or stress, pregnancy or significant weight changes, the dose of the medications should be adjusted.

5. What can you expect from this therapy?

Usually, when an early diagnosis is made, the results are very positive. Recruitment and periodic controls to adjust the doses can lead a normal life.

6. What other complications can Sheehan Syndrome generate?

Some women can live for years without noticing that the pituitary does not work properly. Then, an extreme physical stress factor can trigger an adrenal crisis that puts your life at risk. This may occur as a result of a serious infection or surgery. On the other hand, this ailment can also cause low blood pressure and unintentional thinning, so it is important to be aware of its signs.

Chapter 111. Empty Turkish Chair Syndrome

Empty Turkish Chair Syndrome is a condition in which the pituitary gland shrinks or becomes flattened. This gland is essential for the body, since it controls the activity of the others and coordinates certain functions of the body, such as growth and sexual activity.

In addition, the hormones it produces are essential to maintain the health, development and regulation of metabolism. The pituitary gland is located at the base of the skull, in a depression of the sphenoid bone that, seen in profile, resembles a saddle of horses that the Turks used. That is why it is called a Turkish chair.

When the gland shrinks or becomes flattened, it cannot be seen on an MRI. This makes it appear that the chair is empty.

To learn more about this condition, we consulted Dr. Mario Vega Carbó, an endocrinology specialist, in charge of the Vega & Vado Office.

Doctor Mario,
1. What causes the pituitary to shrink?

Generally, when the Turkish chair looks empty, it is actually filled with cerebrospinal fluid, which surrounds the brain and spinal cord. When it leaks into this area, it puts pressure on the pituitary gland and causes it to shrink or flatten.

On the other hand, gland damage can also be due to a tumor, trauma, radiotherapy or surgery.

2. What disorders causes Empty Turkish Chair Syndrome?

The pituitary gland is responsible for controlling the adrenal glands, thyroid, ovaries and testicles, so any damage you suffer can cause problems in these organs and abnormal hormonal levels in the body. However, in many cases where the Turkish chair looks empty, it may be functioning normally.

3. What are the main symptoms of this syndrome?

When the pituitary gland does not work properly, patients may experience headache, irregular or absent menstruation, impotence, decreased libido, high blood pressure, ringing in the ears, visual disturbances, anxiety, fatigue and decay.

4. How is this condition detected?

Usually, the Empty Turkish Chair Syndrome is discovered during an MRI or a CT scan of the head and brain. To confirm the diagnosis, tests are usually done to control the levels of different hormones in the body.

5. Who is more likely to have it?

Usually, patients suffering from this syndrome are between 40 and 50 years old, although it can also occur in childhood. There is a predominance of women, with a high incidence of obesity.

6. What is the treatment?

The therapy will depend on whether the pituitary presents any damage or not. If it works normally, no treatment is necessary. If instead, this syndrome produces a hormonal deficit in the body, it will be necessary to take medications that replace them. This may include corticosteroids (cortisol), Levothyroxine, growth hormone, sex hormones, thyroid hormone and desmopressin, among other drugs. If pituitary insufficiency is caused by a tumor, it may be necessary to treat it with radiotherapy or remove it with surgery.

7. What other disorders can cause this ailment?

Empty Turkish Chair Syndrome can cause a higher level in the body of prolactin, the hormone that stimulates breast development and breast milk production.

Medications that suppress its preparation, such as bromocriptine, are usually effective in solving this problem. On the other hand, it is believed that this condition may be one of the causes of hypopituitarism.

Chapter 112. Galactorrhea and abnormal breast secretion

Galactorrhea is the secretion of milk through the nipples that is not related to breastfeeding. It usually affects women, although in some cases it can occur in men and even in babies. This disorder is not a disease in itself, but it can be a symptom of some undiagnosed pathology. Breasts can drip on their own or when touched. The secretion is usually white and, less frequently, yellow, green or brown.

To learn more about this topic, we interview Mario Vega Carbó, an endocrinologist with more than 20 years of experience.

Doctor Mario,
1. What causes Galactorrhea?

There are many possible causes. It is usually due to an excess of prolactin in the body, the hormone responsible for milk production when babies are born. It can also occur as a result of excessive breast stimulation, pituitary or thyroid problems, kidney or autoimmune diseases, a tumor, stress, inflammation or the use of clothing that irritates the breasts.

On the other hand, the consumption of certain medications, such as birth control pills, antidepressants or sedatives, or illegal drugs, such as marijuana, cocaine and opiates, can generate it. In some cases its origin is not entirely clear.

2. How does it occur in men and babies?

In men it is usually related to a lack of testosterone and is usually accompanied by an enlarged breast, a disorder known as gynecomastia. In babies, breast tissue enlargement can occur when high levels of maternal estrogen cross the placenta and reach your blood. In this case, secession is usually temporary and resolves on its own.

3. What are the symptoms of Galactorrhea?

In addition to persistent nipple discharge, other signs associated with this disorder are the absence or irregularities in the menstrual period, headaches, vision problems, decreased sexual desire, acne and increased hair. In men there may be erectile dysfunction.

4. How is this condition diagnosed?

In view of their symptoms, the patient's history is usually analyzed and a physical examination is performed. Also a blood test to control hormone levels and other tests to rule out pregnancy. If a tumor or pituitary problem is suspected, an MRI of the brain, mammography and breast biopsy may be necessary.

5. What is your treatment?

The therapy will depend on what causes Galactorrhea. If it is due to excess prolactin production, it can be controlled with medications, the same happens in the case of hypothyroidism. In case of benign tumors, they can be removed by surgery or treated with drugs.

If it is due to the consumption of a certain remedy, the doctor may replace it with another. On the other hand, some creams can treat changes in the skin around the nipple. Many times Galactorrhea disappears on its own over time, without the need for treatment.

6. What complications can this disorder bring?

If the secretion includes blood or is transparent and is linked to a nodule, it may be a symptom of breast cancer and therefore requires urgent control. It may also be due to a pituitary tumor or caused by Paget's disease of the breast, a rare type of cancer that affects the skin of the nipple.

7. What other aspects should be taken into account?

People with Galactorrhea should avoid stimulating their breasts during sexual intercourse and wear tight clothes that rub or irritate the skin.

Hyperprolactinemia is a disorder in which the level of prolactin in the blood is higher than normal. This hormone is secreted by the pituitary gland and is responsible for stimulating the production of breast milk after childbirth. This condition can cause the decrease of estrogen in women and testosterone in men, alter vision and generate Galactorrhea and infertility.

The most frequent cause of Hyperprolactinemia is the presence of a tumor in the pituitary gland, usually benign, known as prolactinoma.

To learn more about this topic, we interview Mario Vega Carbó, an endocrinologist with more than 20 years of experience.

Doctor Mario,
1. What causes Hyperprolactinemia?

Usually this disorder is caused by a tumor in the pituitary gland that produces a high level of prolactin. Other possible causes are the consumption of certain medications for high blood pressure, depression, heartburn, severe mental disorders and pain, or certain problems in the thyroid, pituitary, liver or kidneys.

2. What are your main symptoms?

Among other signs, Hyperprolactinemia can cause infertility and loss of libido and bone mass. In women, vaginal dryness, menstrual problems, acne, hirsutism and breast milk production for no reason are also common. In men, there may be erectile dysfunction, enlarged breasts and decreased body hair.

On the other hand, in case of prolactinoma, large tumors can cause headaches and vision problems.

3. How is hyperprolactinemia detected?

A blood test is usually done to measure blood prolactin levels. In case of being elevated, hypothyroidism and pregnancy will be ruled out, and the medications the patient is taking will be analyzed.

On the other hand, if a tumor is suspected, an MRI of the brain and pituitary gland will be performed. If the prolactinoma is confirmed, vision tests may be necessary to determine if it has been affected.

4. Who has more risks of suffering it?

Hyperprolactinemia derived from a tumor is more frequent in women between 20 and 35 years old, although it can manifest itself in anyone of any age.

5. What is the treatment of Hyperprolactinemia?

Therapy depends on the cause and its symptoms. In certain cases where there are no signs, treatment may not be necessary.

If the condition is caused by a prolactinoma, certain medications such as bromocriptine and cabergoline decrease the production of this hormone and help reduce the size of the tumor. However, these drugs can cause nausea, vomiting, nasal congestion, headaches and drowsiness, among other side effects.

If the tumor needs to be removed, surgery can be performed or treated with radiation. If this disorder is a consequence of the consumption of a certain medicine, the dose should be adjusted or replaced by another. If the cause is hypothyroidism, it is treated with Levothyroxine.

6. What is Galactorrhea and what is its relationship with Hyperprolactinemia?

Galactorrhea is the secretion of milk through the nipples that is not related to breastfeeding. It is usually due to an excess of prolactin in the body, which can be controlled with medication.

Chapter 114. Pituitary Tumors

Pituitary Tumor is an abnormal growth in the pituitary gland, which is usually non-cancerous (benign). This gland is located at the base of the skull and is responsible for controlling the activity of other organs and regulating certain functions of the body, such as growth, metabolism, blood pressure and sexual activity.

Among the substances secreted are corticotropin, growth hormone, prolactin, thyroid stimulating hormone, luteinizing hormone and follicle stimulating hormone. Pituitary Tumors can cause a significant increase or decrease in hormones, generating different complications in the body. In addition, they can grow and exert pressure on other structures.

To learn more about this topic, we interviewed Cuban doctor Mario Vega Carbó, an endocrinology specialist with more than 20 years of clinical experience.

Doctor Mario,
1. How do pituitary tumors originate?

At the moment the reason that causes the uncontrolled cell growth in the gland that generates this condition is unknown, although it is suspected that it has to do with genetic alterations. In a few cases, pituitary tumors are part of an inherited disorder known as Multiple Endocrine Neoplasia.

2. What are your main symptoms?

Sometimes these tumors are very small, do not produce any signs and are never detected during the life of the person. In others, the symptoms depend on the hormonal excess or lack they generate or the pressure they exert on other structures. In the latter case, they can cause vision problems, headache, lack of energy, nausea and vomiting, and loss of sense of smell.

If they produce a hormonal deficit, they can generate weakness, feeling cold, absence or reduction of menstrual periods, sexual dysfunction, more urine, nausea and vomiting, and involuntary loss or weight gain.

Meanwhile, the exaggerated production of hormones can lead to Cushing's syndrome - cortisol excess - whose main signs are obesity in the middle and upper body, rounded and red face, thin arms and legs, purple streaks, Fine and fragile skin, slow recovery of cuts and easy bruising.

It can also cause Acromegaly or Gigantism - growth hormone excess - and show excessive height; large hands, feet, jaw, forehead, nose and tongue; alteration of facial features; hypersudoration with a strong odor on the body; Blood in the stool; muscular weakness; visual and metabolic difficulties; headache and joint pain; Serious voice and sleep apnea.

In very few cases, it can cause hyperthyroidism - excess thyroid stimulating hormone - whose most common symptoms are anxiety, nervousness, fatigue, difficulty concentrating, diarrhea, thin and fragile hair, trembling hands, heat intolerance, increased of appetite, sweating, menstrual irregularities, palpitations, sleep problems and weight loss.

Finally, excess prolactin can cause irregular or absent menstrual periods and galactorrhea in women, and erectile dysfunction, loss of sexual desire and breast growth in men.

3. How are pituitary tumors detected?

A physical exam and blood and urine tests are usually done to measure hormone levels; computed tomography or magnetic resonance imaging of the brain to determine the location and size of the tumor; and vision analysis to see if it has been affected.

4. What is your treatment?

The therapy will depend on the symptoms of the tumor, its size, how much it has grown in the brain and the disorders it generates. The patient's age and health status will also be evaluated.

In some cases, surgery will be necessary to remove it, especially if you are putting pressure on the optic nerves. Radiation therapy or certain medications can also be used to reduce their size. In other cases, if there are no signs, the tumor will be kept under observation by periodic checks to see its evolution.

As for changes in hormonal production, levels will be normalized through the use of medications.

5. What other complications can these tumors bring?

Pituitary Tumors usually do not grow or spread widely. The most serious problem they can cause is blindness if the optic nerve is seriously damaged.

On the other hand, the tumor or its excision can cause hormonal imbalances for life, and the patient must take medications permanently. In addition, damage to the pituitary gland can cause diabetes insipidus, which causes excessive urination and thirst, the need to drink a large amount of fluids, urinary incontinence and confusion due to dehydration and a higher than normal level of sodium.

Also, they can cause a Pituitary Stroke, a rare disease caused by bleeding or infarction of the gland in the context of a tumor. This condition is characterized by sudden and intense headache, meningeal irritation, nausea, vomiting, visual disturbances that can lead to blindness and, sometimes, decrease in the level of consciousness and even coma.

Chapter 115. Acromegaly

Acromegaly is a rare condition that occurs when the pituitary gland produces excess growth hormone during adulthood. This is usually due to a non-cancerous tumor in the gland, which must be treated with radiotherapy or removed by surgery.

When this occurs in childhood, it can cause gigantism, where the bones and body grow too much and make the boy extremely tall for his age. In adulthood, Acromegaly generates larger than normal hands, feet and face. It affects an average of between 5 and 10 people per 100 thousand, without presenting differences between men and women.

To learn more about this condition, we consulted Dr. Mario Vega Carbó, an endocrinology specialist, in charge of the Vega & Vado Office.

Doctor Mario,
1. What are the main symptoms of Acromegaly?

Among other signs, people suffering from this disorder may have hypersudoration with a strong smell in the body, blood in the stool, muscle weakness, fatigue, visual and metabolic difficulties, headache and joint pain, severe voice and sleep apnea.

From a physical point of view, excessive height is common; large hands, feet, jaw, forehead, nose and tongue; alteration of facial features; widely spaced teeth; warts thick lips; Marked wrinkles and swollen fingers.

Many people begin to notice that the rings stop entering their fingers and that their number of shoes increases progressively. Men may have erectile dysfunction and women irregularities in the menstrual cycle.

2. Who are more likely to suffer from this disease?

Acromegaly usually affects middle-aged adults. However, it can manifest at any age. Because it is not a common disease, and because physical changes occur gradually, it sometimes takes time to detect. It is diagnosed between 5 and 15 years after the onset of its symptoms, at an average age of between 40 and 50 years.

3. How is this ailment confirmed?

To corroborate Acromegaly, it is necessary to analyze the patient's medical history, perform a physical examination and blood glucose, prolactin tests and a growth hormone measurement.

Generally, an x-ray of the spine and an MRI of the brain that includes the pituitary gland are performed, among other studies.

4. What is the treatment of Acromegaly?

If it is confirmed that the reason for the condition is a tumor in the pituitary gland, it can be removed by surgery. This usually solves the problem. When the tumor is too large to be completely removed, it can be treated with radiation and medications.

On the other hand, there are specific remedies that inhibit or reduce excess growth hormone secretion.

5. What other causes can cause this disease?

In some people, Acromegaly is caused by tumors in other parts of the body, such as the lungs, pancreas or adrenal glands.

6. What inconveniences can Acromegaly cause?

In addition to changes in appearance, people suffering from this anomaly may suffer colon polyps, high blood pressure, diabetes, osteoarthritis, cardiovascular diseases, spinal cord compression, visual problems, sexual dysfunction, depression and an enlarged Thyroid and heart.

Chapter 116. Craniopharyngioma

Craniopharyngioma is a rare non-cancerous tumor that develops at the base of the brain, near the pituitary gland and the hypothalamus. Although it can occur at any age, it mainly affects children between 5 and 10 years old, and older adults. Its origin is not hereditary nor is it linked to diseases during pregnancy.

Among other consequences, this condition causes an increase in pressure in the brain, alteration of the production of hormones of the pituitary gland and atrophy of the optimal nerve. Its main symptoms are headache, nausea, vomiting, fatigue, increased thirst, excessive urination, visual disturbances and slow growth. In addition, patients may have difficulty sleeping, learning and behavioral problems.

To learn more about this condition, we consult Dr. Mario Vega Carbó, a specialist in clinical endocrinology.

Doctor Mario,
1. How is craniopharyngioma detected?

Usually, when a patient presents these signs, a series of physical evaluations (vision, hearing, balance, coordination and reflexes) are performed, and tests for a tumor. This includes blood tests to measure hormone levels, computed tomography or MRI of the brain and a study of the nervous system.

2. What is a tumor and what risks does it involve in this case?

A tumor is an accumulation of cells that have abnormal growth. In the case of Craniopharyngioma, it is a benign tumor, that is, it does not spread to other parts of the body. However, it can reach a large size and compress various areas of the brain, causing problems for its functioning.

3. If the diagnosis is confirmed, what is the treatment that is applied?

The most common is to perform surgery to remove the tumor, which will depend on its location and size. Because there are many delicate and important structures nearby, sometimes everything is not removed, to ensure a good quality of life after treatment.

A radiation therapy and chemotherapy or a combination of both can also be applied for craniopharyngioma. The medication that is most commonly used to treat brain tumors is temozolomide, which is taken as a tablet.

4. Is surgery very risky?

Surgery to remove the brain tumor carries risks, such as infection or bleeding. They depend on where it is located. For example, if it is near the nerves connected to the eyes, it could involve a risk of vision loss. Anyway, today it is possible to perform a brain surgery without scars and minimally invasive.

5. And in the case of radiotherapy and chemotherapy?

Its applications may cause side effects, which will depend on the type and dose used. In the case of radiation, the most common are fatigue, headaches, memory loss and irritation of the scalp, while chemotherapy can cause nausea, vomiting and hair loss.

6. What is the general prognosis after the intervention?

The results depend on whether the tumor could be completely removed and the problems that the condition causes in the nervous system. The expectations are usually favorable, with a probability of cure of 80 to 90%. However, in many cases hormonal and vision difficulties do not improve with treatment.

7. How is post operative therapy?

After surgery it is essential to carry out studies to verify whether the pituitary or pituitary gland function is normal or is altered. In the case of children, it is advised to monitor their growth and development, and the onset of puberty. If this does not happen in a normal way, we must evaluate the performance of hormonal therapy.

On the other hand, considering that these tumors may occur in parts of the brain that control motor skills, speech, sight and thinking, rehabilitation may be necessary. This may include physical therapy, speech therapy and support to address changes in memory, thinking and mood after surgery.

8. Are there chances that the tumor will come back?

When the tumor is not completely removed, the condition may return. In those cases, it usually occurs within the first 2 years after surgery.

Chapter 117. Pineal Tumors and Early Puberty

Pineal Tumors are a type of brain tumor that forms in the pineal gland, a member of both the nervous and endocrine systems. This organ produces the hormone melatonin, which modulates the patterns of wakefulness and sleep, and the onset of puberty, among other aspects.

In addition, it also participates in the generation of endorphins, the hormones that cause states of happiness and allow pain to be regulated, and others that govern the menstrual cycle in women. Pineal Tumors, which are usually slow growing, can be benign (not cancerous) or malignant (cancerous). In adolescents, they can generate Precocious Puberty.

To learn more about this condition, we consult Dr. Mario Vega Carbó, an endocrinology specialist in charge of the Vega & Vado Office.

Doctor Mario,
1. Why do these tumors appear?

Pineal Tumors are unusual and occur more frequently during childhood. They may arise due to the proliferation of primary pinealocytes, astrocytes or germ cells.

2. What are your main symptoms?

Some common signs are gait disorders, vomiting, headache or eye pain, blurred or double vision, hearing impairment and insomnia.

3. How are Pineal Tumors detected?

Faced with its symptoms, a CT scan or MRI of the head, an electroencephalogram to measure the electrical activity of the brain, and a stereotactic biopsy are usually performed. Early diagnosis is essential to be able to initiate adequate treatment and avoid the development of hydrocephalus and other sequelae.

4. What is your treatment?

The therapy will depend on the tumor histology and its size at the time of diagnosis. Radiation therapy, chemotherapy and surgery will be used alone or in combination. The prognosis is usually delicate because of its location the extraction is complex.

However, the improvement of surgical techniques has allowed good results in many cases. Ventricular drainage may be necessary to decrease hydrocephalus.

5. What other conditions can cause Pineal Tumors?

This condition can cause Precocious Puberty, especially in men; Insipid diabetes and hypogonadism.

6. What other aspects should be taken into account during the illness?

In the case of a malignant tumor, it is recommended to seek psychological support and participation in therapeutic groups with people who are suffering from this same disease, to treat the anxiety, anguish and stress that can cause.

Chapter 118. Pituitary Surgery

The pituitary gland is a gland located at the base of the skull that is responsible for controlling the activity of other organs and regulating certain functions of the body, such as growth metabolism, blood pressure and sexual activity. Abnormal tissue masses may appear there, which are usually non-cancerous. However, these tumors can cause an increase or a significant hormonal decrease, generating different complications in the body.

In addition, they can grow in size and exert pressure on other structures, such as optic nerves. In those cases, surgery may be necessary to remove them. A surgical intervention may also be required to treat a pituitary stroke, a rare disease caused by bleeding or infarction of the gland in the context of a tumor.

To learn more about this topic, we interview Mario Vega Carbó, an endocrinology specialist in charge of the Vega & Vado Office.

Doctor Mario,
1. How is pituitary surgery performed?

For this type of procedure there are two techniques. The most commonly used is endoscopic transsphenoidal transsphenoidal surgery, in which the pituitary tumor is removed through the nose and sinuses. When the intervention cannot be performed in this way, a craniotomy is performed, in which the extraction is performed through the upper part of the skull, by means of an incision in the scalp.

2. How is the preparation for this surgery?

Before the operation it is important to inform the doctor about all the medications that are being taken, if any type of allergy or illness is suffered, or if you are pregnant. In case of taking anticoagulant remedies, such as aspirin and ibuprofen, the patient may have to suspend them temporarily before the intervention.

3. What are the advantages of the transsphenoidal transnasal endoscopic approach?

This procedure offers the advantage that it is minimally invasive and allows the tumor to be removed without making an external incision. In this way, no other part of the brain is affected and leaves no visible scars or sutures.

During this surgery the endoscope, a thin tube with a light and a camera at its end is used as a source of vision. It allows to obtain a panoramic perspective of the interior of the sphenoid sinuses, the Turkish chair and the tumor cavity. In addition, dissection and reconstruction of the septal and nasal structures is avoided with this technique.

4. For what cases is a transcranial approach necessary?

Craniotomy is necessary for large or difficult to treat tumors, such as those that invaded brain tissue or nearby nerves, as it allows better access. In this case, a cut is made on the forehead or on one side of the head and an endotracheal tube may be placed to help the patient breathe during the intervention.

The surgeon will remove a piece of the skull and cut and open the lining of the brain to reach the tumor. Once this is removed, it may be necessary to use metal plates or screws to reattach the part of the bone that was removed. Meanwhile, the head cut will be closed with stitches or staples.

5. What risks does pituitary surgery have?

The success of this procedure depends largely on the type of tumor, its location, its size and whether or not it invaded nearby tissues. During the operation the brain, eyes, bones, blood vessels or nerves can suffer injuries. In addition, the patient may bleed more than expected, get an infection or have trouble breathing.

On the other hand, their hormonal levels can change and cause serious complications, a blood clot can form or there is loss of fluid around the brain and spinal cord. Other risks are loss of vision, taste and smell.

In addition, after surgery, the patient may have diabetes insipidus, a condition that causes excessive urination and thirst, the need to drink a large amount of fluids, urinary incontinence and confusion due to dehydration and a higher than normal sodium level. .

6. What care should the patient follow after surgery?

During the first days you may have congestion and headache and need medications that help regulate hormonal levels, which will gradually reduce.

On the other hand, you may need a nasal spray of saline solution to keep the nasal mucous membranes moist and facilitate healing. You should avoid sneezing, coughing and blowing your nose for at least two weeks.

7. What symptoms require attention after the operation?

If the patient has chest pain, shortness of breath, fever, signs of infection in the wound, dripping clear liquid from the nose or throat, severe and persistent headache, dizziness, sensitivity to light, loss or problems of vision, constant need to urinate or swelling in the legs, it will be necessary to seek medical attention urgently.

8. What other aspects should be taken into account after surgery?

In cases where it is not possible to remove the entire tumor during the intervention, a new operation or radiotherapy may be necessary. It is possible that the levels of certain hormones do not return to normal after surgery, so it will be necessary to take medication to supplant them.

Chapter 119. Pituitary Stroke

Pituitary Stroke is a rare disease, caused by bleeding or infarction of this gland in the context of a tumor. The condition is characterized by sudden and intense headache, meningeal irritation, nausea, vomiting, visual disturbances that can lead to blindness and, sometimes, decrease in the level of consciousness and even coma.

Pituitary infarction is caused by bleeding into the gland or by a blockage in blood flow to it. Early diagnosis, hormone replacement therapy to combat hypopituitarism and transsphenoidal surgery are the basis for treating this condition.

To learn more about this topic, we interview Mario Vega Carbó, an endocrinology specialist, in charge of the Vega & Vado Office in Managua, Nicaragua.

Doctor Mario,
1. What causes a Pituitary Stroke?

The reasons why it develops are not entirely clear, although ischemic necrosis is suspected, due to rapid tumor growth, vascular abnormalities and compression of the superior pituitary artery against the selar diaphragm.

In most patients there is no known precipitating factor, although it is believed that the reduction in vascular supply, acute increase in blood flow, stimulation of the pituitary gland, anticoagulation situations and head trauma could influence its appearance.

2. How is this condition detected?

Given its symptoms, it is important to perform an MRI or CT scan to see if there is hemorrhage or tumor infarction, and tests to control the levels of different hormones in the body.

From the clinical point of view, these patients usually present with a destruction of the pituitary tissue that leads to hypopituitarism, an extension of the bleeding with nerve compression, and headache and signs of meningeal irritation due to the outflow of blood to the subarachnoid space and compression of the seal diaphragm.

3. What symptoms of a headache make you suspect the presence of a pituitary apoplexy?

Along with visual disturbances, some signs of headache alarm are fever that cannot be explained by other causes, severe sudden onset pain, progressive worsening, vomiting and nausea, low blood pressure, decreased awareness, psychomotor agitation, epileptic seizures and behavioral disorders.

4. What is the treatment of this condition?

The therapy consists of urgent transsphenoidal decompressive surgery and hormone replacement therapy with high doses of corticosteroids, thyroid hormone and gonadotropins, among other medications. If vision is not affected, surgical intervention is usually not necessary.

On the other hand, the administration of growth hormone in adults is controversial, although it is recommended in children until the end of the development stage.

5. What is the expected prognosis of this treatment?

When diagnosed early, patients evolve favorably in the vast majority of cases, presenting a significant recovery of visual disturbances. As for hormonal levels, treatment should generally be continued, performing periodic checks to adjust the dose of medications.

6. What other complications can Pituitary Stroke bring?

When presented in acute form it is considered a neuroendocrinological emergency and requires urgent treatment because it is life threatening.

Abrupt corticotropin and cortisol deficiency can cause serious risks of adrenal insufficiency.

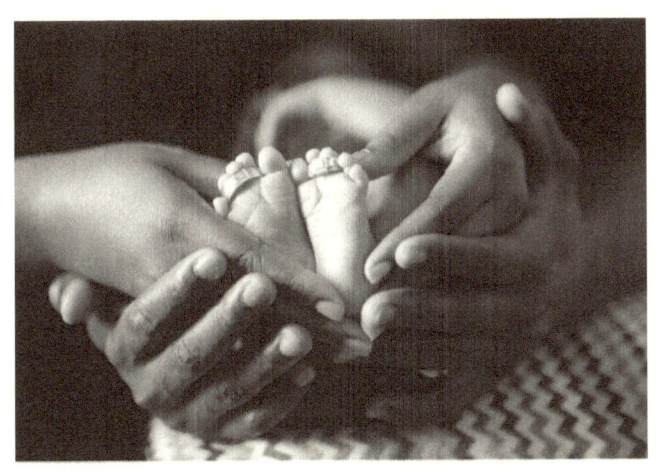

SECTION III REPRODUCTION AND LIFE CYCLE

SECTION III REPRODUCTION AND LIFE CYCLE

The third section of the interview book is divided into 5 large parts which, in turn, group the chapters related to *Reproduction and the life cycle of the individual*.

In the first part, the reader will find discussions on the issues related to the female sexual gland, the Ovary, its functions, and the different alterations derived from its condition. They will answer questions about alterations of the menstrual cycle, so frequent and common among women, as well as polycystic ovary syndrome and other infertility problems.

We continue researching on the male sex glands, the Testicles, and, this part will find interesting topics such as frequent genetic syndromes that affect male sexual function, and androgenic hormone therapy is also discussed.

In the following chapters, we talk about Endocrinology in pediatrics, we will know that specific hormonal conditions or alterations lead to the development of diseases in this first stage of life, addressing issues such as precocious puberty, growth disorders, morphological alterations in the genitals due to hormonal abnormalities, and juvenile diabetes.

The next part tells us about Endocrinology in obstetrics, how the influence of hormones on maternal metabolism is decisive for the conditions in which pregnancy develops, and how alterations in these hormonal levels can lead to situations such as diabetes Gestational, abortion, thyroid dysfunction, among other diseases.

Closing this section and the book of interviews, we present Endocrinology in geriatrics, a set of chapters aimed at educating the elderly and the physiological and pathological changes that are related to this stage of life, with special emphasis on prevention topics for maintain the functionality of the elderly, such as proper nutrition, adequate physical exercise, and for the prevention of prevalent diseases at this age such as sarcopenia, osteoporosis and complications of chronic noncommunicable diseases.

Continue your reading and learn a little more about *Reproduction and life cycle.*

Part VIII Ovary

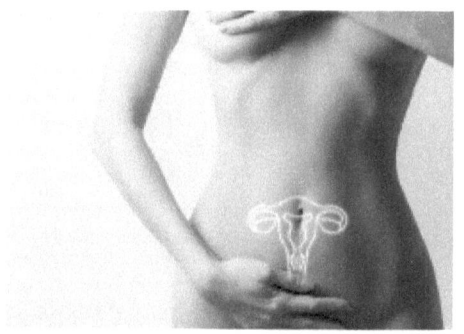

Capítulo 120. Disfunción Sexual Femenina

Sexual Dysfunction is any difficulty that occurs during the different stages of intercourse, including desire, arousal and the relationship itself. These inconveniences can occur at the beginning of a person's sexual life or develop later with the passage of time.

Its causes may be physical, psychological, a combination of both, or due to an external factor. In the case of women, there are several problems that can prevent them from enjoying their relationships. Among them are the lack of libido, the inability to achieve excitement, the inability to reach orgasm or feel pain during encounters.

Sexual dysfunction can be permanent or temporary, and vary depending on the occasion and the couple. The absence of pleasure in intercourse can cause distress and affect the quality of life of a person and their personal relationships.

To learn more about this topic, we consulted Dr. Mario Vega Carbó, an endocrinology specialist in charge of the Vega & Vado Office.

Doctor Mario,
1. What are the main reasons for Female Sexual Dysfunction?

Within the physical causes, this may be due to diseases such as diabetes, heart failure, nervous disorders, hormonal problems, spinal injuries, certain types of cancer, infections, arthritis, gynecological disorders, fatigue or obesity.

Among the psychological ones are stress, anxiety, mood swings, depression, lack of self-esteem, traumatic sexual episodes, strict religious or cultural beliefs, fear of getting pregnant, boredom and partner or other problems that Affect your life.

On the other hand, sexual dysfunction can also occur due to the use of certain medications, excessive alcohol and drug use, after having a baby or during menopause.

2. What are your symptoms?

Depending on its cause, female sexual dysfunction may present various signs. The most common are: lack of desire, absence of fantasies, avoiding relationships with the couple, difficulties in becoming aroused, inability to reach orgasm and pain during stimulation or vaginal contact.

3. What are the main reasons for pain during sex?

The causes are very variable. Among the main ones we can mention inflammatory disorders, gynecological surgeries, tumors or uterine cysts, endometriosis, urinary tract infections, lack of lubrication, vaginismus and sexually transmitted diseases.

In addition, any dermatological condition such as eczema, warts or psoriasis near the sexual organs can cause the skin in the area to retract. On the other, certain soaps, creams or latex condoms can cause allergies and irritations.

4. What is the treatment of Female Sexual Dysfunction?

The sexual response implies a complex combination of physical, emotional components, experiences and ways of thinking and living. The alteration of any of them can cause dysfunction, so a holistic and complete approach is usually necessary for your therapy.

From the medical point of view the treatment should aim to solve the physical causes that cause the condition. If it is a hormonal problem, estrogens or androgens can be applied, according to the patient's need.

From the non-medical point of view, it is recommended to talk openly about the issue with the couple and express the tastes and preferences at the time of love. In some cases it may also be necessary to consult a therapist specializing in sexual problems and relationships.

In case of vaginal pain or dryness, the use of lubricants or moisturizers is advised. On the other hand, some devices incite blood flow to the genital area and increase sensations.

If the problem is a medication, it can be replaced by another. In addition, certain drugs such as flibanserine stimulate sexual appetite, while the use of viagra can help certain women.

5. What other recommendations can be taken into account?

To have a better sex life, it is advisable to eat healthy, exercise daily, maintain an adequate body weight, sleep well, do not smoke and avoid alcohol consumption. Also avoid stress and conflict situations, and learn to improve self-esteem and accept one's body as it is.

On the other hand, relaxation exercises are also recommended.

Chapter 121. Hypoactive Sexual Desire Disorder

Hypoactive Sexual Desire Disorder is known for the repeated and constant absence of sexual fantasies or interest in performing some type of activity of this type. Lack of sexual appetite is relatively common. It is estimated that one in five people lose desire at some time in their lives and in women the figure is even higher.

This condition varies according to each patient but is usually accompanied by anxiety, anguish and difficulties in relating. They are also more common in times of stress, pregnancy, menopause, during an illness or at the beginning or end of a relationship.

To talk about this topic, we interviewed Dr. Mario Vega Carbó, an endocrinology specialist, in charge of the Vega & Vado Office.

Doctor Mario,
1. What are the main causes of Hypoactive Sexual Desire Disorder?

This medical condition can be caused by many factors, which can be both physical and emotional, as well as psychological. Among them we can highlight the hormonal changes. For example, during menopause the estrogen level drops, which decreases desire. For the same reason I could be affected during pregnancy or breastfeeding.

In addition, it can be caused by certain diseases, such as arthritis, cancer, diabetes, high blood pressure or neurological disorders.

As for psychological factors, mood is essential to maintain libido. Anxiety, depression, stress, low self-esteem, partner problems and negative sexual experiences, such as cases of abuse or abuse, can seriously affect desire.

On the other hand, this disorder can also be a consequence of the use of certain medications, such as antidepressants, excessive consumption of alcohol and drugs, or smoking.

2. How is this condition diagnosed?

Faced with its symptoms, the doctor will seek to find the cause that is causing the decrease in libido. For this, the patient's medical history and sexual history will be analyzed.

To rule out physical factors, a pelvic exam and blood tests may be necessary to check hormone levels. On the other hand, a sex therapist can evaluate emotional and psychological factors.

3. What is your treatment?

The therapy will depend on the cause. In some cases a hormonal treatment with application of testosterone or estrogen may be necessary to increase desire and improve vaginal dryness. Some medications, such as flibanserin, can also help increase libido.

On the other hand, psychological counseling or couple therapy can be used to try to solve emotional or relational problems.

4. What other aspects can be taken into account to treat this disorder?

Healthy lifestyle changes, such as exercising regularly and eating properly can help stimulate sexual desire. The same reduce stress.

Similarly, it is important to avoid alcohol, cigarettes and drugs, which can cause a decrease in libido. It is recommended to improve communication with the couple and talk openly about intimate issues. It is also key to give time for sexual encounters and add new experiences that increase desire, such as trying different places, adding sex toys or different fantasies to ignite the flame.

Chapter 122. Hormone Therapy of Feminization

Gender identity disorder (GIT) from male to female occurs when a person who was born with male genitalia identifies with the characteristics of the female sex, feeling the desire and need to live and behave as such. This usually causes great disagreement and affliction, in addition to anxiety and depression, to be inside a body with which they do not feel at ease.

People may feel a strong dislike for their genitals and want to have the physical and sexual characteristics of the other gender. TIG can occur in both children and adults.

To learn how on this subject, we interview Dr. Mario Vega Carbó, who is an endocrinologist with more than 20 years of experience.

Doctor Mario,
1. What is the feminization hormone therapy?

It is a treatment that is used to induce physical changes in the body caused by female hormones during puberty, to promote concordance between gender identity and appearance.

2. What effects does this therapy have on the patient?

This treatment can reduce the severity of gender dysphoria, psychological and emotional distress, and improve social functioning, sexual satisfaction and quality of life

3. How is the treatment of female hormonalization?

In the case of people with male biological sex who feel female, they will be given medications to inhibit the action of the hormone testosterone. They are also given female hormones (estrogens) that cause a decrease in libido and facial and body hair growth, an increase in breast tissue, an appropriate distribution of fat and a slight change in voice tone.

4. At what age is it advisable to start hormonal treatment in these patients?

Children who do not feel identified with their own sex should be evaluated and treated by a mental health specialist. If this condition is maintained over time and the expert considers that it will not be modified, a hormonal treatment can be started after 16 years.

If therapy is started before the first changes in puberty, secondary male sexual characteristics can be avoided, such as increased body hair and changes in voice tone. However, it is important to analyze each case in a particular way. Hormone therapy is not usually used in children.

5. What are the risks of feminizing hormone therapy?

Some of the complications of this treatment are deep vein thrombosis, pulmonary embolism, high triglycerides, gallstones, weight gain, high liver function analysis, decreased libido, erectile dysfunction, high potassium level, hypertension, diabetes and cardiovascular diseases .

On the other hand, the risk of permanent sterility increases with prolonged use of hormones, especially when therapy is started before puberty.

6. With this hormonal treatment is it possible to achieve a complete body modification?

Although many changes are achieved that allow to resemble the desired gender, some physical characteristics cannot be modified and require surgical interventions to complete the transition. In cases of moving from male to female, the external genitalia are removed and an artificial vagina is created, and the breast size is increased by surgery.

It is important to clarify that the autonomy and freedom of the patient to manage his own body is respected at all times, and it is he who decides what medical or surgical stage he wishes to reach.

7. What is the degree of patient satisfaction with these treatments?

Usually, when they are performed with adequate psychological support, these treatments have very good results, with satisfaction rates above 90 percent.

On the contrary, regret rates are below 3 percent and in most cases they are due to the loss of family and social support, personal instability or the occurrence of traumatic events.

Chapter 123. Premenstrual Syndrome

Premenstrual Syndrome is the set of symptoms that occurs in women before menstruation. They usually begin during the second half of the menstrual cycle and disappear one or two days after the period begins.

Its main signs include depression, mood swings, anxiety, breast tenderness, food cravings, fatigue, difficulty concentrating and irritability. These symptoms may be barely noticeable or very intense. It is estimated that 3 out of 4 women suffer some form of Premenstrual Syndrome.

To learn more about this topic, we interviewed the Cuban doctor Mario Vega Carbó, specialist in endocrinology and general general medicine.

Doctor Mario,
1. What are the causes of this condition?

The exact reasons are not known, but it is believed that they are related to cyclic changes in hormonal levels and chemicals in the brain. It is also linked to social, cultural, biological and psychological factors.

2. Who are more likely to have it?

Most women experience symptoms related to Premenstrual Syndrome during their fertile life. These are more frequent among those between 20 and 40 years old, those who have had at least one child and those with a family or personal history of depression.

3. What are your main symptoms?

The most frequent are abdominal inflammation, breast tenderness, constipation or diarrhea, food cravings, headache, poor tolerance to noise and lights, fatigue, feelings of sadness, nervousness, anxiety, depression, irritability, loss of sex drive , crying, low self-esteem, acne, insomnia and trouble concentrating. These signs get worse around age 40, when menopause approaches.

On the other hand, some symptoms of Premenstrual Syndrome are similar to other mood and thyroid disorders, so they should be evaluated in detail so as not to confuse them.

4. When should the doctor be consulted?

If the physical pain and emotional stress are very intense and affect the normal daily life of the person, it may be convenient to visit a specialist.

5. What is the Premenstrual Syndrome Treatment?

Often leading a healthy lifestyle allows you to improve the symptoms of this condition. With headache and back pain, cramps and breast tenderness, these symptoms can be treated with various medications such as acetylsalicylic acid, ibuprofen and other nonsteroidal anti-inflammatory drugs. Hormonal contraceptives can also be used.

For its part, diuretics help prevent fluid retention that causes inflammation, swelling and weight gain. In severe cases, antidepressants, such as selective serotonin reuptake inhibitors, and anxiolytics may be prescribed. The effectiveness of these drugs varies from one woman to another.

Finally, you can also try alternative medicine, such as the consumption of certain herbs and the practice of acupuncture.

6. What changes can be made in lifestyle to improve the symptoms of Premenstrual Syndrome?

It is advisable to do regular aerobic exercise, maintain an adequate body weight, drink plenty of fluids, sleep well, do not smoke and avoid alcohol and drug use. Also eat healthy, with frequent and small meals. It is recommended to add whole grains, vegetables and fruits in the diet, and limit salt, caffeine and sugar.

If necessary, nutritional supplements with vitamin B6, calcium and magnesium may be prescribed. It is important to control stress, practicing relaxation techniques, such as yoga or meditation.

Endometriosis is a fairly common condition in which the tissue that lines the inside of the uterus, called the endometrium, grows outside it and also appears in the ovaries, fallopian tubes, intestines and bladder.

This disease can cause very painful periods, heavy bleeding and fertility problems. Although it has no cure, there are treatments to relieve its symptoms.

Any woman can suffer from it, although it occurs more frequently between the ages of 30 and 50. In addition, people who never had children and those who have intense menstrual periods that last more than 7 days or short cycles less than 27 days are at greater risk.

On the other hand, there is also a greater propensity when a family member already had it and if there is a problem that prevents the normal passage of menstrual flow out of the body.

To learn more about Endometriosis, we consult Dr. Mario Vega Carbó, a specialist in clinical endocrinology.

Doctor Mario,
1. What are the main symptoms of this condition?

The most common sign of Endometriosis is severe pain before and during the menstrual period. There may also be a continuous discomfort in the lower abdomen or back, and during sexual intercourse. Other usual symptoms are bleeding between periods, very heavy periods, infertility, gastrointestinal or digestive problems, fatigue, lack of energy and discomfort at the time of bowel movement or urination.

Depending on each case, the pain caused by this condition may be mild or so acute that the person cannot get out of bed.

2. What is the cause of this disease?

At the moment the exact causes that cause it are not known, but it is believed that its origin is the retrograde menstrual flow. However, it is known that people who exercise regularly and have low body fat are less likely to suffer from it.

The same if they have already given birth and if their menstrual cycles began late in adolescence.

3. How is Endometriosis diagnosed?

To detect it, it is necessary to perform a minor surgical procedure called laparoscopy. To do this, a small cut is made in the abdomen and a thin tube with a camera and light is introduced to look for tissues that grow outside the uterus. Sometimes a small sample is taken for studies.

Before performing this surgery, the professional will probably review the patient's symptoms and medical history and perform a pelvic exam, an MRI and a transvaginal or abdominal ultrasound.

4. How does this condition affect fertility?

When the woman menstruates, the endometrium lining the uterus thickens, breaks down and bleeds. The same goes for the tissue that grows out of it and causes this disease.

However, since here it is out of its usual place, blood has no way out of the body and is trapped. This causes the area to swell and generate pain, and also to form a scar tissue that blocks the fallopian tubes, making conception difficult.

It is estimated that between 30 and 50% of women with Endometriosis have difficulty getting pregnant.

5. What other disorders can cause this ailment?

In women with Endometriosis ovarian cancer occurs more frequently than expected. However, the risks of suffering from it remain relatively low.

6. How is the treatment for this disease?

Endometriosis has no cure, but it is treated with medication and surgery. If the symptoms are mild, non-steroidal pain relievers such as Ibuprofen help fight discomfort.

On the other hand, hormone and contraceptive supplements, such as the pill or IUD, can reduce pain and bleeding. If the discomfort is very intense, it is possible to remove the excess tissue by surgical treatment, which reduces its signs and facilitates pregnancy. However, these can grow back over time.

As a last resort, some people opt for a hysterectomy (removal of the uterus), which in some cases also includes the removal of the ovaries and fallopian tubes.

7. Is there any therapy for infertility caused by Endometriosis?

Yes. In addition to the aforementioned treatments, a laparoscopy can be performed to remove the endometriosis patches, stimulate the ovaries to produce more eggs, or perform in vitro fertilization.

Chapter 125. Treatment of abnormal uterine bleeding

Many women suffer from abnormal uterine bleeding (SUA), which can affect their lives in a negative way, generating anxiety and limiting their activities. Together with chronic pelvic pain and excessive vaginal secretion, it is one of the main causes of gynecological consultation.

SUA is a bleeding that lasts longer than usual and occurs in an irregular time. It can arise between menstrual cycles, after intercourse or after menopause. As various pathologies are involved, in their treatment, in addition to the gynecologist, other specialists usually intervene, among which is the endocrinologist, who investigates the role of hormones in this process.

To learn more about this topic, we talked to Dr. Mario Vega Carbó, who works as an endocrinologist at the Vega & Vado Office.

Doctor Mario,
1. What is the reason for abnormal uterine bleeding?

The causes are very varied. Usually, hormonal changes or imbalances are what cause a menstrual cycle to go ahead or be delayed and in some cases to be more abundant than normal. It can also occur as a result of a thickening of the uterine lining, fibroids, polyps, infections or some type of cancer in the vaginal area, coagulation disorders, pregnancy complications, alterations of the urinary and gastrointestinal tracts, thyroid dysfunction or severe changes of weight.

Similarly, hormonal contraceptives, such as pills or IUDs, tranquilizers or psychotropics can be the cause of this problem.

2. Who are the most likely to suffer from SUA?

Abnormal uterine bleeding is more common in adolescents and in premenopausal or overweight women.

3. What are your main symptoms?

The SUA includes alterations in the menstrual cycle, which can last more than 2 days than usual and have intervals between periods with 4 days less than usual. In turn, it can present intermenstrual bleeding and, as a result of its intensity, cause fatigue, anemia and often prevent the performance of daily activities. For example, women may bleed enough to be absorbed by 1 or more tampons or sanitary pads per hour.

On the other hand, SUA can also generate changes in mood and sensitivity and dryness in the vaginal area.

4. What factors must be taken into account at the time of diagnosis?

In these cases, the first thing to do is rule out a pregnancy and then analyze the patient's age, family planning method, medical history and infertility problems.

Next, a series of tests are usually performed to rule out other possible causes of bleeding, such as a pelvic, hormonal and thyroid exam, a blood coagulation profile and complete liver biometrics.

5. How is the treatment for abnormal uterine bleeding?

It depends on the reason for the bleeding, the patient's age and whether or not she wants to get pregnant in the future. Cases of heavy bleeding are usually treated with high doses of estrogen.

Treatments with hormonal therapy, birth control pills, uterine devices, anti-inflammatories, iron diets and even surgery are also performed. The curettage, for example, is an intervention in which the lining of the uterus is scraped for analysis.

On the other hand, hormonal manipulation with antagonistic substances like LHRH (GnRH), danazol and other substances constitute non-invasive methods that are increasingly used in these cases.

6. What can you expect from these treatments?

Hormone therapy usually relieves symptoms of abnormal uterine bleeding. In turn, when the causes of this discomfort are known, targeted treatments are very effective.

Amenorrhea is the absence of prolonged menstrual periods. This disorder can affect women of any age and its most frequent causes are pregnancy and problems in the genital organs or glands that help regulate hormonal levels.

It is known as Primary Amenorrhea when a teenager reaches the age of 16 if she has begun to menstruate. Meanwhile, Secondary Amenorrhea occurs when, having menstruated regularly, a woman stops having her period for at least three cycles in a row.

To learn more about this topic, we interview Mario Vega Carbó, an endocrinologist with more than 20 years of experience.

Doctor Mario,
1. What are the most frequent causes of Amenorrhea?

There are many possible causes. Among the natural ones are pregnancy, lactation and menopause. Meanwhile, women who take oral or injectable contraceptives may not have periods even for 6 months after they stop using them.

On the other hand, organic problems in the vaginal canal, uterus or ovaries, or the absence of them, can also cause Amenorrhea. The same is the hormonal alterations of the hypothalamus, thyroid and pituitary gland, such as Polycystic Ovarian Syndrome, Hyperthyroidism, Hypothyroidism, pituitary tumors and premature menopause.

In addition, this disorder can be caused by the consumption of certain medications, such as antipsychotics, antidepressants, antiallergics and others for blood pressure and chemotherapy. Other possible causes are related to lifestyle, such as low body weight, obesity, excessive exercise, or stress.

2. Who has more risks of suffering it?

Obese women, those who exercise excessively, those who have very little body fat, those who follow extreme diets, those who suffer from anorexia or bulimia, those who suffer from anxiety or severe emotional distress and those who suddenly lose weight They are more likely to suffer.

The same are those who have a family history with this disorder and those who perform rigorous athletic training, such as elite athletes or dancers.

3. What are your main symptoms?

Along with the lack of menstrual periods, the woman may have milk secretion from the nipple, breast size changes, hair loss, vaginal dryness, headache, vision or voice changes, acne, facial hair excessive and weight gain or loss.

4. How is Amenorrhea diagnosed?

Faced with its symptoms, a pelvic exam and physical exams are usually done to check if there is a problem in the genital organs. Also pregnancy tests and blood tests to measure the levels of thyroid and ovarian functions, prolactin and other hormones.

Other studies include genetic studies, computed tomography in the head in search of tumors, ultrasound in the genital organs, biopsy of the lining of the uterus and ultrasound of the pelvis.

5. What is your treatment?

The therapy will depend on the causes of Amenorrhea. When these are resolved, usually the menstrual periods return to normal. If it is due to a hormonal problem, it can be treated with medication. If it is caused by a tumor or structural blockage, it can be remedied with surgery.

When the reason is eating problems or obesity, the practice of regular exercise and a balanced diet can solve it. If the cause is a certain medication, the dose can be adjusted or replaced by another.

In some cases, birth control pills and other hormonal therapies can restore menstrual cycles.

6. What other complications can Amenorrhea bring?

Depending on the case, if left untreated, the causes of Amenorrhea can also lead to infertility, osteoporosis and sexual problems.

Chapter 127. Hormone Contraception and its different possibilities

There are many methods of Hormone Contraception that can be used to prevent pregnancy. These include the pill, the vaginal ring, the implant, the injection, the intrauterine device and the patch. All these options are effective, although they offer different advantages and disadvantages that must be known before choosing one of them.

To know how each method works, we interview Dr. Mario Vega Carbó, an endocrinology specialist with more than 20 years of experience.

Doctor Mario,
1. What are birth control pills and how do they work?

These pills contain estrogen and progestin, two hormones that prevent a woman's ovary from releasing an egg during menstruation. This is achieved by changing the levels of natural hormones that the body produces. In addition, progestin also causes the cervical mucus to become thick, preventing sperm from entering.

2. How are they used and what are their advantages?

The pills are administered orally once a day. To avoid nausea, it is recommended to eat them with food. If taken periodically they are a very effective and easy to use method of contraception, but they do not provide protection against sexually transmitted diseases.

On the other hand, among other benefits its use improves acne, reduces severe bleeding and the risks of ovarian and endometrial cancer, relieves premenstrual syndrome and the intensity of cramps.

3. What happens if a person forgets to take a pill?

In that case, you may be at risk of becoming pregnant. Therefore it is recommended that you use another method of birth control for a while. However, each product in particular offers precise instructions on what to do in that case, which should be followed.

4. Can the contraceptive pill cause side effects?

Yes, the most common are nausea, vomiting, abdominal distention, diarrhea, weight gain or loss, acne, hair growth in unusual places, vaginal burning, breast tenderness, changes in the flow and menstrual period and others that may be more serious

On the other hand, smokers who use birth control pills may be at greater risk of heart attacks and strokes, so this method is not recommended.

The same goes for people who are breastfeeding, those who have high blood pressure or a history of breast cancer, Diabetes and other diseases.

5. What is the hormonal contraceptive patch and how does it work?

This method is a small patch that contains the hormones estrogen and progestin, which should be placed on the skin once a week, for three weeks, and then not used for one, so that menstrual bleeding occurs. It is usually placed on the shoulder or buttocks and its operation is similar to that of the pills.

6. What is the hormonal intrauterine device?

The IUD is a plastic structure that is inserted into the uterus, where it releases the hormone progestin. It begins to function within seven days after insertion and can remain in the uterus for 3 to 5 years.

Among other advantages, it can be used while breastfeeding, reduces bleeding and menstrual pain and does not have estrogen-related side effects. In addition, it reduces the risks of pelvic infection and endometrial cancer.

7. What are your disadvantages?

One of them is that it must be placed and removed by a professional. In addition, in a few cases it can get out of place or cause perforation of the uterus.

On the other hand, the hormonal IUD is not recommended for patients with a history of pelvic infection, cervical or uterine cancer, liver disease or who have a uterus or very large or very small.

8. What is contraceptive injection?

It is an injection that contains the hormone progestin, which is given every three months in the muscles of the upper arm or in the buttocks. It is estimated that it works better than birth control pills to prevent pregnancy and fertility return is likely to be delayed by 10 months or more when it is discontinued.

9. What is the vaginal ring and how does it work?

It is a flexible plastic ring that is placed inside the vagina and releases estrogen and progestin. It is about 5 centimeters wide and should be used for 3 weeks. Then it is removed, a week is passed, and a new one is placed. Like pills, it prevents pregnancy by releasing hormones in the body.

With estrogen, there is a small risk of high blood pressure, blood clots, heart attack and stroke, which increases among smokers.

10. What are progestin implants?

It is a small bar that is placed under the skin, usually in the upper arm, and releases small amounts of the hormone progestin into the bloodstream. The implant is performed in less than five minutes with local anesthesia and can be used for up to 3 years, although it can be removed when desired.

11. What other aspects should be taken into account when choosing a method of Hormone Contraception?

Because everyone has associated side effects and different risks, it is important that the choice be made jointly with a professional. It is recommended to talk with the specialist about the different methods and, according to personal tastes, the wishes or not to get pregnant in the short or medium term, and the medical history of each patient, choose the best option.

Finally, remember that none of these methods provides protection against sexually transmitted diseases.

Infertility is a medical expression used when a woman fails to conceive or carry a pregnancy to term after a year of frequent sexual intercourse. It is estimated that this problem affects 15 percent of couples. However, with proper treatment, most of them manage to have babies.

In a third of the time infertility is due to female factors. Another third corresponds to male factors, while the rest is a combination of both or its exact cause is unknown.

On the side of women, this disorder may be due to physical and hormonal problems, or be related to their lifestyle or environmental variables.

To learn more about this topic, we consulted Dr. Mario Vega Carbó, an endocrinology specialist, who is in charge of the Vega & Vado Office.

Doctor Mario,
1. What are the main causes of Female Infertility?

In most cases these are problems with ovulation, either because it is not regular or because it does not occur directly. This may be due to several factors, such as Polycystic Ovary Syndrome, which causes the ovaries to not release an ovum regularly or is unhealthy, and Primary Ovarian Insufficiency, when they stop functioning normally before age 40 .

Other causes are excessive prolactin production, a vaginal obstruction, damage to the fallopian tubes, infections, pelvic inflammation and sexually transmitted diseases.

Also genital tuberculosis, Endometriosis, benign polyps or tumors, congenital uterine abnormalities, vaginismus and cervical stenosis. In many cases, infertility is due to the consumption of certain medications. In others, the reason cannot be explained.

2. What other diseases can cause infertility?

Diabetes Mellitus, liver or thyroid problems, Celiac disease, renal or adrenal diseases, Kallman Syndrome, hypothalamic dysfunction, Hyperprolactinemia and Hypopituitarism, among other conditions, can cause or assist in infertility.

On the other hand, there is also a psychological factor, related to emotions, sensations and feelings that can affect reproductive capacity.

3. What are the main symptoms of Female Infertility?

In addition to the inability to conceive or carry a pregnancy to term, other frequent signs are menstrual abnormalities. It may have cycles that are too long (35 days or more) or short (less than 21 days), irregular or absent. On the other hand, there may also be pain or discomfort in the vaginal area.

4. Who is more at risk of suffering it?

Women over 35, smokers, those who are overweight, those who suffered from sexually transmitted infections and those who drink alcohol in excess are more likely to suffer infertility.

5. How is this disorder detected?

In front of its symptoms, an analysis of the clinical history and different studies are carried out to look for its causes. Fertility tests may include genetic and ovulation tests, blood tests to control hormone levels, hysterosalpingography to detect abnormalities in the uterine cavity, pelvic ultrasound and laparoscopy to look at the fallopian tubes, ovaries and uterus.

6. What is the treatment for Female Infertility?

The therapy will depend on the cause, the age of the patient and her personal preference. This may include medications, surgery or the use of techniques that help conception. In many cases, ovulation disorders can be resolved with the use of certain drugs, such as clomiphene citrate, gonadotropin, metformin, letrozole or bomocriptine. For its part, surgery can correct or remove abnormalities.

Within assisted reproduction, artificial insemination or in vitro fertilization can be performed. If the cause is another illness or a psychological or emotional problem, they should be treated. If it is due to the consumption of a certain medicine, the doctor may replace it with another.

7. Can the use of fertility drugs have other consequences?

Its use can increase the risks of multiple pregnancies and cause ovarian hyperstimulation syndrome, which causes inflammation and pain in the ovaries. On the other hand, although the possibilities are few, its prolonged use may also increase the chances of developing ovarian tumors in the future.

8. What other recommendations can be taken into account?

To improve fertility it is advisable to eat healthy, exercise daily, maintain an adequate body weight, sleep well, do not smoke and avoid alcohol consumption. Also avoid stress and limit caffeine.

On the other hand, the inability to get pregnant is often due to psychological and emotional issues and can lead to depression. Therefore, psychological support is recommended, if necessary.

Chapter 129. Fertility: ovulation inducers

Most cases of female infertility are due to problems with ovulation, either because it is not regular or because it does not occur directly. This may be due to several factors, such as polycystic ovary syndrome, primary ovarian insufficiency, excessive prolactin production, vaginal obstruction, damage to the fallopian tubes, infections, pelvic inflammation or sexually transmitted diseases.

It can also be a consequence of genital tuberculosis, endometriosis, benign polyps or tumors, congenital uterine abnormalities, vaginismus, cervical stenosis, eating disorders or the consumption of certain medications.

In many cases, ovulation disorders can be resolved with the use of certain drugs, such as clomiphene citrate, gonadotropin, metformin, cabergoline or bromocriptine.

To talk about this topic, we interview Mario Vega Carbó, an endocrinologist with more than 20 years of experience.

Doctor Mario,
1. What patients are prescribed ovulation inducers?

These medications are used to treat women who do not ovulate on a regular basis. In general, patients who have irregular menstrual cycles or who present with amenorrhea usually have ovulatory dysfunction.

However, before starting to use these drugs, it is convenient to perform a diagnostic evaluation to determine the causes of this condition.

2. How do these medications work?

These drugs stimulate the ovaries to produce the growth of one or several mature follicles per cycle, with the aim of at least one of them being fertilized and getting a pregnancy.

3. What is the most frequently used drug to induce ovulation?

The most commonly used is clomiphene citrate, which works in the same way as estrogen, a female hormone that causes the ovaries to produce eggs and release. This medicine comes as a tablet and is usually taken once a day for 5 days, starting the third day after menstruation. The standard dose is 50 to 100 milligrams per day.

Clomiphene citrate is generally indicated for patients with polycystic ovary or with sterility of unknown origin. In addition, it is also used to treat menstrual abnormalities, fibrocystic breasts and persistent breast milk production.

4. What side effects can clomiphene citrate have?

This medicine may cause a higher incidence of multiple pregnancies, hot flashes, thick and dry cervical mucosa, blurred vision, headaches, nausea, depression, breast tenderness, mood swings, vaginal bleeding, ovarian cysts and pelvic discomfort.

Clomiphene citrate should not be used for more than six consecutive menstrual cycles.

5. What are gonadotrophins and how do they work?

Gonadotrophins are hormones naturally secreted by the pituitary gland, which are responsible for follicular development and ovum maturation. In assisted reproduction treatments they are used to produce the controlled growth of one or several follicles.

This medicine is given by subcutaneous injections once a day. Treatment usually begins on the third day of the ovarian cycle and usually lasts between 7 and 12 days, depending on each case. The normal starting dose is usually between 75 and 150 units per day.

6. What side effects can gonadotrophins cause?

385

This medicine may cause mild abdominal distension, breast tenderness, mood swings and rashes in the injection area. In addition, it can generate ovarian hyperstimulation syndrome, which causes pain and swelling of the ovaries, and an increased risk of multiple pregnancies.

7. How can bomocriptine and cabergoline induce ovulation?

In many cases, patients ovulate irregularly because the pituitary gland secretes too much prolactin. Hyperprolactinemia can cause the decrease of estrogen and generate galactorrhea and infertility.

Bromocriptine and cabergoline are two drugs that reduce the amount of prolactin released by the pituitary gland. The first is taken orally every day, while the second is ingested in the form of one or two pills, twice a week. In addition, bromocriptine can also be administered vaginally.

8. What side effects can bomocriptine and cabergoline cause?

These drugs can cause nausea, vomiting, nasal congestion, headaches, tiredness, fainting, dizziness, decreased blood pressure and drowsiness, among other side effects. To avoid them, treatment with low doses is usually started and gradually increased.

9. What other aspects should be taken into account during the use of these drugs?

Before starting the treatment it is important to inform the doctor about any other medication, vitamin or supplement that is being used, so that it evaluates whether the combination can be harmful.

You should also notify if you suffer from allergies or other conditions, such as hypertension or kidney, heart or liver problems; or vaginal bleeding.

On the other hand, during the treatment it is very important to carry out ultrasound controls to strictly monitor the follicular growth, as well as to diagnose an excessive number of developing follicles that can raise the risk of multiple gestation.

Finally, these medications should be stored in a suitable place, at room temperature and out of the reach of children.

Chapter 130. Female Androgenic Alopecia

Female Androgenetic Alopecia is the most common type of hair loss in women. Also known as female pattern baldness, it causes the hair to become short, very thin and without progressive pigmentation.

The thinning of the hair occurs mainly in the upper part of the head, generating the loss of density and the appearance of cleared areas. Although it can occur at any age, it is more common after age 50. Its manifestation can cause low self-esteem and depression.

To learn more about this topic, we consulted Dr. Mario Vega Carbó, an endocrinology specialist in charge of the Vega & Vado Office.

Doctor Mario,
1. What is the cause of Female Androgenic Alopecia?

This condition can be caused by the presence of certain male hormones, such as testosterone, androsterone and dihydrotestosterone (DHT) at elevated levels. These can cause depletion of hair follicles, generating greater fragility and less hair growth.

Androgenic Female Alopecia can also be due to aging, genetic and hereditary reasons, the use of certain medications, stressful situations, poor diet, oxidation and micro inflammation, thyroid disease and excessive use of treatments and hair products. It usually manifests once menopause is reached.

2. What medications can cause this medical condition?

Androgenic Female Alopecia can be caused by drugs to reduce cholesterol; to treat Parkinson's, stomach ulcers, arthritis, depression and hypertension; and anticonvulsants.

3. What are your main symptoms?

In women, the hair is thinned especially in the upper part of the head and begins with a widening through the central area. Unlike men, in very few cases alopecia progresses to baldness, but generates a loss of density.

4. What is the treatment of Female Androgenic Alopecia?

Among the medications used to treat this condition are minoxidil, finasteride, spironolactone, cimetidine, birth control pills and ketoconazole.

In turn, the plant drugs Serenoa repens and Pygeun africanum help to inhibit the activity of the enzyme 5α-reductase, which reduces the passage of testosterone to dihydrotestosterone, responsible for the miniaturization of hair follicles.

Methylsulfonylmethane (MSM), which has antioxidant and anti-inflammatory effects, is also used and is an essential source of organic sulfur for the life cycle of the hair. If necessary it is also possible to perform a hair transplant, which usually gives very good results. To do this, small portions of hair are removed from areas where it is thicker and placed in others that have baldness.

Another option is the stimulation of the scalp by applying carbon dioxide through subcutaneous injections.

5. What other aspects are recommended in these cases?

To help alleviate the problem, it is important to adopt a healthy diet and good eating habits. Also consume vitamin supplements and antioxidants, rest properly and exercise regularly. In addition, scalp massages are recommended to activate circulation and avoid the use of dryers, irons and dyes.

On the other hand, it is important to avoid stress and treat problems of depression, anxiety, anemia and insomnia quickly.

6. What other complications can Female Androgenic Alopecia bring?

Hair loss can lower self-esteem and cause depression and anxiety, as well as affect family, work and social relationships. Extensions, the use of wigs, hats or scarves, or a change of hairstyle can help hide its effects and improve the appearance.

Chapter 131. Hyperandrogenism, Hirsutism and Acne

Hyperandrogenism is a disorder in which women produce an excess of androgens, the male sex hormones. This is a fairly common problem, which affects between 5 and 10 percent of women of reproductive age.

It can lead to the development of male characteristics in the body, such as exaggerated hair growth (hirsutism), decreased breast size, absence of menstrual periods, seborrhea and acne.

To learn more about this topic, we interview Mario Vega Carbó, a specialist in clinical endocrinology.

Doctor Mario,
1. What are the main causes of hyperandrogenism?

This disorder is usually the result of excessive androgen production of the ovaries and adrenal glands. This may be due to Congenital Adrenal Hyperplasia, tumors, Cushing's Syndrome, Polycystic Ovary Syndrome or the consumption of certain medications, such as danazol, systemic corticosteroids and fluoxetine, among other possibilities.

2. What are your main symptoms?

Hyperandrogenism can cause severe acne, decreased breast size, increased body and facial hair, absence of menstrual periods, infertility, thickening of the voice, clitoral size growth, increased muscle mass, male pattern baldness and oily skin.

On the other hand, in newborns it can manifest itself in the form of ambiguous genitals, while in girls it occurs with premature appearance of pubic or axillary hair before age 9, acne, increased body odor and growth acceleration.

3. How is this disease detected?

A physical exam and different tests are usually done to measure the level of certain hormones and other substances in the blood, including testosterone, prolactin, cholesterol, insulin, glucose and thyroid stimulants, among others.

Diagnostic imaging tests may also be necessary to detect abnormalities of the ovaries, pituitary gland and adrenal glands, and a pelvic exam to look for tumors.

4. What is the treatment of hyperandrogenism?

Therapy may include the use of antiandrogens, such as cyproterone acetate, spironolactone and flutamide. If the cause of this disorder is an ovarian or adrenal tumor, surgery, radiation therapy and other treatments may be necessary.

On the other hand, if it is caused by any medication, the dose can be lowered or changed to a similar one that does not produce these symptoms.

If the patient suffers from obesity, she seeks to normalize her weight through a low-calorie diet and physical activities. This helps improve the condition and effectiveness of medications. In the case of girls born with genitals of male appearance, repair surgery can be performed to normalize their appearance and function.

5. What is Hirsutism and what causes it?

Hirsutism is a disorder that causes women to grow excessively dark and thick hair on the face, chest and back. It is usually caused by an excess of androgens, although it may also be due to inherited traits.

6. How is it treated?

Hormonal contraceptives that contain estrogen and progestin, and antiandrogen medications are often used to treat hirsutism caused by the production of male hormones.

On the other hand, topical creams can also be prescribed to treat excessive facial hair on the face or use laser therapy to permanently remove it. For these cases, hair removal with tweezers, wax or chemicals, or shaving is not recommended.

7. What is Acne and what causes it?

Acne is a skin condition that occurs when hair follicles become clogged with fat and dead cells, causing the appearance of blackheads or pimples. This can be caused by the abundant production of fat, the obstruction of the hair follicles, bacteria or the excess of androgens.

8. How is it treated?

Therapy usually combines the use of topical and oral medications. There are several drugs to restrict the production of fat or androgens, to accelerate the renewal of dermal cells, to fight bacterial infection and to reduce inflammation.

In severe cases, laser treatment, chemical peel, comedone extraction and steroid injection can be used.

9. What other complications can Hyperandrogenism bring?

This disorder may be accompanied by infertility and problems during pregnancy. In turn, women with Polycystic Ovarian Syndrome have an increased risk of diabetes, high cholesterol and blood pressure, uterine cancer and obesity.

To prevent these inconveniences, they are recommended to adopt a healthy lifestyle by controlling weight, exercising regularly and following an appropriate diet.

On the other hand, women taking medication to treat hirsutism should avoid becoming pregnant, due to the risk of birth defects.

Finally, those who suffer from this condition may suffer from lack of self-esteem, shame and depression as a result of severe hirsutism and acne, so it is advisable to accompany the treatment with psychological and family support if necessary.

Chapter 132. Clitoromegaly or clitoral hypertrophy

Clitoromegaly or clitoral hypertrophy is a disorder in which this organ has a larger than normal size, which can resemble a small penis.

The clitoris is located inside the vagina and is visible from the top of the vulva. It is responsible for providing sexual pleasure to women and has no reproductive functions or related to the secretion of urine. The size of its visible part can vary between 2 and 6 millimeters wide, and 2 and 9 millimeters long. Clitoromegaly appears when these measures are exceeded.

To learn more about this topic, we interviewed Cuban doctor Mario Vega Carbó, a specialist in clinical endocrinology.

Doctor Mario,
1. What causes clitoromegaly?

This condition may be due to congenital causes, caused by an exaggerated increase in testosterone levels or other hormonal disorders. This causes the external genitals to become masculinized, causing the clitoris to lengthen.

Another reason may be congenital adrenal hyperplasia, an inherited disorder that affects the production of hormones in the adrenal glands. People with this condition generate more androgens, a hormone that causes early or inappropriate appearance of male characteristics.

Clitoromegaly may also be due to maternal tumors that secrete androgens, the consumption of anabolic steroids during pregnancy and a traumatic swelling of the genitals during labor.

On the other hand, it can also appear during male hormone therapy.

2. What disorders can generate clitoromegaly?

This condition can cause painful sexual intercourse and emotional disorders due to its appearance, generating shame and complexes due to the appearance of a small penis. In addition, in almost all cases the clitoromegaly is accompanied by a hypertrophy of the cap, that is, an enlargement of the fold of skin that covers the clitoris.

3. How is this condition treated?

It can be treated by surgery to reduce its size. During it, the excess tissue is removed and the clitoris is put back in its correct position.

In cases where there is also hypertrophy of the cap, this can be corrected in the same operation. Usually this surgery is performed on an outpatient basis with local anesthesia.

4. What consequences can this intervention have?

After surgery, the patient may have discomfort or swelling in the area, which disappear in a few days. In cases of pain, anti-inflammatories and analgesics indicated by the doctor can be taken.

The person can quickly resume their activities after 48 hours of rest, but must wait at least one month to have sex. This operation does not affect the erogenous sensitivity of the organ at all.

5. How are cases of congenital adrenal hyperplasia treated?

In these cases, the therapy used seeks to normalize hormonal levels, through the application of hydrocortisone to replace cortisol, mineralocorticoids to replace aldosterone and other medications.

The objectives are to maintain a balance of liquids and salts, blood sugar levels, avoid an adrenal crisis and ensure physical growth and habitual sexual development. For this, it is essential to undergo periodic analysis to see if the doses used should be adjusted.

In the case of girls born with genitals of male appearance, repair surgery can also be performed to normalize their appearance and function. It is usually done between 2 and 6 months of age and, sometimes, new procedures are required during puberty or later.

If hyperplasia is detected before birth, it is also possible to prevent the effect of androgens on female genitals by prenatal treatment, using the synthetic hormone dexamethasone.

Chapter 133. Symptoms and Treatment of Polycystic Ovary Syndrome

Polycystic Ovary Syndrome (PCOS) is a common disorder in women of reproductive age, who have an elevated level of hormones in their body.

Its main symptoms include irregular menstruation, excessive hair growth in rare areas (upper lip, sideburns, chin, neck, breast areolas, chest, navel, groin, thighs and back), severe acne and male pattern baldness .

In addition, it usually causes metabolic disorders such as hyperinsulinemia, insulin resistance, high cholesterol and triglyceride levels, and obesity; skin changes, infertility and an increase in the number of cysts in the ovaries. The exact cause of PCOS is unknown, but it could involve a combination of intrauterine and extrauterine genetic and environmental factors.

To learn more about this disorder, we interview Mario Vega Carbó, an endocrinologist with more than 20 years of experience.

Doctor Mario,
1. What causes Polycystic Ovary Syndrome?

PCOS is generally associated with changes in the hormone levels of estrogen and progesterone, which contribute to the release of the ovules; and androgens, a male hormone found in small amounts in women. It is also related to excess insulin.

In many cases, when this disorder occurs, the ovules are not released and remain in the ovaries, which can contribute to sterility. The other symptoms related to this pathology are due to the high level of male hormones in the body.

2. Who are more likely to suffer from PCOS?

Usually the syndrome is diagnosed in women between 20 and 30 years old, although it can also affect adolescent girls. Symptoms usually begin when menstrual periods begin.

Its signs are usually more severe in obese people. On the other hand, the families of women who suffered from this disorder have a higher risk of suffering from it.

3. What other complications do you have for health?

Women with PCOS are more likely to suffer from endometrial cancer, diabetes, infertility, spontaneous abortions, non-alcoholic steatohepatitis, sleep apnea, depression, anxiety and eating disorders.

4. How is Polycystic Ovary Syndrome diagnosed?

First, it is necessary to make an analysis of the patient's medical history and a series of physical studies, including the review of weight and body mass index, and measuring the size of his abdomen.

In addition, it is customary to perform pelvic exams to look at the ovaries, and blood tests to check hormone and glucose levels. Also tests of pregnancy and thyroid function. With all this information, plus family history consultation, it is possible to make an accurate diagnosis.

5. What is the treatment?

PCOS treatment usually includes birth control pills and progesterone therapy to regularize menstruation, metformin to prevent diabetes, statins to control high cholesterol levels, hormones to increase fertility, spironolactone to block androgens, and procedures to decrease and eliminate excess hair, such as electrolysis and laser hair removal.

In general, the patient is also expected to normalize his weight, through a low-calorie diet and physical activities. This helps improve the condition and effectiveness of medications.

6. What results are expected?

With proper care, PCOS symptoms usually disappear. In addition, women may become pregnant, although there is an increased risk of miscarriages and gestational diabetes.

Once the treatment is finished, patients are advised to perform periodic checks of weight, blood pressure, glucose levels and lipids.

Chapter 134. Antiandrogens: Finasteride, Spironolactone and Flutamide

Antiandrogens are a group of medications that inhibit the biological effects of male sex hormones androgens on body tissues. They are used for the treatment of cancer or benign prostatic hyperplasia; acne and hirsutism in women; androgenic alopecia; and serious sexual disorders, such as hypersexuality or paraphilias in men.

The administration of these medications can cause a waning in development and an involution of secondary sexual characteristics in men. It can also reduce the function of the sexual organs and decrease libido. Among the most commonly used antiandrogens are Finasteride, Spironolactone and Flutamide.

To learn more about this topic, we interviewed Cuban doctor Mario Vega Carbó, a specialist in clinical endocrinology.

Doctor Mario,
1. What is Finasteride and what is it used for?

Finasteride is an antiandrogen that inhibits 5 alpha reductase, a primary enzyme in the conversion of testosterone to dihydrotestosterone in the prostatic epithelium.

This medicine is used to treat an enlarged prostate and some of its symptoms, such as excessive urination or difficulty urinating. Its use may decrease the need for surgery. In addition, this drug is used to treat male androgenic alopecia.

2. How is this medicine used?

Finasteride comes in tablets that are taken orally, usually once a day.

3. What side effects can Finasteride cause?

This medicine can cause impotence, decreased libido, reduced ejaculation volume, pain in the testicles and gynecomastia. Also, depression and the increase of suicidal ideas.

4. What is spironolactone and what is it used for?

Spironolactone is a synthetic steroid that reduces the effects of aldosterone and androgens. This medicine is used to treat hyperaldosteronism, a hormonal disorder in which the adrenal glands produce an excessive amount of aldosterone in the blood. It helps the kidneys eliminate unnecessary water and sodium in the urine, but reduces the loss of potassium from the body.

In addition, it is also used to treat heart failure and hypertension, and in patients with edema caused by liver or kidney disease. Spironolactone is used to control these conditions, but it does not cure them.

On the other hand, it is also used in combination with other medications to treat precocious puberty and hirsutism.

5. How is this medicine used?

Spironolactone comes in tablets and suspension that are taken orally, usually once or twice a day. It is possible that you first start with a low dose and then gradually increase it.

6. What side effects can Spironolactone cause?

This medicine can cause vomiting, diarrhea, stomach pain, enlargement or pain in the breasts, irregular menstrual periods, vaginal bleeding, testicular atrophy, erectile dysfunction, increased hair growth in the body, drowsiness, tiredness, cramps and nausea.

7. What is Flutamide and what is it used for?

Flutamide is a non-steroidal antiandrogen that blocks the activity of testosterone. It is used to treat certain types of prostate cancer, by stopping the multiplication and spread of malignant cells.

8. How is this medicine used?

Flutamide comes in pills that are taken orally three times a day, every 8 hours.

9. What side effects can Flutamide cause?

This medicine can cause serious liver damage. In addition, among its side effects there may be swelling in the chest, diarrhea, nausea, vomiting, loss of appetite, erectile dysfunction, decreased libido, hot flashes and excessive sweating, gynecomastia and depression.

On the other hand, pregnant women should not take this medicine as it could cause harm to the fetus.

10. What should be done if you forget to take a dose of these medications?

You should ingest it as soon as you remember. However, if it is almost time for the next dose, it is better to skip it and continue with the regular dosage. In no case should a double dose be taken to compensate for the one that was forgotten.

11. What other aspects should be taken into account while using these antiandrogens?

Before starting the treatment it is important to inform the doctor about any other medication, vitamin or supplement that is being used, so that it evaluates whether the combination can be harmful.

You should also notify if you suffer from allergies or other conditions, such as hypertension or kidney, heart, liver or prostate problems; if you are pregnant or planning to conceive in the short term, or if you are breastfeeding.

Finally, these medications should be stored in a suitable place, at room temperature and out of the reach of children.

Chapter 135. Primary Ovarian Insufficiency

Primary Ovarian Insufficiency, also known as Premature Ovarian Failure, is a disorder that occurs when the ovaries stop functioning normally before age 40.

When the four decades of life pass, women become less fertile and may begin to have irregular menstrual periods as they enter menopause.

However, when they suffer from this condition, this begins to occur early, when they are still young, and even during adolescence.

Primary Ovarian Insufficiency is not the same as premature menopause, where periods stop before 40 and the woman can no longer get pregnant. In this case, the person still has occasional menses and may even conceive.

To learn more about this issue, we interview Cuban doctor Mario Vega Carbó, an endocrinology specialist.

Doctor Mario,
1. What is the cause of Primary Ovarian Insufficiency?

In most cases, the exact reason for this failure is unknown, but it is believed to be related to problems in the follicles that contain immature eggs. These cease to function properly, either due to genetic diseases (Turner syndrome and Fragile X chromosome syndrome), chemotherapy or radiotherapy treatments, metabolic disorders or exposure to some toxins.

Similarly, certain medications for autoimmune diseases or to prevent organ transplant rejection may also be related.

2. What are your symptoms?

The first sign of Primary Ovarian Insufficiency is irregular or absent periods. In addition, women may have symptoms similar to those of menopause, such as sudden hot flashes, night sweats, irritability, lack of concentration, decreased sexual desire, pain during intercourse, vaginal dryness, difficulty sleeping and infertility.

3. What other disorders can cause this condition?

As a consequence of hormonal changes, patients may suffer from anxiety, depression, eye problems, hardening of the arteries and heart disease, hypothyroidism and osteoporosis.

4. How is Premature Ovarian Failure diagnosed?

To confirm this condition, it is necessary to analyze the patient's medical history, see if she has a family history with this same problem, and perform a physical exam to rule out other diseases that may be causing the symptoms.

On the other hand, a blood test is usually performed to check hormone levels, a pelvic ultrasound to control the ovaries and follicles, and a chromosome test known as a karyotype. During diagnosis, pregnancy must also be ruled out.

5. What is the treatment of Primary Ovarian Insufficiency?

At the moment there is no treatment to restore the normal functioning of the ovaries. What there are therapies to mitigate your symptoms. For example, a hormone replacement treatment with estrogen and progesterone improves sexual health and decreases the risks of heart disease and osteoporosis.

Generally this therapy is recommended until age 50, since after that age can increase the risk of breast cancer and stroke.

To treat the decrease in bone tissue density, calcium and vitamin D supplementation, regular physical activity and weight control are also advised.

If the patient wishes to have children, she may consider the option of in vitro fertilization with donor eggs or adopt. However, a small percentage of women with this problem may conceive spontaneously, as a result of intermittent ovarian function in the early stages of the disorder.

On the other hand, after hormonal stimulation, human oocytes or embryos of people at risk of primary ovarian failure can be cryopreserved.

6. What other aspects must be taken into account in the face of Primary Ovarian Insufficiency?

In some cases, the loss of ovarian function and the inability to get pregnant can lead to depression. Therefore, psychological support is recommended, if necessary.

On the other hand, to mitigate the symptoms of this disorder, it is also advisable to make improvements in lifestyle. This includes no smoking, the acquisition of healthy eating patterns, the practice of constant physical activity, and avoiding alcohol and drinks containing caffeine.

Chapter 136. Hormone replacement therapy during menopause

Menopause is the period of a woman's life in which she stops having periods. It usually occurs naturally, most often between 45 and 55, when the ovaries stop producing estrogen and progesterone.

The signs and symptoms that occur during this stage are known as Climaterio Syndrome. The most common are sudden warming of the body (hot flashes), mood swings, decreased bone mass density (osteoporosis), increased cardiovascular risk and genitourinary disorders.

During this phase, women may also experience difficulty sleeping and concentrating, night sweats, pain during sexual intercourse, vaginal dryness, hair loss, increased facial hair and depression.

To learn more about the treatment of this problem, we interview Dr. Mario Vega Carbó, an endocrinology specialist with more than 20 years of experience.

Doctor Mario,
1. What can a woman do during menopause?

During the pre and post menopause years, female hormonal levels usually rise and fall, causing all kinds of disorders. To relieve these symptoms, it is possible to carry out a hormone replacement treatment, in which estrogens and exogenous progestogens are applied to replace hormones that are not being produced naturally.

This procedure also helps protect women against osteoporosis and prevent recurrent urinary tract infections. In addition, estrogens improve the mood of patients with depressive symptoms.

2. For whom is this treatment recommended?

For some women the symptoms of menopause are mild and disappear on their own. But in others its signs are more powerful and can be very annoying. For those cases, a hormone replacement treatment is recommended.

However, it is important to clarify that this procedure is not suitable for people with vaginal bleeding problems or who have had certain types of cancer, strokes, heart attacks, blood clots or liver diseases.

Therefore, before starting therapy, it is important to review the patient's medical history and family history, consider their characteristics and risk assessment.

3. At what age is this treatment recommended?

Hormone replacement therapy can be initiated within the first 10 years of menopause or in women under 60 who do not have contraindications. For this, it is advisable to make a thorough prior analysis and begin its implementation when the best therapeutic option for your symptoms is considered, since its use is not advised for a prolonged period.

4. How is the administration of these hormones?

There are different forms of administration. The most common are through oral pills, but there are also skin patches, vaginal creams, gel and tablets. All are equally effective.

The dosage is variable according to the route of administration selected, the type of estrogen and progesterone and the therapeutic schemes used. It is recommended to start with low doses and increase if the symptoms persist.

5. In general, how long is the hormone replacement treatment?

Its duration varies from patient to patient, but it is generally advised that the combination therapy be maintained for a period of less than 3 years and simple estrogenic therapy for about 7 years.

6. What other initiatives can be implemented to relieve the symptoms of menopause?

Both before, during and after this period, it is advisable to make improvements in the patient's lifestyle. This includes not smoking, acquiring healthy eating patterns, practicing constant physical activity, and avoiding alcohol and drinks containing caffeine.

On the other hand, in recent years the use of the so-called naturopathic medicine, which uses herbs, homeopathy, acupuncture and other alternatives, has been increasing to relieve symptoms related to menopause.

Chapter 137. Treatment with estrogen and progesterone

In women, the ovules primarily generate estrogen and progesterone, and a small amount of testosterone. These hormones regulate the menstrual cycle and pregnancy, secondary sexual characteristics, and act on other organs and systems of the body.

In patients with hypogonadism, a condition that occurs when the gonads do not generate the proper amount of these substances, hormone replacement therapy is one of the available alternatives.

There are different ways to apply estrogen and progesterone, such as injections, skin patches, vaginal creams, gel and tablets, all being equally effective.

To learn more about this topic, we interview Dr. Mario Vega Carbó, specialist in clinical endocrinology.

Doctor Mario,
1. What disorders generate hypogonadism in women?

This medical condition can affect breast development and height and cause absent menstrual cycles, hot flashes, vaginal dryness, mood swings and infertility. His condition is normal during menopause.

On the other hand, hypogonadism can also cause mental and emotional changes, and abnormal genitalia.

2. In which cases is estrogen and progesterone therapy used?

During the pre and post menopause years, female hormonal levels usually rise and fall, causing all kinds of disorders. The most common are sudden warming of the body (hot flashes), mood swings, decreased bone mass density (osteoporosis), increased cardiovascular risk and genitourinary disorders.

411

During this phase, women may also experience difficulty sleeping and concentrating, night sweats, pain during sexual intercourse, vaginal dryness, hair loss, increased facial hair and depression. To relieve these symptoms, it is possible to carry out a hormone replacement treatment to replace those that are not occurring naturally.

In girls and adolescents its use can stop growth and affect the speed of sexual development. In those with hypogonadism, therapy allows puberty to evolve normally and secondary sexual characteristics appear.

In men, it can cause a decrease in libido and facial and body hair growth, an increase in breast tissue, an appropriate distribution of fat and a slight change in voice tone.

Estrogen and progesterone are also used in female hormonal therapy for cases of gender identity disorder. Its use during pregnancy could harm the baby.

3. What benefits does the treatment offer?

Hormone replacement therapy can stimulate the development of breasts, pubic hair and other sexual characteristics during adolescence.

During pre and post menopause, estrogen reduces the sensation of heat in the upper body and hot flashes, burning and vaginal itching and difficulty urinating, and helps protect against osteoporosis. For its part, progesterone reduces the risk of uterine cancer and is also used to produce menstruation in women of childbearing age who have had normal periods and then it has stopped.

4. How is the administration of these hormones?

There are different forms of administration, such as injections, skin patches, vaginal creams, gel and tablets. All are equally effective. The dosage is variable according to the route of administration selected, the type of estrogen and progesterone and the therapeutic schemes used. It is recommended to start with low doses and increase if the symptoms persist.

5. In general, how long is the hormone replacement treatment?

Its duration varies from patient to patient, but it is generally advised that the combination therapy be maintained for a period of less than 3 years and simple estrogenic therapy for about 7 years.

6. What side effects can the use of estrogen and progesterone have?

Hormone replacement therapy may increase the risk of heart attacks, strokes, breast and endometrial cancer, and gallbladder diseases. In addition, side effects may include headache, vomiting, diarrhea, constipation, changes in appetite and weight, nervousness, acne, drowsiness, swelling of the hands and legs, darkening of the skin, vaginal discharge, changes in the menstrual flow and difficulty wearing contact lenses.

In severe cases there may be headache, trouble speaking, total or partial loss of vision, numbness of the arm or leg, coughing up blood, difficulty thinking clearly and lumps, or other breast changes.

Progesterone can also cause clotting abnormalities and cut off the blood supply to the brain, heart, lungs or eyes and cause serious problems.

7. What other aspects should be taken into account during use?

Before starting the treatment it is important to inform the doctor about any other medication, vitamin or supplement that is being used, so that it evaluates whether the combination can be harmful.

You should also notify if you suffered or suffer from allergies or other conditions, such as hypertension, breast lumps, vaginal bleeding, heart attack, stroke, clots, high cholesterol, diabetes or kidney problems, in the gallbladder or heart. If you are pregnant, if you plan to conceive in the short term or if you are breastfeeding.

On the other hand, during hormonal therapy it is recommended to perform breast exams frequently. These medications should be stored in a suitable place, at room temperature and out of the reach of children.

Part IX Testicles

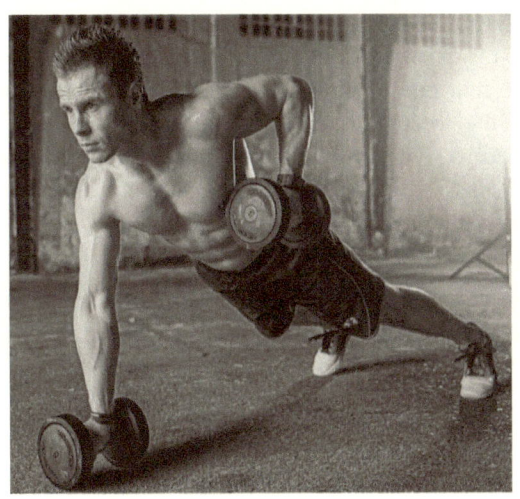

Chapter 138. Gender Identity Disorder

Gender identity disorder (GIT) is a condition whereby a person with a specific biological sex identifies with the characteristics of the opposite sex, feeling the desire and need to live and behave as such. This situation can occur both from male to female, and from female to male.

The TIG refers to the identity and not to the sexual orientation, since the homosexual, for example, does not reject his biological state, but feels attraction for someone of the same gender. The main symptom of this condition is the discomfort and discomfort that patients suffer from finding themselves within a body with which they do not feel comfortable. This causes great emotional suffering by having to play a role in society other than the desired one.

To learn how endocrinology can help them improve their quality of life, we interview Dr. Mario Vega Carbó, who is an endocrinologist with more than 20 years of experience.

Doctor Mario,
1. Is there a specific reason that causes gender identity disorder?

At the moment the cause of TIG is not yet known. The studies carried out highlight that the psychosocial conditions would not be conclusive, the upbringing and the environment in which the person develops would not play a decisive role in this aspect. There are no hormonal factors that differentiate them from those without this condition.

2. What is the procedure followed with a patient who has a gender identity disorder?

First a psychiatrist or a psychologist evaluates the patient and makes a diagnosis to see if the symptoms he refers are compatible with the GIT. If so, a sexual reassignment therapy is carried out, where through a series of psychiatric, medical and surgical treatments a gradual transition is achieved from the sex with which the patient was born to the one with whom he identifies.

3. How does endocrinology enter this whole process?

Endocrinology is the science that studies the endocrine system and the hormones responsible for regulating our body. In the case of a patient with TIG, a hormonal treatment is performed according to the gender to which you want to belong, decreasing or increasing the male or female hormones in your body. This helps to significantly improve the quality of life of the person, by getting an acceptance of himself.

4. What effects do these types of treatments have on patients?

In the case of people with male biological sex who feel female, they are given female hormones (estrogens) that cause a decrease in libido and growth of facial and body hair, an increase in breast tissue, a consistent distribution of the fat and a slight modification in the tone of voice.

Otherwise, they are given male hormones (testosterone) that cause the cessation of menstruation, increased facial hair and libido, the appearance of acne, increased muscle development and severity in the voice, and decreased tissue mammary.

5. How long does it take to have perceptible effects?

The treatment will begin to have visible results from 3 to 6 months and should be maintained for life, since otherwise its effects will be lost..

The endocrinologist will be responsible for providing the appropriate hormonal dose, to ensure its success and avoid the occurrence of unwanted sequelae.

6. At what age is it advisable to start hormonal treatment in patients with TIG?

Children who do not feel identified with their own sex should be evaluated and treated by a mental health specialist. If this condition is maintained over time and the expert considers that it will not be modified, a hormonal treatment can be started after 16 years. However, it is important to analyze each case in a particular way.

7. With a hormonal treatment is it possible to achieve a complete body modification?

Although many changes are achieved that allow to resemble the desired gender, some physical characteristics cannot be modified and require surgical interventions to complete the transition. In cases of moving from male to female, the external genitalia are removed and an artificial vagina is created, and the breast size is increased by surgery.

Otherwise, the breast tissue, uterus, ovaries and vagina are removed, and a penis and artificial testicles are created that fulfill their sexual function.

It is important to clarify that the autonomy and freedom of the patient to manage his own body is respected at all times, and it is he who decides what medical or surgical stage he wishes to reach.

8. What is the degree of patient satisfaction with these treatments?

Usually, when performed with adequate psychological support, these treatments have very good results, with satisfaction rates above 90%.

On the contrary, regret rates are below 3% and in most cases they are due to the loss of family and social support, personal instability or the occurrence of traumatic events.

Chapter 139. Hormone therapy of masculinization

Hormone therapy of masculinization is related to the behavior to follow in the presence of gender identity disorder (GIT).

To learn what male hormone therapy is like, we interview Dr. Mario Vega Carbó, who is an endocrinologist, with more than 20 years of experience.

Doctor Mario,
1. Is there a specific reason that causes gender identity disorder?

At the moment the cause of TIG is not yet known. The studies carried out highlight that the psychosocial conditions would not be conclusive and the upbringing and the environment in which the person develops would not play a decisive role in this aspect.

On the other hand, there are no hormonal factors that differentiate them from those without this condition.

2. What is the procedure followed with a patient who has a gender identity disorder?

First a psychiatrist or a psychologist evaluates the patient and makes a diagnosis to see if the symptoms he refers are compatible with the GIT. If so, a sexual reassignment therapy is carried out, where through a series of psychiatric, medical and surgical treatments a gradual transition is achieved from the sex with which the patient was born to the one with whom he identifies.

3. How does endocrinology enter this whole process?

Endocrinology is the science that studies the endocrine system and the hormones responsible for regulating our body. In a patient with TIG, a hormonal treatment is performed according to the gender to which you want to belong, decreasing or increasing the male or female hormones in your body. This helps to significantly improve the quality of life of the person, by getting an acceptance of himself.

4. How is the treatment of male hormonalization?

In the case of people with female biological sex who feel male, they are given male hormones (testosterone) that cause the cessation of menstruation, increased facial hair and libido, the appearance of acne, increased muscle development and severity in the voice, and decreased breast tissue.

5. How long does it take to have perceptible effects?

The treatment will begin to have visible results from 3 to 6 months and must be maintained for life, otherwise its effects will be lost.

The endocrinologist will be responsible for providing the appropriate hormonal dose, to ensure its success and avoid the occurrence of unwanted sequelae.

6. At what age is it advisable to start hormonal treatment in these patients?

Girls who do not feel identified with their own sex should be evaluated and treated by a mental health specialist. If this condition is maintained over time and the expert considers that it will not be modified, a hormonal treatment can be started after 16 years.

If therapy is started before the first changes at puberty, female secondary sexual characteristics, such as breast development, can be avoided. However, it is important to analyze each case in a particular way. Hormone therapy is not usually used in girls.

7. What are the risks of masculinization hormone therapy?

Some of the complications are overproduction of red blood cells, weight gain, acne, male pattern baldness, sleep apnea, high liver function analysis, abnormal amount of blood lipids, worsening of a pre-existing psychotic or manic disorder and hypertension.

On the other hand, the risk of permanent sterility increases with prolonged use of hormones, especially when therapy is started before puberty.

8. With a hormonal treatment is it possible to achieve a complete body modification?

Although many changes are achieved that allow to resemble the desired gender, some physical characteristics cannot be modified and require surgical interventions to complete the transition.

In cases of moving from woman to man, the breast tissue, the uterus, the ovaries and the vagina are removed, and an artificial penis and testicles are created that fulfill their sexual function.

It is important to clarify that the autonomy and freedom of the patient to manage his own body is respected at all times, and it is he who decides what medical or surgical stage he wishes to reach.

Chapter 140. The micropenis and its treatment

A penis with a normal structure, but whose size is smaller than the common range for a baby, is defined as micropenis. Usually, the length of this organ in a newborn male ranges between 2.8 and 4.2 centimeters, with a circumference of 0.9 to 1.3 centimeters.

When it has a length of less than 1.9 centimeters, it is considered a micropenis. Usually, this medical condition is a consequence of alterations in the hypothalamic-pituitary-testicular axis, which causes abnormal levels of hormones that participate in the development of the sexual organs.

To learn more about this condition, we consulted Dr. Mario Vega Carbó, an endocrinology specialist, who currently works at the Vega & Vado Office.

Doctor Mario,
1. What are the causes of the micropenis?

This disorder is due to a hormonal abnormality produced from the twelfth week of gestation. The most frequent cause is idiopathic, followed by hypogonadism, iatrogen, genital malformations and polymorphic syndromes.

2. How is this condition detected?

After a physical examination, in which it is constant that the penis is less than 1.9 centimeters, a complete endocrinological study of the hypothalamic-pituitary-testicular axis should be performed. In some cases, this medical condition may be accompanied by a low sperm count, the consequence of which may be infertility or a decrease in it.

On the other hand, it is also important to differentiate the micropenis from those situations in which the organ is normal, but seems smaller due to other factors. For example, the buried penis is hidden in suprapubic fat, which can appear in obese children or secondary to major phimosis.

Similarly, the downed penis is due to an alteration of the suspensory ligament, while in the webbed penis the scrotal skin extends to the ventral side of the organ, which causes it to be fixed to the scrotum.

3. What is the treatment for the micropenis?

The therapy will depend on the age of the patient, his general state of health and medical history, the severity of the disease and tolerance to medications. One of the options is hormonal treatment with testosterone to stimulate penis growth. It is recommended to start it during the first months of life, because at this stage there is a greater endowment and affinity of androgenic receptors, followed by higher doses at the beginning of puberty.

On the other hand, pituitary hormone injections can help produce sperm. If this treatment is not satisfactory, reconstructive surgery can be performed once you reach adulthood.

Chapter 141. Gynecomastia and enlarged breasts in men

Gynecomastia is a disorder in which man's breast tissue swells, as a result of a reduction in male hormones (testosterone) or an increase in female hormones (estrogen).

In some cases this condition can occur during puberty and resolve spontaneously. It can also occur in babies born, elderly people or be the result of the consumption of certain drugs or medications. This medical condition can affect one or both breasts, sometimes unevenly.

Gynecomastia is usually not a serious problem, but it can damage the patient's self-esteem and make him feel uncomfortable and ashamed.

To learn more about this problem, we interview Dr. Mario Vega Carbó, specialist in clinical endocrinology.

Doctor Mario,
1. What are the main symptoms of gynecomastia?

Its characteristic signs are inflammation of the tissue of the mammary glands and pain to the touch, which can be mild or constant. In some cases there may also be secretions from the nipple of one or both breasts.

2. What are its causes?

Gynecomastia is caused by a decrease in the amount of testosterone compared to the amount of estrogen in the body. This may be a consequence of hormonal changes or other external factors.

In newborn babies, it is usually due to the effects of the mother's estrogen and her symptoms usually disappear two to three weeks after birth.

At puberty it occurs quite frequently and dissipates without treatment. In adults, it affects 1 in 4 men between 50 and 70 years old, as a result of hormonal changes that occur during aging.

On the other hand, among the medications that can cause this ailment are the antiandrogens used to treat enlarged prostate, anabolic steroids and androgens used to improve athletic performance, efavirenz, anxiolytics such as diazepam, tricyclic antidepressants, antibiotics and some remedies for the ulcer and the heart.

3. What diseases can affect the normal balance of these hormones?

There are several conditions that can cause gynecomastia. Among them are hypogonadism, in which the body does not produce enough testosterone; Klinefelter syndrome, a genetic condition suffered by men who have two or more X chromosomes; some tumors such as those affecting the testicles, adrenal glands or pituitary gland; hyperthyroidism; renal or hepatic impairment; cirrhosis; the obesity; Malnutrition and starvation.

4. What other substances can cause gynecomastia?

Drinking alcohol and drugs such as marijuana, heroin, methadone and amphetamines can also cause this condition. Some herbs, such as lavender, tea tree oil and dong quai that are used in shampoos, soaps and lotions have also been linked to this disorder.

5. How is this condition diagnosed?

To confirm your symptoms, the doctor usually performs a physical exam that may include an evaluation of breast tissue, abdomen, armpit and genitals. Blood tests, mammograms, and other tests may be indicated to determine its cause and rule out other conditions that may cause the same signs, such as adipose tissue in the chest, breast cancer, or mastitis.

In addition, studies may be necessary to determine if the liver, kidneys and thyroid are functioning properly.

6. What is the treatment of gynecomastia?

The treatment will depend on the cause that causes it. If it is a consequence of a pre-existing disease, such as hypogonadism or certain tumors, these conditions should be treated with their respective therapies.

If the condition is due to a medication, the professional who follows the therapy may recommend that you stop taking it or replace it with another. In very annoying and notorious cases, it is possible to perform surgery to remove excess breast tissue, either through a liposuction or a mastectomy.

On the other hand, androgens, anti-estrogens, aromatase inhibitors and danazol can also be used to treat this condition. Low dose radiation therapy may be effective for some particular cases.

In any case, in most cases, Gynecomastia resolves over time without doing anything.

7. What other aspects must be taken into account during treatment?

Gynecomastia can cause emotional and psychological problems. It is a difficult condition to hide that damages the patient's self-esteem and, especially during adolescence, can generate many conflicts, social isolation, anxiety, stress and depression. Therefore, it is recommended to accompany the treatment with psychological and family support.

8. Can this ailment be prevented?

In some cases yes and in others no. To reduce your risks it is recommended to lead a healthy life and diet, to exercise regularly, not to consume alcohol or illegal drugs and to control the medications that are taken to see if Gynecomastia is among its side effects.

Chapter 142. Klinefelter syndrome

Klinefelter Syndrome (SK) is a genetic condition suffered by men who have two or more X chromosomes in their sex chromosomes. The vast majority of those affected have small and firm testicles, which have their diminished functions and produce less testosterone.

Other common symptoms are infertility, abnormal breast enlargement, short hair, tall stature, reduced penis size and infrequent body proportions, such as wide hips and long legs and arms in relation to the trunk.

During adolescence there may be an absent, delayed or incomplete puberty, although the signs vary from one person to another. This medical condition occurs in 1 in 500 to 1,000 babies born.

To learn more about this topic, we interview Dr. Mario Vega Carbó, specialist in clinical endocrinology.

Doctor Mario,
1. What are the causes of Klinefelter Syndrome?

Most humans have 46 chromosomes, which contain their genetic information. The two sex chromosomes, known as X and Y, determine whether they will be male or female.

Men usually have 1 X chromosome and another Y. Klinefelter Syndrome occurs when they have more than one X chromosome between sex chromosomes, which occurs for unknown causes that are not inherited.

2. How is the SK discovered?

In general, Klinefelter Syndrome is diagnosed in adulthood, when there are sexual and infertility problems, because in childhood there are usually no signs of differences.

To confirm the condition, an analysis of the chromosomes known as karyotype and hormonal tests of blood, urine and semen is performed.

3. Are there any special features that can be perceived during childhood and adolescence?

Children with SK usually have learning problems, especially in the areas of communication and verbal expression.

In adolescence, this behavior is associated with an increase in aggression and irritability, difficulties for socialization and a tendency to conduct and solitary activities.

4. Does a child with Klinefelter syndrome have mental retardation?

Although there is no mental retardation, as I said before, it is very possible that you have learning problems in some areas, which is good to treat on time. On the other hand, many patients with SK have different talents that are important to look for and develop.

5. If confirmed, what is the treatment of Klinefelter Syndrome?

In general, a hormonal treatment with testosterone is used to promote the growth of body hair, a serious voice, increased body mass, concentration, self-esteem, energy and sexual drive. This can also improve bone density and reduce the risk of fractures.

Together with an endocrinologist, therapy should also include the consultation of a physiotherapist, a specialist in reproductive medicine and psychological or psychiatric support.

Most men with Klinefelter Syndrome will continue to be infertile, but today's assisted reproduction procedures allow some to have children.

On the other hand, people who have an enlarged breast may remove excess tissue through surgery.

6. What other complications can this ailment bring?

People with SK may have an enlarged tooth known as taurodontism, which is characterized by the elongated shape of the pulp chamber. These are more likely to suffer from hyperactivity and attention deficit disorders, breast cancer, anxiety, depression, dyslexia, diabetes, hypothyroidism, leukemia, lupus, rheumatoid arthritis, lung and heart disease, osteoporosis and testicular tumors.

7. Does the SK affect the gender identity and sexual preferences of the patient?

The extra amount of X chromosomes is not related to sexual identification, orientation and preferences, which are determined by other factors.

As for the physical appearance, beyond the already mentioned signs that can be avoided with the administration of testosterone, the body conformation is almost identical to that of an unaffected male.

Chapter 143. Kallmann syndrome and the sense of smell

Kallmann syndrome is a rare genetic disorder that affects the normal functioning of the hypothalamus and sex glands. It is characterized by the deficiency of gonadotropin-releasing hormone (GnRH) and loss of sense of smell.

This condition is one of the causes of hypogonadism, a disease that appears when the gonads do not secrete the proper amount of hormones, causing sterility and other disorders. The symptoms of Kallmann syndrome vary depending on age.

To learn more about this problem, we interview Dr. Mario Vega Carbó, specialist in clinical endocrinology.

Doctor Mario,
1. What causes Kallmann syndrome?

This disorder has a genetic origin, mainly associated with the genes KAL1, FGFR1, FGF8, PROK2 and PROKR2. Patients usually have mutations in one or more of these genes, due to environmental and hereditary factors.

2. What are your main symptoms?

The main characteristic of Kallmann syndrome is the partial or total loss of the sense of smell. When it occurs in childhood, children also usually present micropenis and the absence of one or two testicles in the scrotal bag. Meanwhile, in adolescence there is an incomplete sexual maturation and signs of hypogonadism.

In adulthood, there may be growth problems in men; low bone and muscle mass; poor development of the genitals, body hair and voice; infertility; erectile dysfunction and loss of sexual desire.

In women it can affect the development of breasts and height and cause absent menstrual cycles, hot flashes, vaginal dryness, mood swings and sterility. Other less frequent symptoms are dental defects, cleft lip, hearing and kidney problems, and color blindness.

3. How is this disease detected?

In the face of its symptoms, a physical examination is usually done in search of alterations in sexual development, and tests to measure hormone levels and olfactory capacity. Neuroimaging studies may also be necessary to evaluate brain structures and genetic tests.

4. What is your treatment?

Generally a hormone replacement therapy is applied, with the aim of inducing puberty and, subsequently, fertility. In men the most common is the administration of testosterone, chorionic gonadotropin and follicle-stimulating hormone to achieve a complete development of male sexual characteristics and stimulate sperm production.

In women, estrogens, gonadotrophins and progestogens are applied to stimulate breast development, pubic hair and other female sexual characteristics, in addition to the endometrial cycle.

5. How is the administration of these hormones?

There are different forms of administration. The most common are through oral pills, but there are also skin patches, creams, gels, injections and tablets. All are equally effective.

6. What can you expect from this therapy?

Proper hormonal treatment will cause the onset of puberty, sexual maturation and can restore fertility. However, at the moment there is no therapy to treat loss of smell.

7. What other complications can Kallmann syndrome bring?

Among other inconveniences this ailment can cause a delay of puberty, sterility, low bone density and sexual and emotional problems. If necessary, psychological support is recommended.

Chapter 144. Causes and main symptoms of Noonan Syndrome

Noonan syndrome is a genetic disorder that causes abnormal development in various parts of the body. In many cases it can be transmitted from parents to children, although it can also be caused by a spontaneous mutation, without family history. This condition can cause unusual facial features, short stature, heart problems and possible developmental delays.

To learn more about this topic, we interview Mario Vega Carbó, an endocrinology specialist, in charge of the Vega & Vado Office in Managua, Nicaragua.

Doctor Mario,
1. What causes Noonan Syndrome?

This disorder is caused by a genetic mutation. In general, these defects cause certain proteins to become hyperactive and disrupt the normal process of growth and cell division.

Mutations can be inherited or present randomly. The children of a father with Noonan Syndrome have a 50 percent chance of getting it.

2. What are your main physical symptoms?

The signs vary from one person to another and can be mild or severe. Most have differences in the shape of the face and head, which are more noticeable in infants and young children. Some characteristic features are widely separated blue or green eyes, thick ears and low implantation, a deep groove between the nose and mouth, small lower jaw, short neck, droopy eyelids and crooked teeth.

In addition, they may have short stature, sunken sternum, separate nipples, small penis and undescended testicles.

3. What other features do they usually have?

Those who suffer from Noonan Syndrome usually have a delay in puberty, vision and hearing impairments, bruises and excessive bleeding, and slow weight gain.

On the other hand, they may have heart defects, skin diseases, growth and feeding problems, learning difficulties and a slight intellectual disability. Also emotional and behavioral disorders.

4. How is Nooman Syndrome detected?

In view of its symptoms, the patient's clinical and family history is usually analyzed and a physical examination is performed to confirm the diagnosis. In addition, depending on the case, a platelet count, hormonal level measurement, chest radiography, echocardiogram, audiometry and genetic tests, among other studies, can be carried out.

5. What is your treatment?

Nooman Syndrome has no cure, since there is no way to repair the changes it produces in genes. However, different therapies can be followed to relieve your symptoms. For example, a treatment with growth hormone can treat short stature, while some drugs can fix bleeding and bleeding.

On the other hand, certain medications and surgery can solve some heart problems and correct undescended testicles. The use of glasses solves most vision problems and educational programs can help a child who has learning difficulties. The same speech therapy and physiotherapy.

6. What other complications can Nooman Syndrome cause?

This condition can cause a buildup of fluid in body tissues, developmental delays, urinary infections, increased risk of leukemia and other cancers, male infertility and problems with the structure of the heart. In addition, as a consequence of physical symptoms, there may be depression, low self-esteem and social problems.

Chapter 145. Erectile Dysfunction

Erectile Dysfunction is the frequent inability that a man has to get or maintain an erection in order to have satisfactory sex. This may occur at any age, but it is more common after age 65.

In most cases it is due to physical problems, although it can also be due to psychological or emotional issues, a combination of both or an external factor, such as the intake of certain medications. Some men may have sporadic inconvenience to get an erection. If this occurs continuously, it is advised to consult a doctor.

In addition to sexual discomfort, Erectile Dysfunction can be a sign of other health problems, such as clogged blood vessels or a nerve injury.

To talk about this topic, we interview Dr. Mario Vega Carbó, an endocrinology specialist with more than 20 years of clinical experience.

Doctor Mario,
1. What are the main reasons for Erectile Dysfunction?

Among the physical causes, this may be due to diseases such as Diabetes, high blood pressure, heart or thyroid conditions, clogged blood vessels, low testosterone levels, spinal cord injury, Parkinson's, multiple sclerosis, high cholesterol, obesity or nervous system disorders.

Among the psychological ones are stress, anxiety, depression, lack of self-esteem, previous traumatic sexual episodes, fear of failure, sleep disorders, poor communication and relationship problems.

On the other hand, Erectile Dysfunction may also occur due to the use of certain medications such as antidepressants or sleeping pills, or excessive alcohol and drug use. Physical causes are more common in older men and emotional causes in young people.

2. What are your symptoms?

The most frequent signs are persistent problems to achieve or maintain an erection, or that this is not firm enough to have a sexual relationship. There may also be lack of desire and less interest in sex.

3. How are the causes of this disorder detected?

In front of its signs, physical, blood and urine tests will be performed to measure the hormonal level, cholesterol and glucose, and look for conditions such as diabetes or heart problems.

On the other hand, an ultrasound of the penis may be necessary to look for circulation problems and psychological tests to analyze possible emotional causes. If the patient has erections in the morning or at night while sleeping, it is probably not a physical problem.

4. What is your treatment?

The therapy will depend on the cause of the problem. If it is a hormonal difference, testosterone can be applied through skin patches, gel or intramuscular injections. In the case of diabetes, heart problems or other chronic diseases, they must be controlled.

Certain oral medications, such as sildenafil (Viagra), avanafil, vardenafil and tadalafil are very effective in treating Erectile Dysfunction. Other drugs that are placed in the urethra or injected into the penis (alprostadil) improve blood flow. Some patients prefer the use of penile pump, a device that helps erection.

If these treatments do not work, by surgery implants can be placed in the penis. If the inconvenience is a medication that is being taken, it may be replaced by another.

From an emotional and psychological point of view, it is recommended to talk openly about the issue with the couple and, if necessary, consult a therapist specializing in sexual and relationship problems.

5. Can Viagra and other related medications have serious side effects?

Yes, these drugs can cause from muscle and headaches, nasal congestion, redness, visual disturbances and stomach upset, to a heart attack. Therefore, they are not recommended for patients who have severe heart disease or who have had a stroke or a recent heart attack.

Nor is it recommended for people with uncontrolled diabetes or with very low or very high blood pressure. It is important that they be prescribed by a doctor. On the other hand, if the use of these medications causes an erection that lasts more than 4 hours, help should be sought urgently.

6. What other recommendations can be taken into account?

To have a better sex life it is advisable to eat healthy, exercise daily, maintain an adequate body weight, sleep well, do not smoke and avoid alcohol and drugs. Also avoid stress and conflict situations, and learn to improve self-esteem and accept one's body as it is. If you have Diabetes, it is important to keep your blood sugar level well controlled.

Chapter 146. Male Infertility

Male Infertility is a medical term used when a man has difficulty getting a woman pregnant, after a year of frequent sexual intercourse without protection. This can be due to various reasons, such as physical or hormonal problems, injuries, illnesses, environmental factors or related to lifestyle.

Once the cause is found, it can be treated with medication, surgery or the use of assisted reproduction techniques.

To learn more about this topic, we consulted Dr. Mario Vega Carbó, an endocrinology specialist, who is in charge of the Vega & Vado Office.

Doctor Mario,
1. What are the main causes of Male Infertility?

There are many reasons that can cause it. In the vast majority of cases the problem is in the testicles, which are responsible for producing sperm and testosterone, the male sex hormone.

Injuries, infections, radiation, chemotherapy, surgeries or certain genetic diseases can damage them and affect their functioning. Heat can also impair sperm production, as is the case with varicoceles (enlarged veins around the testicles).

Infertility can also be due to an obstruction of the vas deferens, tubes that lead semen to the penis. This may be the result of an infection, a vasectomy or cystic fibrosis. Other possible causes are hormonal deficiencies, ejaculation problems, undescended testicles, chronic diseases, tumors, obesity, the use of certain medications and drug use.

In addition, excessive exposure to certain environmental elements, such as heat, toxins and chemicals, can also reduce sperm production or function.

2. What other diseases can cause infertility?

Some inherited conditions, such as Klinefelter Syndrome, suffered by men who have two or more X chromosomes, can cause abnormal development of the reproductive organs. Celiac disease, cystic fibrosis, Kallmann syndrome and Kartagener syndrome can also cause infertility.

3. What are the main symptoms of Male Infertility?

In addition to the inability to conceive, other frequent signs include difficulties in ejaculation, reduced libido, erectile dysfunction, pain or swelling in the testicle area, inability to feel odors, abnormal breast growth and decreased body hair.

4. Who is more at risk of suffering it?

Men who smoke tobacco, those who are overweight, those who suffered sexually transmitted infections, those who drink alcohol excessively and those who use illegal drugs are more likely to suffer infertility. Also those who suffer from stress or depression, those who are exposed to certain toxins, those who had trauma to the testicles or pelvic surgery and those who have certain diseases.

5. How is this disorder detected?

In view of its symptoms, an analysis of the patient's medical history and various studies are performed to look for its causes. Tests may include physical and blood tests to control hormone levels; genetic, semen and urine tests; ultrasound of the scrotum and transrectal to detect enlarged veins, tumors or obstructions; and testicular biopsy.

6. What is the treatment for Male Infertility?

The therapy will depend on the cause. This may include medications, surgery or the use of techniques that help conception. Surgery can repair obstructions and varicoceles, and reverse vasectomies. Meanwhile, if there is a hormonal deficiency, treatment can improve sperm production.

Antibiotics can cure infections in the reproductive tract and certain medications can treat erectile dysfunction. Within assisted reproduction, artificial insemination or in vitro fertilization can be performed.

If the cause is another illness or a psychological or emotional problem, they should be treated. If it is due to the consumption of a certain medicine, the doctor may replace it with another.

7. What other recommendations can be taken into account?

To increase the chances of success, it is recommended to lead a healthy lifestyle. It is advisable to eat healthy, exercise daily, maintain an adequate body weight, sleep well, do not smoke and avoid drinking alcohol. Also avoid stress, exposure to toxins and situations in which the testicles may be exposed to heat for a long time.

On the other hand, male infertility is often due to psychological and emotional issues and can lead to depression. Therefore, psychological support is recommended, if necessary.

Chapter 147. Spermatogram

The spermatogram is an analysis that is performed to measure the quantity and quality of a man's semen and sperm. It allows you to check your reproductive capacity and find abnormalities that hinder conception.

During the study, macroscopic and microscopic parameters of sperm are evaluated, including ejaculate volume, color, viscosity, pH and liquefaction. The way in which the semen solidifies and then becomes liquid, its thickness, acidity and the presence of binders and white blood cells is also analyzed.

Likewise, a sperm count is performed and their mobility, vitality and morphology are studied.

To learn more about this topic, we interviewed Cuban doctor Mario Vega Carbó, a specialist in clinical endocrinology.

Doctor Mario,
1. What is a spermatogram done for?

This study is done to evaluate a man's fertility and determine if any inconvenience in sperm production or quality is causing problems to conceive. Their results are very useful to indicate personalized treatments to the couple.

On the other hand, the test can also be performed after a vasectomy to confirm that there is no sperm in the semen and thus ensure the success of the intervention. This test is done to diagnose Klinefelter Syndrome, a genetic condition suffered by men who have two or more X chromosomes.

2. What is the preparation for this exam?

Before the study, the patient should avoid any sexual activity that generates an ejaculation for 3 days, to ensure sperm quality.

3. How is the sample collection done?

The person should masturbate and ejaculate in a sterile jar or cup. It is recommended that the sample be examined by a specialist within half an hour, since the faster it is analyzed, the more accurate the results will be.

On the other hand, taking into account the daily fluctuations in semen quality, it is advisable to evaluate two or three samples of different days, to have a more reliable diagnosis.

4. What are the expected results during this study?

In general, within the normal values the semen volume varies from 1.5 to 5 milliliters per ejaculation and it must be fully liquefied after 60 minutes.

As for sperm, the number per milliliter must be greater than 15 million, at least 60% must be alive and have normal movement, and the morphology must be greater than 4 percent. Meanwhile, the pH value must be greater than 7.1.

However, an abnormal result does not always mean that the patient cannot conceive.

5. What can the abnormal results mean?

In these cases, if the sperm count is too low or too high, it may mean that the person is less fertile. On the other hand, the acidity and the presence of white blood cells can mark the existence of an infection, while a pH lower than 7.1 could indicate the absence of sperm or chronic inflammatory processes.

Meanwhile, if the sample is very viscous, it may be due to prostate dysfunction. Also, if more than 50 percent of the sperm are attached to other cells or particles, there may be an immune problem.

6. What aspects can affect a man's fertility?

There are many reasons that can affect it. In the vast majority of cases the problem is in the testicles, which are responsible for producing sperm and testosterone, the male sex hormone. Injuries, infections, radiation, chemotherapy, surgeries or certain genetic diseases can damage them and affect their functioning.

Heat can also impair sperm production, as is the case with varicoceles (enlarged veins around the testicles). Infertility can also be due to an obstruction of the vas deferens, tubes that lead semen to the penis. This may be the result of an infection, a vasectomy or cystic fibrosis.

Other possible causes are hormonal deficiencies, ejaculation problems, undescended testicles, chronic diseases, tumors, obesity, the use of certain medications and the consumption of alcohol and drugs.

In addition, excessive exposure to certain environmental elements, such as heat, toxins and chemicals, can also reduce sperm production or function.

Chapter 148. Hypogonadism and the sex glands

Hypogonadism is a condition that occurs when the sex glands, known as gonads, do not secrete the proper amount of hormones.

In men these glands are the testicles and produce testosterone, which influences the development of sexual organs, the maintenance of bones and muscles, the production of sperm and white blood cells, and libido. In women it is the ovules, which primarily generate estrogen and progesterone, and a small amount of testosterone.

These hormones regulate the menstrual cycle and pregnancy, secondary sexual characteristics, and act on other organs and systems of the body.

Hypogonadism can have various causes, be congenital or appear over the years. One of its main consequences is sterility.

To learn more about this disorder, we interview Mario Vega Carbó, an endocrinologist with more than 20 years of experience.

Doctor Mario,
1. What causes hypogonadism?

This condition can occur for various reasons. On the one hand there may be some specific problem in the testicles and ovaries that prevent them from functioning properly. It can be a consequence of inconveniences in the immune system, infections, liver and kidney diseases, trauma and exposure to surgery, radiation or chemotherapy.

There may also be genetic and developmental disorders, such as Turner, Kallman and Klinefelter Syndromes, or due to other diseases, such as a problem in the hypothalamus or pituitary gland, anorexia nervosa, tumors and trauma, as well as certain medications, nutritional deficiencies and Excess iron are other triggers.

2. What are your symptoms?

In women, hypogonadism can affect breast development and height and cause absent menstrual cycles, hot flashes, vaginal dryness, mood swings and infertility. His condition is normal during menopause. In men it also causes growth problems and afflicts muscle, genital, body hair and voice development. In addition, it can cause breast growth, infertility, erectile dysfunction and loss of sexual desire.

On the other hand, hypogonadism can also cause mental and emotional changes, and abnormal genitalia.

3. How is this disease detected?

In the face of their symptoms, a physical examination is usually performed; tests to measure hormone levels and the function of the pituitary and thyroid; blood and chromosome analysis; sperm count and other studies to confirm your diagnosis.

4. What is your treatment?

In these cases a hormone replacement therapy is usually applied, to replace those that are not occurring naturally.

For women, estrogens and progesterone are used, which stimulate the development of breast and pubic hair, and other sexual characteristics. These hormones also help protect against osteoporosis and some types of cancer, prevent urinary infections and improve mood. In some cases, injections or pills may be used to stimulate ovulation.

In men, testosterone is used to promote the growth of body hair, serious voice, increased body mass, concentration, energy and sexual drive. Pituitary hormone injections can help them produce sperm

5. How is the administration of these hormones?

There are different forms of administration. The most common are through oral pills, but there are also skin patches, creams, gels, injections and tablets. All are equally effective.

6. What other complications can this disease bring?

Hypogonadism can increase the risks of osteoporosis and heart disease. In some women, prolonged use of hormonal therapy may increase the chances of breast cancer, blood clots and heart ailments.

7. What other recommendations are provided for these cases?

A good physical condition, with a normal body weight and healthy eating habits can help in the prevention of some cases of hypogonadism.

Chapter 149. Andropause or "male menopause"

Andropause is called the fall in the hormonal level in men that occurs with aging. Although they are not quite similar, it is usually associated with female menopause due to some similar symptoms. This disorder begins to manifest from the age of 40, although its signs are not as defined as in the case of women.

All men have a decrease in testosterone levels starting at age 30. When they go down a lot Andropause appears. Apart from physical factors, psychological, social and emotional aspects also influence its appearance.

To learn more about this topic, we interview Mario Vega Carbó, an endocrinologist with more than 20 years of experience.

Doctor Mario,
1. What is testosterone and what is its function?

Testosterone is a hormone produced in the testicles that influences many physical, biochemical and mental functions of man. It is essential in the development and growth, and when you reach adulthood it is responsible for maintaining strong bones and muscles, desire and sexual capacity, and producing red blood cells and sperm, among other tasks.

2. What are the symptoms of Andropause?

Its main signs are progressive tiredness, decreased sexual desire and alterations in ejaculation. Also less strength and physical endurance, more dry hair and skin, cold hands and feet, and loss of memory and concentration.

On the other hand, vision, testicular size and semen amount are reduced; and increases sweating, muscle weakness and body fat. There may be erectile dysfunction and a tendency to moodiness, signs of depression, prolonged headaches and increased anxiety, irritability and insomnia.

3. Can some diseases increase your risks?

Yes, people suffering from metabolic syndrome, Diabetes Mellitus, cardiovascular system disorders or high blood pressure are more likely to suffer from Andropause.

4. What is your treatment?

With aging it is normal for these symptoms to occur gradually. If testosterone levels are very low and the decrease occurs suddenly, a hormone replacement treatment can be performed and applied orally, in gel or through intramuscular injections.

5. What benefits does this therapy offer?

Testosterone treatment allows the patient to achieve an increase in desire and sexual activity, an increase in erection and feel more energized. This can also increase muscle mass and improve bone density and general mood.

6. What is the danger of self-medication with high doses of testosterone?

Elevated testosterone levels can cause an increase in the prostate, red blood cells and cholesterol. Its use also contributes to sleep apnea and the formation of blood clots in the veins. On the other hand, it increases the risks of prostate cancer, heart attack and stroke.

That is why it is important to consult a doctor to see if hormonal treatment is adequate and really necessary.

7. What other recommendations can those who suffer from Andropause take into account?

To improve your symptoms it is advised to lead a healthy life. This includes a balanced diet, exercising daily, maintaining an adequate body weight, sleeping well, not smoking and avoiding the consumption of caffeine, alcohol and drugs.

Also avoid stress and, in case of depression, seek therapeutic help and discuss the issue with the couple and with friends of the same age.

Chapter 150. Testosterone Treatment

In men, the testicles are responsible for secreting testosterone, a hormone that influences the development of sexual organs, the maintenance of bones and muscles, the production of sperm and white blood cells, and libido.

In patients with hypogonadism, a condition that occurs when the gonads do not generate the proper amount of this substance, hormone replacement therapy is one of the available alternatives. There are different ways to apply testosterone. The most common through oral pills, but can also be supplied by creams, gels, injections and tablets, all being equally effective.

To learn more about this topic, we interview Dr. Mario Vega Carbó, specialist in clinical endocrinology.

Doctor Mario,
1. In which cases is testosterone therapy used?

This treatment is generally used in adult men with low levels of the hormone caused by disorders in the testicles, pituitary gland or hypothalamus.

In children and adolescents its use could stop the growth of bones and cause early puberty. In those with hypogonadism it allows puberty to evolve normally and secondary sexual characters appear.

In women, it can cause a serious voice, hair growth in unusual places, genital enlargement, decreased breast size, male pattern hair loss and irregular menstrual cycles. Its use during pregnancy or breastfeeding could harm the baby.

2. What benefits does testosterone treatment offer?

Depending on what it is used for, it can promote hair growth and increase body mass, concentration, energy and sex drive. It can also improve bone density, erections and general mood.

3. How is this medicine used?

Testosterone through pills is usually taken with meals twice a day. The topical gel presentation is applied once a day in the morning and must be expected to dry. It should not be placed on the penis or scrotum or in areas of the skin with sores, cuts or irritation. You should also avoid contact with the eyes.

Meanwhile, subcutaneous injections are applied every 10 or 20 days, while intramuscular injections are placed every 3 months.

4. What should be done if you forget to take a dose of this medicine?

You should ingest it as soon as you remember. However, if it is almost time for the next dose, it is better to skip it and continue with the regular dosage. In no case should a double dose be taken to compensate for the one that was forgotten.

5. What side effects can testosterone use have?

Elevated testosterone levels can cause an increase in the prostate, red blood cells and cholesterol. Its use also contributes to sleep apnea and the formation of blood clots in the veins. On the other hand, it increases the risks of heart attack and stroke.

Other possible side effects are stroke, liver disease, heartburn, diarrhea, gas, headache, breast enlargement, shortness of breath, decreased sperm count, seizures and changes in mental health, such as depression, aggressive behavior or hostile and hallucinations.

That is why it is important to consult a doctor to see if hormonal treatment is adequate and really necessary. If yes, testosterone should be taken exactly as directed by the doctor.

6. What other aspects should be taken into account during use?

Before starting the treatment it is important to inform the doctor about any other medication, vitamin or supplement that is being used, so that it evaluates whether the combination can be harmful. You should notify if you suffer from allergies or other conditions, such as hypertension or kidney, heart or prostate problems.

On the other hand, topical testosterone products can cause harmful effects to people who touch the skin in the area where the gel or solution was applied.

In turn, the injection can cause serious breathing problems and allergic reactions during or immediately after application.

Finally, these medications should be stored in a suitable place, at room temperature and out of the reach of children.

Chapter 151. Anabolic Steroids and their dangers

Anabolic Steroids are male sex hormones, or synthetic substances based on them, that are used for different purposes.

Within the field of medicine, they are used to treat hormonal problems, late puberty and loss of muscle mass as a result of various diseases. In sports and athletics, they are used to improve performance. However, its consumption is illicit and can cause serious health problems.

Among other harmful effects, Anabolic Steroids can cause cardiovascular problems and the development of liver or testicular tumors.

To talk about this topic, we interviewed Dr. Mario Vega Carbó, an endocrinology specialist, in charge of the Vega & Vado Office.

Doctor Mario,
1. Why do some people use Anabolic Steroids for non-medical purposes?

These substances promote muscle development and increased strength. They also reduce damage to muscles and help athletes recover faster after an arduous training session. Some people like the muscular appearance generated by the consumption of these steroids.

2. What unwanted effects can its use generate?

Anabolic Steroids can cause serious heart problems, including heart attack, and the development of liver or testicular tumors. Other unwanted effects are intense acne, increased blood pressure, aggressive and violent behavior, abnormal cholesterol levels, psychiatric disorders and drug dependence.

In women it can also cause thickening of the voice, growth of the clitoris and body hair, baldness and menstrual problems. In men, infertility, breast augmentation, reduction of the testicles and enlargement of the prostate. In adolescents, growth inhibition and risk of future health problems.

3. What is Creatine and what risks does it have?

Creatine is a natural body compound that helps muscles release energy. It is sold as a nutritional supplement and is used to increase muscle mass and strength.

Among other side effects it can cause stomach and muscle cramps, weight gain, water retention and dehydration.

4. What is Androstenedione?

It is a hormone that the body converts into testosterone and a form of estrogen. It is used to increase muscle mass and achieve rapid recovery after training, although scientific studies do not confirm that it is effective for it.

Among other risks, this substance can damage the heart and blood vessels. In addition, it can generate acne, reduced sperm production, breast augmentation and decreased testicle size in men, and male baldness and voice in women.

5. How is it possible to detect if a teenager is using Anabolic Steroids?

Some signs are accelerated muscle growth, increased aggression and acne and needle marks on the buttocks or thighs. Also the emotional and psychological changes.

In men there may be an increase in the breasts and a shrinking of the testicles. In women, a decrease in breasts, thickening of the voice and excessive growth of body hair.

6. How do you get these substances?

In most countries its sale is prohibited for sports use. This is why they are usually acquired illegally and in many cases they are made in clandestine laboratories, which further increases their risks.

Chapter 152. Male Androgenic Alopecia

Androgenic Male Alopecia is the most common type of hair loss in men and is related to male sex hormones and genes. It is characterized by a pattern of hair implantation line that regresses and thinning and loss of hair in the temporal, fronto-parietal and vertex regions. It is estimated that it affects 45% of men and its most frequent causes are hereditary factor and age.

To learn more about this topic, we consulted Dr. Mario Vega Carbó, specialist in clinical endocrinology.

Doctor Mario,
1. What causes Male Androgenic Alopecia?

This medical condition can be generated by various factors, including genetic predisposition, age, hormonal changes and chronic diseases, such as insulin resistance and metabolic syndrome. Androgens, especially dihydrotestosterone, have a very important role in the cause of this type of baldness.

On the other hand, it can be caused by the use of certain medications, such as those used to treat cancer, arthritis, depression, heart problems, gout and hypertension; radiotherapy; stress situations; poor diet and excessive use of treatments and hair products.

2. How does this condition occur?

Androgenic Male Alopecia can appear in many ways, depending on the reason that causes it. It can arise suddenly or gradually, and only affect the scalp or the entire body. In a few cases it is temporary, while in the majority it is permanent.

The typical pattern of male baldness begins in the hair implantation line, which gradually recedes and forms an "M". Then the hair becomes thinner and drifts in a horseshoe around the sides of the head.

When hair loss occurs in patches, there is redness, peeling, pus or pain, it can be caused by other causes. In these cases it is recommended to perform skin biopsy, blood tests or other procedures to detect other disorders.

3. What is the treatment of Male Androgenic Alopecia?

Among the medications used to treat this condition are minoxidil in 5% lotion and 5% foam, and finasteride, in doses of 1 milligram per day.

In a few cases, the latter has side effects such as decreased libido, reduced semen, erectile dysfunction, cataracts and soft iris syndrome.

Vegetable drugs Serenoa repens and Pygeun africanum help to inhibit the activity of the enzyme 5α-reductase, which reduces the passage of testosterone to dihydrotestosterone, responsible for the miniaturization of hair follicles.

On the other hand, other topical and systemic antioxidants are also effective and safe to combat hair loss. It is possible to perform a hair transplant, which usually gives very good results. To do this, small portions of hair are removed from areas where it is thicker and placed in others that have baldness. Another option is low intensity light therapy.

If the person is comfortable with their appearance, treatment is not necessary.

4. What other aspects are recommended in these cases?

Hair loss can lower self-esteem and cause depression. Hair extensions, the use of toupees, hats or bandanas, or a change of hairstyle can help hide its effects and improve the appearance.

Massages in the scalp are recommended to activate circulation, avoid stress and treat problems of depression, anxiety, anemia and insomnia quickly, to avoid possible triggers of Androgenic Alopecia.

Part X. Endocrinology in Pediatrics

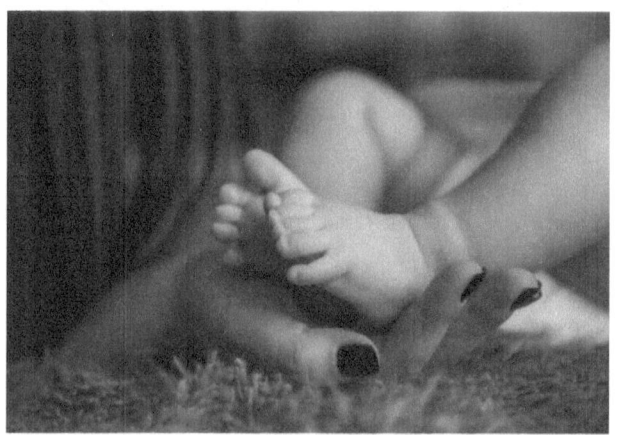

Capítulo 153. Endocrinología Pediátrica

Pediatric Endocrinology is a medical specialty that treats diseases related to the endocrine system in children and adolescents. This includes the set of organs and tissues of the body responsible for hormonal secretions, substances that regulate several of the body's main functions.

The alterations in this system can cause problems in growth and development, metabolism, sleep and aspects related to behavior, among other inconveniences. That is why the importance of being attentive to your symptoms, performing periodic checks and consulting a specialist for any anomaly.

To learn more about this specialty, we interview Mario Vega Carbó, an endocrinologist with more than 20 years of experience.

Doctor Mario,
1. What is the main function of Pediatric Endocrinology?

The main function is to restore the hormonal balance in the body of the child, in case it has been altered by some factor. For this, important glands such as the thyroid, the parathyroid, the pancreas, the adrenal glands, the pituitary gland, the ovaries and the testicles, and the substances that they generate are controlled and treated.

2. What abnormal symptoms should parents of children and adolescents be alert to?

It is important to pay attention to signs such as obesity and growth problems, either because the child is short or very tall for his age, or in relation to the size of his parents. Be alert to puberty abnormalities, such as the appearance of pubic hair and breast development in women and testicular in men before age 9, or by their absence exceeding 13.

Other symptoms that should not be missed are loss or exaggerated weight gain, fatigue, sleepiness, poor school performance, sadness, nervousness, polyuria, palpitations and tremors.

3. How is the first consultation with a Pediatric Endocrinologist?

Usually the child's medical history and family history are analyzed first, and then he is interrogated about possible discomfort. An anthropometric evaluation is then carried out in which its size, weight, head circumference and other body proportions are measured, and a physical examination.

In case of detecting abnormalities other studies and tests are requested and, based on their results, a diagnosis is made and then a treatment is carried out.

4. What are the main causes of consultation of children and adolescents?

The most common are related to growth problems and obesity, an increasingly common disorder in childhood. An obese child is more likely to be also in adulthood.

In addition, this condition is related to the metabolic syndrome, a series of conditions that occur jointly and include high blood pressure, high blood sugar levels, excess body fat around the waist and abnormal cholesterol and triglyceride levels. This increases the risks of suffering from heart or kidney disease, a stroke or diabetes.

5. What other diseases does a Pediatric Endocrinologist treat?

In addition to obesity and short stature, other common ailments are Diabetes, Hypoglycemia, Hypothyroidism, Hyperthyroidism, Rickets, Hypocalcaemia, Hypoparathyroidism, Hyperparathyroidism, Hirsutism, Polycystic Ovary, Congenital Adrenal Hyperplasia, Pituitary Syndrome, Puberty Syndrome, Genital Syndrome of Turner and other hormonal alterations due to tumors located in the endocrine glands.

6. What other aspects are important in Pediatric Endocrinology?

At this stage of life, prevention and education are fundamental, since the habits acquired in childhood are often maintained throughout life. Healthy practices that are initiated and acquired in childhood reduce the risks of osteoporosis, overweight, obesity and other disorders in adulthood.

Chapter 154. Diagnosis and care of Congenital Adrenal Hyperplasia

Congenital Adrenal Hyperplasia (HAC) is an inherited disorder that affects the production of hormones in the adrenal glands, which are found in the upper part of the kidneys. These hormones, such as cortisol and aldosterone, are essential for life, allowing normal growth and regulating metabolism, among other essential functions.

Cortisol adjusts energy levels, blood pressure, blood glucose concentrations, the immune system and the stress response, while aldosterone helps maintain the right amount of sodium in the body by regulating its elimination by urine, sweat glands and intestine. People with HAC also generate more androgens, a hormone that causes early or inappropriate appearance of male characteristics.

To learn more about this condition, we consult Dr. Mario Vega Carbó, an endocrinology specialist, in charge of the Vega & Vado Office.

Doctor Mario,
1. What are the causes of Congenital Adrenal Hyperplasia?

People with HAC lack one of the enzymes used by the adrenal glands to produce hormones, in the vast majority of cases, 21-hydroxylase. It is an inherited disorder where both parents usually have HAC or are carriers of the genetic mutation that causes it.

2. What are the symptoms of a person with Congenital Adrenal Hyperplasia?

Symptoms may vary, depending on the type of HAC the patient has and the age at which it is detected. In childhood, if the condition is mild, it is possible that the person has no signs and is newly diagnosed in adolescence.

In more severe cases, girls usually have abnormal genitals at birth, while in boys the symptoms appear at 2 or 3 weeks and include poor feeding, vomiting, dehydration, abnormal sodium and potassium levels and altered heart rhythm.

3. How is it detected in adolescence?

Women with mild conditions usually have normal reproductive organs and, during adolescence, may begin to experience infrequent or non-existent menstrual periods, excessive body hair, severe acne and clitoral enlargement. Males, on the other hand, may suffer from precocious puberty and have a thick voice, early hair growth on the body and well-developed muscles.

In both cases they will be tall as children, but lower than normal as adults.

4. What is the main complication that this disorder can bring?

People with severe HAC run the risk of having an adrenal crisis, as a result of very low blood cortisol levels. This causes diarrhea, vomiting, dehydration and a drop in sugar in the body that require immediate attention.

5. What is the treatment of Congenital Adrenal Hyperplasia?

The therapy used seeks to normalize hormone levels, by applying hydrocortisone to replace cortisol, mineralocorticoids to replace aldosterone and other medications.

The objectives are to maintain a balance of liquids and salts, blood sugar levels, avoid an adrenal crisis and ensure physical growth and habitual sexual development. For this, it is essential to undergo periodic analysis to see if the doses used should be adjusted.

In the case of girls born with genitals of male appearance, repair surgery can be performed to normalize their appearance and function. It is usually done between 2 and 6 months of age and, sometimes, new procedures are required during puberty or later.

If HAC is detected before birth, it is also possible to prevent the effect of androgens on female genitals by prenatal treatment, using the synthetic hormone dexamethasone.

6. How do you perform these hormones?

There are different forms of administration, it can be via tablets or by intramuscular or intravenous injection.

7. Can they cause side effects?

Treatment usually does not cause unwanted effects, such as obesity or weak bones, since the dose used is to supplant hormones that the body does not naturally produce.

However, if the amount of steroids is high and remains high for a long time, it can cause decreased growth speed and excessive weight gain.

8. What are the expected results of the treatment?

With proper therapy, people with HAC can usually lead a normal life, although they should always be medicated. The majority will not present special or different risks to those of the general population. In situations of significant illness or stress, they may need to take higher doses of the medications.

Chapter 155. Ambiguous Genitals

The term Ambiguous Genitals refers to the fact that the external genital organs of a newborn do not have the typical appearance of a boy or a girl.

It is a rare congenital disorder, which means that doctors cannot immediately determine the sex of the baby. In these cases the genitals may be incompletely developed or have both female and male characteristics. It can also happen that the external sexual organs do not coincide with the internal ones or with the genetic sex of the baby.

In order to learn more about this topic, we interview Mario Vega Carbó, an endocrinology specialist with more than 20 years of experience.

Doctor Mario,
1. Why are Ambiguous Genitals generated?

The first thing to note is that a person's genetic sex is established at the same time of conception. If the father's sperm contains an X chromosome, the baby will be female, and if it has a Y chromosome, it will be male.

On the other hand, the male and female reproductive organs develop from the same tissue in the fetus, and their determination depends on the chromosomes and the presence or absence of male hormones. When this process is altered or interrupted by some circumstance, such as hormonal abnormalities or the mutation of certain genes, Ambiguous Genitalia may appear.

2. What characteristics can these genitals have?

In the case of people of female genetic sex, the enlarged clitoris may have the appearance of a small penis, the urethral opening may be poorly located and the vaginal lips may be closed and look like a scrotum with undescended testicles.

Meanwhile, people of male genetic sex may have a small penis that looks like an enlarged clitoris; the urethral opening may be poorly located; the scrotum may be small and separate, looking like vaginal lips; and the testicles are usually not descended.

3. What are the causes of Ambiguous Genitals?

Among other reasons, this may be a consequence of hermaphroditism, where the child may have parts of male and female genitals, or pseudohermaphroditism, where some physical characteristics of the other sex appear.

It can also be caused by a Congenital Adrenal Hyperplasia, an inherited disorder that affects the production of hormones in the adrenal glands. Other reasons are chromosomal abnormalities, such as Klinefelter and Turner syndromes, lack of production of certain hormones or consumption of certain medications during pregnancy.

On very rare occasions, the mother may also have a tumor that generates male hormones and causes Ambiguous Genitals.

4. Who has more risks of suffering from this disorder?

Since many causes of the Ambiguous Genitals have a hereditary genetic origin, it is important to pay special attention to family history. Among the factors that must be taken into account are unexplained deaths in early childhood, infertility, lack of menstrual periods, genital problems, abnormal physical development during puberty and Congenital Adrenal Hyperplasia.

5. How are Ambiguous Genitals detected?

The medical staff who perform the delivery usually diagnose this disorder at the time of birth. Against their physical signs, genetic tests can determine if a baby is genetically male or female.

In more complicated cases, a chromosomal analysis and other tests such as endoscopy, abdominal radiography and ultrasound of the pelvis can be performed to determine the presence of internal genital structures and the functioning of the reproductive organs. A laparoscopy or a biopsy of the gonads may also be necessary.

6. How is the definitive sex of a baby with Ambiguous Genitals determined?

The decision is made once all the exams and tests mentioned above are finished. Taking into account the cause of this disorder, the genetic sex, the anatomy and the possible sexual and reproductive future of the baby, the medical team recommends to the parents the sex and they must decide whether they are raised as a man or as a woman.

This is a difficult decision, whose long-term social and psychological impact is unpredictable. As the child grows, he can make another decision regarding his sexual identity.

7. What is the treatment of Ambiguous Genitals?

Once the baby's sex is chosen, therapy can begin, which will seek to preserve future sexual activity, fertility and stable identity. Surgery can normalize the aesthetic appearance and function of the genitals. Doctors may suggest operating some patients during childhood. In other cases, the parents can postpone the intervention until the child is old enough to help decide.

On the other hand, hormonal therapy during puberty can solve imbalances in that aspect.

8. What other complications can this disorder bring?

In many cases, the Ambiguous Genitals can cause infertility, sexual and psychological problems, and greater risks of certain types of cancer. On the other hand, some repair surgeries may have imperfect aesthetic and functional results.

9. What other aspects should be taken into account during this disorder?

Given the complexity of the situation, therapeutic support is recommended for the parents and for the child at all times. Also the periodic medical checks to monitor the evolution.

Chapter 156. Cryptorchidism or undescended testicle

Cryptorchidism is a developmental disorder in which one or both testicles fail to get down to the scrotum before birth. This condition is rare and affects about 3% of men. However, the figure increases to almost 30 percent in premature babies.

In most cases the undescended testicle moves spontaneously to its correct position, within the first 4 months of life. When this does not happen it can be relocated by surgery.

To learn more about this disorder, we interview Mario Vega Carbó, an endocrinologist with more than 20 years of experience.

Doctor Mario,
1. What causes cryptorchidism?

The causes that cause it are not known exactly, but it is estimated that it is due to a combination of genetic, environmental and health factors of the mother, which alter hormones and nervous activity that influence the development of the testicles.

2. Who has more risks of having it?

Premature babies, with low birth weight, with a family history of cryptorchidism or other genital development problems, or with Down syndrome have a higher risk of suffering from it. Also the children of mothers who consume alcohol or smoke during pregnancy or of parents who were exposed to pesticides.

3. Can the undescended testicle occur during childhood or pre-adolescence?

In children who did not have cryptorchidism at birth, when their symptoms appear later, it could be due to a retractable testicle, which can move from side to side between the scrotum and groin. The retractable testicle does not require treatment.

4. How is cryptorchidism diagnosed?

This condition is usually detected on a physical exam after birth. In cases where the doctor cannot find the testicles in the scrotum, imaging tests may be performed to determine if they are not present or did not descend.

5. Why is treatment necessary?

In these cases, being located higher in the body, the undescended testicles are exposed to a higher temperature than usual. This could inhibit their development and their ability to make sperm in the future, causing sterility. In addition, there are more risks of developing tumors and cancer, suffering injuries and developing inguinal hernias.

6. What is the treatment?

This disorder is usually corrected with surgery in which the testicle is relocated within the scrotum. In cases where the baby has an inguinal hernia associated with cryptorchidism, it is also treated during the intervention. It is recommended to perform the operation between 6 and 12 months of life, since early treatment reduces the risks of future complications.

Another option is to carry out hormone therapy to relocate the testicle, although it is less effective than surgery.

7. What complications can cryptorchidism bring?

As I said, this disorder can generate testicular damage, sterility and increased cancer risks. After surgery, patients with only one descended testicle usually have an almost normal fertility. In cases where cryptorchidism affects both testicles, the risks of having low sperm numbers, poor quality sperm and sterility are much greater.

Chapter 157. Diagnosis and treatment of Congenital Hypothyroidism

Congenital Hypothyroidism (HC) is a condition in which the thyroid gland is absent or not functioning properly. This condition occurs in 1 in 2,500 to 4,000 babies born, is usually permanent and requires lifelong treatment.

Thyroid hormone is essential for brain development and growth, so if the patient is not treated on time, he may suffer intellectual disabilities and a maturational delay. However, with timely and adequate therapy, they can lead a normal life.

To talk about this topic, we interviewed Dr. Mario Vega Carbó, an endocrinology specialist in charge of the Vega & Vado Office in Managua, Nicaragua.

Doctor Mario,
1. What are the causes of Congenital Hypothyroidism?

Typically, HC occurs when the thyroid gland does not develop properly, either because it is absent, because it is too small, or because it is in an inappropriate part of the neck. In some cases, the gland is developed but does not produce hormones conveniently or does not capture the signal from the pituitary gland.

On the other hand, this condition may also be due to a lack of iodine or medications taken by the mother during pregnancy. His condition is not usually hereditary.

2. What are the main symptoms of HC?

In the first weeks of life it is not easy to detect it without studies. However, in severe cases, the baby may have a swollen face, poor diet, excessive sleep, weak crying, constipation, large tongue and a yellowing of the skin.

However, due to the difficulty of diagnosing in newborns, tests are usually performed to discover the disease. This test is known as neonatal screening and is practiced in medical centers in most Spanish-speaking countries.

3. What is the function of the thyroid?

This gland is responsible for producing and sending thyroid hormones to the blood, which participate in the regulation of metabolism, that is, the speed with which the body uses food to produce the energy necessary for it to perform its daily functions.

That there are usual levels of this hormone in the body is essential for normal growth and development in childhood, and for the functioning of the brain throughout life.

4. What is the treatment of Congenital Hypothyroidism?

HC is treated with Levothyroxine, a pill that contains thyroid hormone. In the case of babies, it should be crushed and administered mixed with water or breast milk using a dropper or syringe.

The dose administered will depend on the size of the body and its degree of maturation, and will have to be adjusted regularly based on the test results. With this medication and periodic checks, the patient will have normal growth and brain development. In most cases, Levothyroxine should be taken for life.

5. What happens if a larger than adequate dose is given?

If ingested more than necessary, the patient may have an accelerated pulse, weight loss, tiredness and hyperactivity. That is why periodic checks are essential for its administration correctly, since in the proper dose it has no side effects.

6. Can levothyroxine be applied together with other medications?

Yes, there is no limitation for the application of vaccines in children or problems with taking other medications.

7. What can happen if HC is not treated on time?

Brain and nervous system development are very important during the first months of life. Therefore, if it is not treated, the HC can cause irreversible damage, such as serious intellectual disability and growth problems.

8. Is a patient with Congenital Hypothyroidism more prone to other diseases?

In general. The majority will not present special or different risks to the rest of the population.

Chapter 158. Children with growth problems

It is common for parents to compare the height of their children with that of friends or classmates of the same age. When they notice that the size differs from the average, they tend to worry and go to the doctor to corroborate if there is a growth problem. However, only 20 percent of children who go to the pediatrician for a short stature suffer from some type of illness.

In most cases, they are developing normally and the differences are due to hereditary issues or a passing pubertal delay. Current growth depends on the combination of a number of factors, including good health, proper nutrition and normal genetic characteristics.

Developmental problems may result from chromosomal abnormalities, hormonal or systemic diseases, malnutrition, congenital disorders or disturbances in the bones and cartilage.

To learn more about this topic, we interview Mario Vega Carbó, an endocrinology specialist, with more than 20 years of experience.

Doctor Mario,
1. What is the importance of periodically controlling the size of children?

Growth represents a very sensitive indicator to assess the general health status of a child, and any deviation from normal parameters represents an alarm.

That is why it is important to evaluate weight, height and developmental speed on a regular basis, to avoid possible diseases. In case of finding any anomaly, it is essential to look for the cause and resolve it.

2. How do you define if a child has growth problems?

Before making a diagnosis, the doctor performs a series of studies in which he measures the size, weight and perimeter of the child's head; and analyzes their body proportions, their general state of health and the parents' height. You can also carry out tests of hormonal function; chromosomal, urine and blood tests; and a blood count.

3. What is the treatment for these cases?

The type of therapy that is implemented depends on the causes that are causing the growth problem. For example, in cases where it is a consequence of gastrointestinal, cardiovascular or renal diseases, a gluten intolerance or a hormonal deficiency, the determined pathology is treated to favor the normal development of the patient.

4. What is the main reason for short stature in childhood and puberty?

One of the most frequent causes is due to what is known as constitutional growth retardation, where there is a slower maturation rate, inherited from one or both parents.

In these cases there is usually a history of family members who were relatively short in childhood, started puberty later and took longer to finish growing, but eventually managed to reach a normal size as adults.

5. What are the causes of a growth hormone deficiency?

Its insufficiency may be due to damage to the pituitary gland or the hypothalamus, whether as a result of a tumor, inherited disorders, blows to the skull or an inflammation or infection in the brain. In some cases it is not possible to determine the exact cause.

6. When is it recommended to use a hormonal treatment?

This therapy is indicated for cases of growth hormone deficiency, renal insufficiency or Turner Syndrome (a genetic condition that some women suffer, caused by the absence or abnormality of the X chromosome).

Also for children born small and do not recover the normal level of development or those with short stature without cause to explain.

7. How are these hormones applied?

The growth hormone is applied through injections, usually at night once a day, either in the front of the thigh, the back of the arms, the abdomen or the buttocks. This treatment is long-term and often lasts several years, in which periodic controls are necessary to adjust the dose to ensure its effectiveness.

The same should be followed until the patient reaches the adult bone age, at which time the bone can no longer grow. In some cases, when there is a hormone deficiency, therapy continues throughout life.

8. What is the expected effect?

The earlier treatment is started, the greater the probability that the patient will reach an adult height close to normal. With hormonal therapy, children generally grow about ten centimeters during the first year and about 7.5 centimeters in the next two. Then the rate decreases progressively.

Growth hormone has been used for many years with great success. One of the best known cases is that of Argentine soccer player Lionel Messi.

9. Can this therapy cause side effects?

Hormonal treatment is safe and has no serious side effects. In some cases there may be skin irritation, headache, fluid retention, joint and muscle aches, and changes in the hip bones.

10. What is the case of children who produce growth hormone greater than normal?

Too much growth hormone can cause gigantism, in which case the bones and body grow too much. This is usually due to a non-carcinogenic tumor in the pituitary gland, which must be treated with radiotherapy or removed through surgery. In adults, this disorder can cause acromegaly, which makes the hands, feet and face larger than normal.

Chapter 159. Precocious Puberty

Puberty is the period of life in which the sexual and physical characteristics of a person develop, and the ability to reproduce is achieved. It is called Precocious Puberty when these changes happen earlier than normal.

This is considered to occur when the body of a child begins to become that of an adult before 8 years of age in the case of women and 9 years in the case of men. Sometimes Precocious Puberty is simply a variant of normal growth. In others, it may be due to infections, hormonal or genetic disorders, tumors or brain abnormalities.

To talk about this topic, we interviewed Dr. Mario Vega Carbó, an endocrinology specialist who currently works as an endocrinologist at the Santa Fe Medical Center and the Vega & Vado Office.

Doctor Mario,
1. What are the main signs of Precocious Puberty?

Some of the frequent signs are the appearance of pubic and underarm hair, rapid growth of height, acne and body odor as an adult. In the case of girls there may be an advanced development of the breasts and vaginal bleeding, and in boys a growth of the testicles and penis, muscle growth, thickening of the voice and facial hair.

2. Why is Precocious Puberty generated?

In some cases the process of body development occurs normally, only earlier than usual. This is called Central Precocious Puberty and usually has no apparent cause or hidden medical problem.

Rarely it may be due to a tumor, a brain or spinal cord injury, radiation exposure, inflammation or diseases such as meningitis, McCune-Albright Syndrome, Congenital Adrenal Hyperplasia or Hypothyroidism.

On the other hand, if the early development of the body is a consequence of premature production of sex hormones, this is known as Peripheral Precocious Puberty. It may be due to problems in the ovaries, testicles, pituitary glands or adrenal glands.

Another cause may be external exposure to sex hormones, such as the use of estrogen or testosterone creams or ointments.

3. How is this condition detected?

In view of its symptoms, the patient's clinical and family history is usually analyzed, and a physical and blood test is performed to check hormone levels. A CT scan or MRI of the brain or abdomen may be done to rule out tumors, and an x-ray to see if the bones are growing too fast.

4. What is your treatment?

Therapy will depend on the cause of Precocious Puberty. If it is a consequence of a tumor, it will be removed by surgery. If it is due to an early secretion of sex hormones, medications may be prescribed to delay its development.

If it is a consequence of the use of estrogen or testosterone creams, its use should be avoided.

5. What other complications can Precocious Puberty bring?

Children with this condition may be short when they reach adults. This is because their bones mature faster than normal and stop their growth early. Early treatment can help them be taller.

On the other hand, Precocious Puberty can generate social and emotional problems in the child, by feeling different from developing before their peers. This can affect your self-esteem and increase depression risks. If necessary, it is recommended to seek psychological support.

Chapter 160. Delayed Puberty

It is called Delayed or Delayed Puberty, when it does not start before the age of 13 in girls and 14 in boys. Puberty is the period of life in which the sexual and physical characteristics of a person develop, and the ability to reproduce is achieved.

In the case of Delayed Puberty these changes may not occur or progress very slowly. This is more common in men than in women.

In most cases the child develops later than his peers, but then sexual maturation occurs normally. In others, the delay may be due to infections, hormonal or genetic disorders, tumors, eating problems or other diseases.

To talk about this topic, we interviewed Dr. Mario Vega Carbó, an endocrinology specialist in charge of the Vega & Vado Office.

Doctor Mario,
1. What are the main signs of a Delayed Puberty?

In men, typical signs include the absence of testicular growth at age 14, the penis is small and immature, there is little hair growth, the body remains thin and short, and the voice remains sharp.

In women, the main symptoms are the absence of breast development at 13 years and menstruation at 16. Generally there is no pubic hair, the uterus has not developed, height is short and growth is slow.

2. Why does Delayed Puberty occur?

Sometimes it is simply a variant of normal growth, which can be inherited. In others it can be caused by chronic conditions, such as Diabetes, Hypogonadism, Celiac disease, inflammatory bowel disease, renal or hepatic deficiencies, autoimmune or genetic disorders, anemia, cystic fibrosis or tumors in the pituitary gland or the hypothalamus.

In men it can also be caused by trauma, infections or lesions in the testicles, or by their absence. In women, being a consequence of eating disorders, such as bulimia or anorexia, or extreme thinness.

Finally, it can also occur in adolescents who exercise excessively, or who received radiotherapy or chemotherapy in cancer treatments.

3. How is this condition detected?

In view of its symptoms, the patient's clinical and family history is generally studied, and a physical and blood test is performed to check hormone levels and a chromosomal analysis. A CT scan or MRI of the brain or abdomen may be performed to rule out tumors, ultrasound of the genital organs, and an x-ray to determine the level of bone maturity.

4. What is your treatment?

Therapy depends on the cause of delayed puberty. If there is a family history of maturational delay, treatment is often not needed and it starts on its own over time. If necessary, sex hormones (testosterone or estrogen) can be applied to start the process.

If the delay is a consequence of a tumor, it will be removed by surgery. If it is caused by another underlying disease, it should be treated.

5. What other complications can Delayed Puberty bring?

The low level of hormones can cause erection problems or early menopause, infertility and osteoporosis. This disorder can generate social and emotional problems in the child, feeling different because they do not develop in the same way as their peers, which can affect their self-esteem and increase the risks of depression. If necessary, it is recommended to seek psychological support.

Chapter 161. Turner Syndrome care and treatments

Turner Syndrome (ST) is a genetic condition that some women suffer, caused by the absence or abnormality of the X chromosome. It is a frequent pathology that affects 1 in 2,500 people of the female sex, without knowing their Causes.

Among other symptoms, those who suffer from it usually have a shorter than normal height and ovarian insufficiency, with a lack of secondary sexual characteristics. They may also have congenital heart disease, kidney abnormalities, diseases of the middle and inner ear and skeletal abnormalities.

From the physical point of view, other visible signs of Turner Syndrome are the low implantation of the ears, short or winged neck, broad chest, narrow palate, small fingers and nails, plump hands and feet, lower lower jaw and droopy eyelids.

To learn more about this condition, we consulted Dr. Mario Vega Carbó, an endocrinology specialist, in charge of the Vega & Vado Office.

Doctor Mario,
1. How is Turner Syndrome detected?

ST can be diagnosed at any stage of life, even before birth if a chromosomal analysis is performed during a prenatal exam. Short stature is its most frequent manifestation. However, in many cases the anomalies derived from the syndrome can become very subtle and may not be noticed before 11 years of age.

In general, if this happens, the analysis is carried out late, when the adolescent consults for example the absence of menstruation or an adult woman due to infertility.

2. In addition to the visible physical signs, what other symptoms do women with ST have?

When they reach adolescence, they can present sexual infantilism, not develop breasts and have absent or very light menstrual periods. Also suffer from vaginal dryness, pain during sexual intercourse and infertility.

In general, patients with TS have normal intelligence, although in some cases they may show some intellectual disability and learning deficit.

3. Does the ST also have other health consequences?

Women with Turner Syndrome are more susceptible to heart, kidney, thyroid and fertility problems. In addition, they may have a particular neurocognitive development and higher incidence of autoimmune diseases.

On the other hand, they are more prone to hearing loss, high blood pressure, diabetes, osteoporosis, cataracts, strabismus, obesity and depression.

4. What is the treatment of ST?

Growth hormone can help a girl with Turner syndrome increase her height. In turn, estrogen and other hormones also stimulate the development of breast and pubic hair, and other sexual characteristics.

Its use also improves fine motor activity, verbal and working memory, attention span, visualization, self-perception and memory. In short, in these patients a hormone replacement therapy is essential to guarantee a convenient feminization and social adaptation, improve cognitive function and avoid the metabolic syndrome derived from early ovarian failure.

5. Can women with TS have children and lead a normal life?

There are reproduction techniques available that can allow them to get pregnant. In any case, pregnancy should be discussed with the attending medical specialist, due to the high incidence of fetal malformations and cases of maternal mortality.

However, through special assisted fertility techniques and using a donated egg, it is already possible for them to carry a pregnancy in their own uterus.

On the other hand, with the right controls, women with Turner Syndrome can have a completely normal life.

Chapter 162. Hyperhidrosis and excessive sweating

Hyperhidrosis is a condition for which a person sweats excessively, even when the temperature is low and he is not doing any physical activity.

Perspiration is the way in which the body regulates body temperature. Through it we eliminate water, mineral salts and toxins. Sweat occurs mainly under the arms, feet and palms. When mixed with the bacteria found on the surface of the skin, it can generate a bad smell.

People sweat more when it's hot, when they exercise, when they have a fever or in response to situations that make them feel nervous, angry, anxious, embarrassed or afraid. However, if you sweat excessively, it may be due to a thyroid or nervous system disorder, a decrease in blood sugar or another health problem.

To learn more about this topic, we consulted Dr. Mario Vega Carbó, an endocrinology specialist, with more than 20 years of experience.

Doctor Mario,
1. What is the cause of this condition?

Hyperhidrosis is an exaggerated sweating that occurs for no apparent reason. When it affects the hands, feet and armpits, it is known as primary hyperhidrosis and, in most cases, its cause is unknown, which seems to be hereditary. If perspiration is a consequence of other diseases, it is called secondary hyperhidrosis and can occur throughout the body or only in a particular area.

2. What other ailments can cause this disorder?

Acromegaly, anxiety conditions, cancer, carcinoid syndrome, abuse of certain medications and substances, alcohol consumption, diabetes, thyroid problems, menopause, Parkinson's disease, tuberculosis, infections and some lung, nerve or heart disease can cause hyperhidrosis.

3. What are your main symptoms?

In addition to excessive sweating, the patient may have a strong body odor, weight or appetite loss, chest pain, rapid and very intense heartbeat, nausea, shortness of breath, dizziness, skin infections and fever.

4. How do you distinguish normal sweating from excessive sweating?

In the case of Hyperhidrosis, excessive sweat occurs even at moderate temperatures and without any physical activity. The person usually has perspiration haloes under the arms, moisture stains on the clothes and perspiration drops run down his face, affecting his normal life. The hands become sticky, cold and wet, and the feet and shoes also get wet and smell bad. For those who suffer from this condition this happens at least once a week.

5. How is this disease diagnosed?

To corroborate the signs of visible sweat, starch and iodine tests, or paper tests can be performed to confirm the diagnosis. Blood and urine tests and other studies can also be done to analyze the functioning of the thyroid gland and look for tumors and other conditions that may be the cause of this problem.

6. What is the treatment for Hyperhidrosis?

If there is a preexisting condition, that disease should be treated. Excessive perspiration can be controlled with powerful antiperspirants, which plug the sweat ducts. These products must contain high doses of aluminum chloride, which is applied to the affected areas and can irritate the skin.

Certain medications that prevent the stimulation of the glands that cause perspiration may also be prescribed. These usually have side effects, such as dryness, blurred vision, bladder problems, and are not suitable for all people. Some glycopyrrolate creams can help control sweating of the face and head.

Another available therapy is known as Iontophoresis, which uses electricity to temporarily deactivate the sweat glands.

For its part, Botox injections are used for the treatment of the armpits, feet and hands, blocking the nerves that stimulate perspiration.

In severe cases, it is possible to perform surgery to remove the axillary glands, or a sympathectomy to disconnect the nerves responsible for sweat overproductionr.

7. What other recommendations are provided for these cases?

Intense hyperhidrosis can cause disruption of the patient's normal activities and cause emotional distress, depression, anxiety and social withdrawal. Therefore, it may be necessary to accompany the therapy with a psychological treatment.

In addition to the use of antiperspirants and bathing regularly, it is also recommended to wear light clothing made of natural materials, such as cotton, wool and silk, and leather shoes, which allow the skin to breathe.

It is important to ventilate the feet, change the socks frequently, avoid spicy foods and sun exposure, and the consumption of alcohol and coffee. In addition, axillary patches that absorb sweating and protect clothing can be used.

Finally, the practice of relaxation techniques, such as yoga or meditation, that help control the stress caused by perspiration is advised.

Chapter 163. Type 1 Diabetes or Juvenile Diabetes

Type 1 Diabetes, also known as Juvenile Diabetes, is a chronic disorder in which the pancreas does not produce enough insulin. This hormone is responsible for regulating sugar in the body and its use as a source of energy in muscles and other tissues.

Its lack causes an excess of glucose to remain in the blood, which can cause serious problems in the heart, eyes, kidneys, nerves and feet.

Type 1 diabetes usually appears during childhood, although it can also occur in adolescence and adulthood. While it has no cure, it can be controlled with treatment, proper diet, regular exercise, weight loss and medications.

To learn more about this topic, we interview Mario Vega Carbó, an endocrinologist, with more than 20 years of experience.

Doctor Mario,
1. What causes Type 1 Diabetes?

The reasons that cause it are not known exactly. In most cases the immune system mistakenly attacks the pancreas and destroys the cells that produce insulin. The disease may be due to exposure to certain viruses and genetic and environmental factors.

2. What are your main symptoms?

Its main signs are an increase in hunger, thirst and the need to urinate. Other common symptoms are the permanent feeling of tiredness, weight loss for no apparent reason, the presence of sores that take time to heal, dry skin, blurred vision, itching, tingling in the feet, irritability and other changes in mood.

3. How is this disease detected?

In view of their symptoms, an analysis of the patient's medical history, a physical examination and blood glucose, hemoglobin and lipid levels are usually performed. It is also possible that urine, osmolarity, heart rate, blood pressure and other tests to confirm the diagnosis may be carried out.

4. What is the treatment of type 1 diabetes?

The therapy involves the application of three or more daily injections of insulin to maintain a normal blood sugar level. Another option is the use of an insulin pump, a device the size of a mobile phone that administers the hormone continuously for 24 hours. To do this, a tube connects the insulin reservoir to a catheter, which is inserted under the skin of the abdomen.

The patient must learn to measure his blood sugar level and perform periodic checks. Based on these results, the treatment will be adjusted according to the needs to maintain an appropriate range.

If necessary, medications for high blood pressure and lowering cholesterol, and the use of daily aspirin to protect the heart, may also be prescribed.

It is important that the patient adopts a healthy lifestyle. In that sense, you should control your weight and eat a well-balanced diet with fewer calories, refined carbohydrates and saturated fats, and more fruits, vegetables and fibers. Also do physical activity on a regular basis and avoid smoking and consuming excess alcohol. This treatment should be followed throughout life.

5. What other complications can this disease bring?

People with Type 1 Diabetes have a higher risk of circulatory and heart disease; nerve injuries; kidney, eye and foot damage; skin and mouth infections; and complications in pregnancy.

6. What other aspects should these patients take into account?

People with Type 1 Diabetes are recommended to measure their glucose levels before driving or operating a machine. Also that they wear a bracelet or special card that indicates their condition, to notify others in emergency situations.

Similarly, it is good to alert family, friends and coworkers and tell them how to act in a crisis. Finally, living with Diabetes can be very stressful and cause depression and distress. That is why it is also important to take care of emotional health.

In that sense, they are advised to practice meditation to free the mind from worries, do yoga and other relaxing activities. If necessary, psychological and therapeutic support is also recommended.

Chapter 164. Obesity in childhood

Obesity is a chronic disease that is characterized by excessive accumulation of fat in the body, which produces a clear increase in health risk. This disorder is increasingly common among children and adolescents and is causing them to acquire diseases that were previously considered exclusive to adults, such as Diabetes.

Overweight is related to metabolic syndrome, a series of conditions that occur together and include high blood pressure, high blood sugar levels, excess body fat around the waist and abnormal cholesterol and triglyceride levels. Prevention, education and the acquisition of healthy lifestyle habits are essential to treat obesity in children.

To learn more about this topic, we interview Dr. Mario Vega Carbó, an endocrinology specialist, with more than 20 years of experience.

Doctor Mario,
1. What are the main causes of childhood obesity?

This disorder can be due to many reasons, including genetic, hormonal, nutritional, social, cultural and hereditary factors. However, the main cause of obesity in childhood is related to lifestyle.

In recent decades, the consumption of foods and beverages with many calories, poor physical activity and excessive time invested in cell phones, computers, televisions and video consoles have generated an increase in this condition in children and adolescents.

On the other hand, certain diseases, the consumption of certain medications and emotional disorders are also some of the possible causes of Obesity.

2. Who has more risks of suffering from this disease?

Children who do not do daily physical activity, who eat fast, frozen or high-calorie foods, and who consume sweets, soda and other sugary drinks have a higher risk of being obese.

The same goes for those who lead a sedentary life, those who come from a family of overweight people and those who suffer emotional and psychological problems.

3. What role does the environment play in these cases?

The environment surrounding the child is very important. It is essential that you have the possibility of following a healthy lifestyle model, with access to adequate food and places with spaces to recreate and exercise. One of the best strategies to reduce childhood obesity is to improve the habits of the whole family group.

At this stage of life, prevention and education are fundamental, since the practices acquired in childhood are often maintained throughout life.

Healthy habits that begin in childhood reduce the risks of osteoporosis, overweight, obesity and other disorders in adulthood. By contrast, an obese child is more likely to be too when he grows up.

4. How is Obesity diagnosed?

Usually the doctor performs a physical examination of the child and compares their values with the Body Mass Index (BMI), to see if their weight is exceeded based on their height and age. It also analyzes your medical history, your family history, your eating habits and your level of physical activity.

On the other hand, a blood test may be necessary to measure cholesterol, sugar, vitamin D and hormonal levels.

5. What is your treatment?

Therapy generally points to the adaptation of healthy lifestyle habits. The first thing to do is for the child to follow a balanced diet in which soft drinks and junk food such as french fries, hamburgers, sausages, cookies and ice cream are reduced, and the consumption of fruits, vegetables, legumes, cereals is increased.

It is also important that you perform daily physical activity, for which parents should encourage him to play, run, swim, ride a bike and play some sport in his spare time. If Obesity is a consequence of another disease, it must be treated.

In severe cases, surgery may be an option for adolescents who fail to lose weight with changes in lifestyle. Usually weight loss medications are not recommended for children.

6. What other complications can Childhood Obesity bring?

Children with this disorder are more likely to have diabetes; hypertension; abnormal cholesterol and triglycerides; heart, liver and kidney diseases; bone and joint problems; Asthma and sleep apnea.

On the other hand, Obesity also usually generates low self-esteem, depression and social and behavioral problems. If necessary, it is recommended to seek psychological support.

7. What other aspects can be taken into account to improve this disorder?

To guarantee the success of the treatment, family support is important and that everyone is involved in therapy and in the adoption of healthy habits.

Part XI Endocrinology in Obstetrics

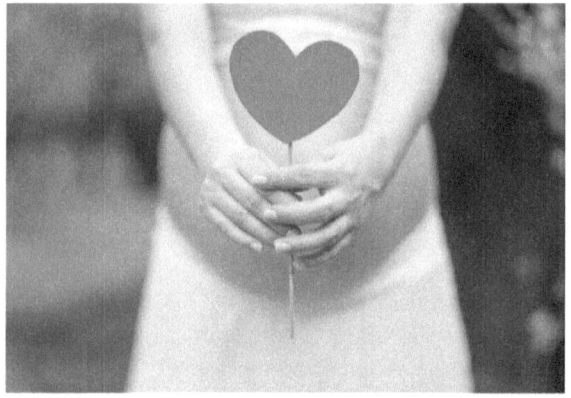

Chapter 165. Nutrition and pregnancy

Pregnancy requires a series of special care among which is the need for a healthy diet. Everything the mother eats impacts on the baby and its normal development, since the nutrients it needs reach through the placenta.

An inadequate diet increases the risks of preterm birth, low birth weight and congenital defects. On the contrary, proper feeding is one of the fundamental pillars of the well-being of both mother and baby.

To learn more about this topic, we interview Dr. Mario Vega Carbó, an endocrinology specialist, in charge of the Vega & Vado Office.

Doctor Mario,
1. Why is nutrition so important during pregnancy?

A healthy and balanced diet allows the body to receive the nutrients it needs to function and grow. This includes proteins, carbohydrates, fats, vitamins, minerals and water. During pregnancy, feeding is more important than ever since the need for nutrients increases.

Deficiencies of calcium, iron, vitamin A or iodine can endanger both the mother and the baby. On the contrary, healthy eating helps it develop normally.

2. How does nutrition change during pregnancy?

At this stage the woman needs to consume more folic acid, iron, calcium and vitamin D than before pregnancy. Folic acid helps prevent certain birth defects; iron is essential for the child's growth and brain development; Calcium reduces the risk of sudden hypertension and, together with vitamin D, are important for the formation of bones and teeth.

On the other hand, during pregnancy the need for protein and water also increases, so it is essential to always stay well hydrated.

3. How many kilos should be gained during pregnancy?

That will depend on the mother's health and condition before becoming pregnant. If you had a normal weight, it is generally estimated that you should gain between 11 and 14 kilos. If she was very thin, she should climb more. If you were overweight, you should climb less. Weight gain should occur gradually throughout pregnancy.

4. What foods are recommended during pregnancy?

Eating well during pregnancy does not simply mean eating too much. It is important to pay attention to what you eat, always looking for healthy foods.

Fortified bread and whole grains are important to get enough folic acid. Also spinach, lettuce, orange, lemon, mango, tomato, kiwi and legumes, some of which also provide vitamin C.

Fruits and vegetables contain different essential vitamins and minerals, in addition to fiber to aid in digestion. Meanwhile, meats, fish, shellfish and eggs provide protein, vitamin B and iron, while milk and milk products provide calcium.

Similarly, fish, nuts, seeds and avocados provide healthy fats such as Omega-3. On the other hand, it is advisable to drink 3 liters of water per day.

5. What foods should be avoided?

At this stage it is important to avoid alcohol, fish with high levels of mercury, processed meats such as sausages and sausages, milk and unpasteurized cheeses, raw eggs and caffeine.

6. Are nutritional supplements recommended?

In most cases they are recommended, to ensure that the nutritional needs during pregnancy are well met. However, these supplements do not replace a healthy diet, but complement it.

Chapter 166. Obesity and pregnancy

Obesity during pregnancy can seriously affect the health of both the mother and the baby. In addition to impairing fertility, excessive accumulation of fat in the body increases the risks of high blood pressure, gestational diabetes and miscarriages.

On the other hand, children of obese mothers can be born with overweight, congenital defects and suffer injuries during childbirth. Proper diet, physical exercise and regular medical check-ups can help avoid these disorders.

To learn more about this topic, we interview Dr. Mario Vega Carbó, an endocrinology specialist, with more than 20 years of experience.

Doctor Mario,
1. When is someone considered obese?

Obesity is a chronic disease that is characterized by excessive accumulation of fat in the body. Someone is considered obese when the percentage of fat exceeds 25 percent of body weight in men and 33 percent in women. Obesity can also be classified according to body mass index (BMI).

2. How does obesity affect fertility?

This disorder can contribute to the appearance of ovulation problems, irregular menstrual periods and spontaneous abortions. Obese women have a lower response to infertility treatments, such as in vitro fertilization. On the other hand, Polycystic Ovary Syndrome is also related to overweight and sterility.

3. How does this disorder affect pregnancy?

During pregnancy, obesity increases the risks of miscarriages and births of dead fetuses. Women with this disorder are more likely to have

Gestational Diabetes, a condition in which blood sugar levels are elevated and that increases the chances of developing Diabetes Mellitus later.

Other possible complications are Preeclampsia, a type of hypertension associated with pregnancy that affects important organs such as liver, kidneys and causes protein loss; cardiac dysfunction and sleep apnea.

On the other hand, obesity makes vaginal delivery difficult and increases the need for a C-section.

4. How does obesity affect the baby?

The children of women with this disorder are usually born with more body fat than normal, which increases the risks of metabolic syndrome and childhood obesity.

They may also have neural tube defects, in which the brain or spine does not form properly in the early stages of development; heart problems or injuries during childbirth as a result of its larger size.

5. How many kilos should be gained during pregnancy?

That will depend on the mother's health and condition before becoming pregnant. In the case of obese women, the recommended weight gain is between 5 and 9 kilos.

6. What is recommended to an obese woman before becoming pregnant?

You are generally advised to perform a preconception check, so that your doctor can recommend a special treatment of healthy food and specific physical exercise for her. That way you can lose weight before you get pregnant.

7. What is recommended to an obese woman during pregnancy?

In these cases it is important that regular checks be carried out from the beginning of pregnancy. Among other studies, the doctor may recommend performing tests for early detection of gestational diabetes and obstructive sleep apnea.

On the other hand, having good nutrition, staying active and increasing the right amount of weight are important ways to promote a healthy pregnancy.

During this stage diets are not recommended to lose weight, as they can reduce the nutrients that the baby needs to develop normally. Therefore, it is essential to speak with a nutritionist to follow an appropriate meal regime.

In turn, it is advisable to follow a routine of safe physical exercises, such as walking, swimming, stationary cycling or yoga.

Chapter 167. Diabetes and pregnancy

Pregnancy is a time in life when you have to be especially careful with blood sugar levels. Uncontrolled diabetes can lead to serious health complications during pregnancy and childbirth, both for the mother and the baby.

In addition to the conventional disease, there is another variant of it that appears at this stage, known as Gestational Diabetes. This condition begins when the body cannot produce or use all the insulin it needs for pregnancy.

To learn more about this topic, we interview Mario Vega Carbó, an endocrinologist, with more than 20 years of experience.

Doctor Mario,
1. What is Gestational Diabetes and what causes it?

It is a condition in which a woman who has never had diabetes begins to have a high blood glucose level during pregnancy.

It is not known for sure what causes it, but it is known that placental hormones, which contribute to the development of the baby, also block the action of insulin, causing sugar to accumulate more easily in the blood. Gestational diabetes usually occurs in the last stage of pregnancy.

2. What are the symptoms of Gestational Diabetes?

It usually has no symptoms, but is detected during prenatal checkups.

3. Who has more risks of having it?

Women who had gestational diabetes in a previous pregnancy; those who have given birth to babies over 4 kilos; those with cardiovascular disease, hypertension or obesity; Those who have relatives with diabetes or are over 30 years of age are more likely to suffer from it.

Also those with disorders associated with insulin resistance, such as Polycystic Ovary Syndrome or Acanthosis Nigricans.

4. What should a person with diabetes before pregnancy do?

If the person already has diabetes, it is important that he control the disease before becoming pregnant. On the other hand, during pregnancy, regular check-ups and follow a healthy eating plan, safe physical activity and treatment established by a specialist doctor should be carried out. It is possible that diabetes medicines change during pregnancy.

5. What disorders can Diabetes generate during pregnancy?

Previous diabetes can increase the risks of abortions, birth defects and preeclampsia, a type of high blood pressure that damages the kidneys and causes protein loss

In the case of gestational diabetes, as it appears at the end of pregnancy, when the baby's body has already formed, the damage is minor. However, both cases can cause the child to be excessively large (macrosomia) and have an enlargement of the organs, shoulder dystocia, hypoglycemia, respiratory problems and metabolic complications.

In addition, very large babies have more risks of getting stuck in the birth canal, suffering birth injuries or needing a C-section. Diabetes can cause premature births.

6. What is the treatment of Diabetes during pregnancy?

Generally the first thing that is done is to implement an adequate nutritional plan and a routine of safe physical exercises, such as walking, swimming, stationary cycling or yoga.

The distribution of calories is very important and you should avoid carbohydrates that have a high glycemic index and stimulate the consumption of whole grains, fruits and vegetables. It is advisable to distribute food throughout the day. In addition, the patient must learn to measure her blood sugar level and perform permanent controls.

If necessary, insulin will be applied or medications that help lower blood sugar, such as metformin and glibenclamide, will be recommended, however, there is insufficient scientific evidence to support the safety of these medications during pregnancy.

7. What other complications can this ailment bring?

In cases of gestational diabetes, blood glucose usually returns to normal after delivery. However, these women have more risks of getting diabetes mellitus in the future, so they should continue with the care.

During pregnancy usually increases the production of ketones, acids present in the blood. In severe cases, this can cause a buildup of fluid in the brain, heart attack and kidney failure, so it must be monitored.

Finally, babies of mothers with gestational diabetes are also more likely to suffer from obesity and diabetes mellitus later.

Chapter 168. Recurring Abortions

It is defined as recurrent abortion when 3 or more consecutive miscarriages occur before 20 weeks of gestation. It is estimated that between 1 and 3% of couples of reproductive age suffer from this disorder. In most cases, natural abortions are due to chromosomal problems, which cause the fetus to not develop normally. They can also be a consequence of uncontrolled systemic diseases, such as diabetes or hypothyroidism.

To learn more about the subject, we interview Dr. Mario Vega Carbó, an endocrinology specialist, with more than 20 years of experience.

Doctor Mario,
1. What causes recurrent abortions?

In many cases they occur without apparent cause and then the couple manages to conceive normally without the need for any treatment. In others they can be caused by a congenital defect of the fetus or chromosomal problems related to the father's or mother's genes, exposure to certain environmental toxins, serious injuries, infections or structural abnormalities in the reproductive organs.

Other possible causes are being overweight; diabetes, hypothyroidism, celiac disease or an uncontrolled chronic kidney disease; hormonal or immune problems; smoking; and the use of drugs or alcohol.

2. What percentages of spontaneous abortions occur?

It is estimated that about 50 percent of the fertilized eggs die spontaneously, usually before the woman discovers she is pregnant. In the case of those recognized, the percentage is between 10 and 15 percent. Most natural abortions occur during the first 12 weeks of gestation.

3. Who has more risks of suffering them?

Women over 35 years; those who suffered previous miscarriages; those with abnormalities in the uterus, chronic uncontrolled conditions or overweight; and those who smoke, drink alcohol or use drugs are more likely to suffer them.

4. What are your main symptoms?

Some of the most common signs are pain or cramping in the abdomen and hemorrhages, including bleeding and fluid or tissue leakage from the vagina.

5. How is it detected?

Through a pelvic exam I can see if the cervix has dilated or become thinner. In turn, an ultrasound can verify the development of the baby and his heartbeat.

6. What is your treatment?

After a miscarriage, the tissue that leaves the vagina is usually examined to investigate abnormalities. It is also important to detect if remnants of the placenta and embryo still remain in the uterus. If they are not removed from the body naturally, medical or surgical treatment may be necessary to remove them.

Generally women can get pregnant again during the next menstrual cycle after spontaneous abortion. However, they are advised to evaluate with their partners if they are physically and emotionally prepared to face it.

7. What other complications can this disorder bring?

In some cases, what is known as septic abortion, a serious intrauterine infection, may occur. Among its usual signs are fever, chills, vaginal discharge with a bad smell and peritonitis.

On the other hand, after spontaneous abortion some women usually feel sadness, anxiety, guilt and depression. If necessary, therapeutic support is recommended.

8. What is advised in case of recurrent abortions?

Faced with two or three spontaneous abortions in a row, it is important to carry out studies to try to find the reasons that are causing it, such as chromosomal problems or uterine abnormalities.

If they are a consequence of a systemic disease, it must be controlled and treated before becoming pregnant again. On the other hand, in these cases it is advisable to avoid any type of risk factor, such as alcohol and drug consumption, caffeine, smoking and exposure to X-rays.

In most cases where there is no apparent cause, spontaneous abortion does not recur and the next pregnancies come to fruition.

Chapter 169. Hypothyroidism and pregnancy

Hypothyroidism is a disease in which the thyroid gland does not produce enough thyroid hormone. This disorder can occur during pregnancy, so it is important to be alert to its symptoms, because if it is not treated it can cause infections, heart problems, infertility, spontaneous abortion, premature birth and babies with congenital defects, among other complications.

Thyroid conditions are particularly common in women of reproductive age. As its signs are similar to those of other pathologies, sometimes hypothyroidism can go unnoticed.

To talk about this topic, we interviewed Dr. Mario Vega Carbó, an endocrinology specialist, in charge of the Vega & Vado Office.

Doctor Mario,
1. What are the main symptoms of hypothyroidism?

The most common signs are constipation, difficulty concentrating, pale dry skin, swelling in the front of the throat, fatigue, brittle hair and nails, irregular menstruation, increased sensitivity to cold, weight gain, depression, joint pain and muscle weakness.

If left untreated, in more severe cases there may be a decrease in the sense of taste and smell, hoarseness, thickening of the skin, slow heart rate and swelling of the face, hands and feet.

2. How can this disorder affect before and during pregnancy?

Before pregnancy, hypothyroidism may be the cause of infertility, since it prevents the production of ovules, causes irregularities in the menstrual cycle and increases prolactin levels.

After conception, the risk of spontaneous abortion, premature delivery and preeclampsia increases, a type of high blood pressure that damages the kidneys and causes protein loss

3. How can hypothyroidism affect the baby?

In the first months of pregnancy, the baby depends on the mother to receive thyroid hormones. These play a very important role in the normal development of the brain and the growth of the fetus. Therefore, the lack of these hormones can cause birth defects and that over time children have a low intelligence index and other learning difficulties.

4. How is hypothyroidism detected?

A physical exam and various studies are usually done to measure thyroid hormone levels, thyroid stimulating hormone, cholesterol and glucose, and an antibody test. Other specialized tests of the gland may also be necessary.

5. What is your treatment during pregnancy?

The therapy is similar to that used in non-pregnant people and consists of replacing the thyroid hormone that is missing in the body with Levothyroxine. This oral medication restores adequate levels and reverses the signs and symptoms of the disease.

On the other hand, periodic controls are essential during treatment, since at the appropriate dose this drug has no side effects.

In turn, the requirements of Levothyroxine generally increase during pregnancy, sometimes by 25 or 50 percent.

6. Can prenatal vitamins influence hypothyroidism?

Yes. Both prenatal vitamins and iron supplements and certain foods interfere with the absorption of thyroid hormone. Therefore it is recommended to take Levothyroxine on an empty stomach, one hour before meals, and then wait for a period of two hours to ingest vitamins or supplements.

7. Will babies of mothers with hypothyroidism also be born with the disease?

This disorder is very rare in babies and children. If it is transmitted genetically, in general it does not manifest until the person is an adult.

Chapter 170. Hyperthyroidism and pregnancy

Hyperthyroidism, or overactive thyroid, is a condition in which the thyroid gland produces too much thyroid hormone. When it occurs during pregnancy it can cause premature labor and other complications, so it is important to treat it properly.

As its initial symptoms can be confused with the physiological changes characteristic of conception, it sometimes goes unnoticed or is diagnosed late. The most common reason for hyperthyroidism during pregnancy is Graves' disease, a condition in which the immune system produces antibodies that attack and damage the thyroid.

To talk about this topic, we interviewed Dr. Mario Vega Carbó, an endocrinology specialist, in charge of the Vega & Vado Office.

Doctor Mario,
1. What are the main symptoms of hyperthyroidism?

Its most common signs are anxiety, nervousness, fatigue, difficulty concentrating, diarrhea, thin and fragile hair, hand tremor, heat intolerance, increased appetite, sweating, palpitations, sleep problems and weight loss.

Other symptoms include abnormal swelling or growth of the thyroid, high blood pressure, eye irritation, nausea, vomiting, hot skin and redness, nail changes, depression and skin rashes.

2. How does this disorder affect fertility?

Hyperthyroidism can affect your menstrual periods, causing them to become irregular, not very abundant or directly present. Women with this disease take longer to get pregnant and have more risks, so it is ideal that it be controlled before conceiving.

3. How does hyperthyroidism affect pregnancy?

If the disease is not treated correctly, it can increase the chances of miscarriage, premature delivery, fetal tachycardia and low birth weight babies.

In addition, it can generate other complications in the mother, such as preeclampsia and, in severe cases, a thyroid storm, in which there is an acute increase in symptoms of hyperthyroidism.

The latter can appear as a result of a situation of stress, infection, surgery or labor and requires immediate attention, as it can cause high fever, diarrhea, tachycardia, shock and death.

4. How is hyperthyroidism treated during pregnancy?

The therapy will depend on the cause and the severity of your symptoms. If the disease is mild, no treatment is necessary. Moderate cases are usually treated with antithyroid medications, seeking to use the minimum possible dose, so as not to cause hypothyroidism in the baby.

On the other hand, beta-blockers can help improve heart rhythm disorders, tremors and anxiety, although they should be discontinued a few weeks before pregnancy ends.

During conception the use of radioactive iodine or surgical treatment is not recommended. In all cases, permanent monitoring of thyroid levels is essential.

5. Can therapy affect the baby?

In tight and controlled doses, antithyroid medications do not affect the baby, or they do so in a transitory manner that does not affect their development.

6. How does hyperthyroidism affect a newborn?

The mother with hyperthyroidism during pregnancy can transmit it to her child. However, the symptoms usually disappear in a few months. A baby with this disease may have irritability, a rapid heartbeat, premature closure of the fontanelles, low weight gain, fever, vomiting, diarrhea, goiter and intracranial hypertension.

Chapter 171. Prolactinoma and pregnancy

A prolactinoma is a non-cancerous (benign) pituitary tumor that usually causes a higher level of blood prolactin. This hormone is responsible for stimulating breast milk production after birth.

These tumors appear more frequently in people under 40 years of age and are more common in women, which may present with galactorrhea, breast tenderness, decreased sexual interest, headache, infertility and changes in the menstrual cycle and in the view. During pregnancy, estrogen production increases. This can cause an increase in prolactinoma and its associated symptoms.

To learn more about this topic, we interviewed Cuban doctor Mario Vega Carbó, a specialist in clinical endocrinology.

Doctor Mario,
1. What is the treatment of Hyperprolactinemia?

If the condition is caused by a prolactinoma, certain medications such as bromocriptine or cabergoline decrease the production of this hormone and help reduce the size of the tumor. However, these drugs can cause nausea, vomiting, nasal congestion, headaches and drowsiness, among other side effects.

These may decrease if low-dose therapy is started and the pills are taken overnight with food. In cases where the tumor needs to be removed due to its progressive growth, surgery or radiation treatment can be performed.

2. Can women with prolactinoma get pregnant?

Yes, medications for the treatment of these tumors are very effective in restoring fertility. However, it is important to plan the conception with medical care. In the case of macroprolactinomas, pregnancy should not be authorized until there is strict control of prolactinemia and tumor development.

3. How is the treatment of prolactinomas during pregnancy?

In cases where the pituitary tumor is less than 10 millimeters, medication treatment should be discontinued during pregnancy since the risk of prolactinoma growth is minimal.

If older, it is recommended to continue bromocriptine therapy, the use of which is not associated with fetal malformations or increased frequency of abortions or multiple pregnancies.

With cabergoline at the moment there is no evidence that it causes deleterious effects, but since there is much less experience in its use, it is advisable to move to bromocriptine during this period. In cases of very large tumors, some specialists recommend surgery prior to pregnancy.

4. Is it possible to perform excision surgery during pregnancy?

Yes, in cases where the use of bromocriptine does not work and the tumor continues to grow, a transsphenoidal resection is possible. Studies conducted so far do not indicate that there is a significant increase in risk to the mother and the fetus during surgery.

5. What happens to the pituitary gland during pregnancy?

This gland increases in size during pregnancy, but it is normal that does not cause inconvenience. In the months after childbirth, the pituitary gland quickly involves and returns to its previous size.

6. What other aspects should be taken into account in the treatment of prolactinoma in these cases?

Women who have a prolactin-secreting macroadenoma should undergo strict control throughout pregnancy, performing periodic campimetries to assess visual field abnormalities and confirm any enlargement of the tumor by magnetic resonance imaging.

Chapter 172. Cushing Syndrome and Pregnancy

Cushing's syndrome is a disorder caused by prolonged exposure to an excess of the hormone cortisol, produced by the adrenal glands. Among other conditions, this disease usually causes sterility and irregular or non-existent menstrual periods in women, so it is not common to occur during pregnancy.

However, when it appears dangerously increases the risks of mortality, both of the mother and the baby, so it is important to detect it in time and control it properly.

To learn more about this topic, we interview Mario Vega Carbó, an endocrinology specialist with more than 20 years of experience.

Doctor Mario,
1. What causes Cushing Syndrome?

The cause of this condition is usually due to a benign tumor in the pituitary gland or chronic use of glucocorticoids and other medications to treat inflammatory diseases, such as asthma and rheumatoid arthritis. Another cause is abnormalities in the adrenal glands.

2. What are your main symptoms?

The usual signs of this disorder are obesity in the middle and upper body and the rounded and red face. Other symptoms are thin arms and legs, purple streaks, thin, fragile skin, slow recovery of cuts and easy bruising.

3. How is this medical condition detected during pregnancy?

Its diagnosis is sometimes difficult, because many of its clinical features such as hypertension, gestational diabetes and edema are confused with the changes in pregnancy.

In this context, it is important to pay special attention to dermatological manifestations, such as thick violet streaks, acne, hirsutism, alopecia and poor healing, which are related to Cushing's Syndrome, but not so much with pregnancy.

4. How does this disease affect fertility?

Cushing syndrome can cause sterility in both partners. In women, high cortisol levels interfere with the functioning of the ovaries and may cause menstrual periods to be interrupted or become irregular. Therefore, patients with this disorder often have difficulty getting pregnant.

5. How does Cushing syndrome affect pregnancy?

This disease dangerously increases the risks of both the mother and the baby. In these cases there are more possibilities of spontaneous abortions and premature births.

In addition, the risks of preeclampsia, gestational diabetes, pulmonary edema, heart failure and infections with a slower wound healing process increase in the mother. In the baby, there may be intrauterine growth restriction and post natal infection.

6. What is the treatment during pregnancy?

The therapy will depend on what is causing the excess cortisol in the body. If the reason is a tumor, in mild cases it is recommended to defer removal surgery after delivery. If necessary, it will be carried out as soon as possible to reduce the risks.

If the syndrome is caused by any medication, the dose can be lowered or changed to a similar one that does not produce these symptoms.

There are different drugs to control the excessive production of cortisol, which would be safe for both the mother and the fetus.

7. If the mother has Cushing Syndrome during pregnancy, will the baby also have it?

Very rarely people inherit a tendency to suffer tumors in their endocrine glands, which affects cortisol levels and causes this disease.

Part XII Endocrinology in Geriatrics

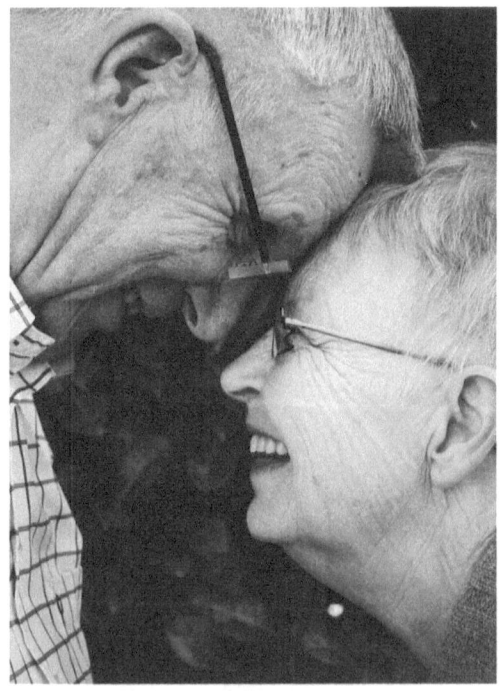

Chapter 173. Endocrinopathies in the elderly

Aging is a gradual, heterogeneous and irreversible process that implies a decrease in the capacities of the different organs and systems of the body, and a general physiological decline. It implies a series of morphological, functional, biochemical and psychological modifications that also affect the endocrine glands and their normal performance.

Over the years the organs become less sensitive to hormones and the amount of substances produced may vary. This can lead to the emergence of chronic diseases, such as diabetes, hypothyroidism, hyperthyroidism, hypogonadism, sarcopenia and obesity, which can cause serious damage to health.

To learn more about this topic, we interview Mario Vega Carbó, an endocrinologist and master in satisfactory longevity with more than 20 years of experience.

Doctor Mario,
1. What natural changes occur with aging?

As we get older there are several progressive changes among which are the decrease in protein synthesis; the loss of muscle mass and power, with the consequent decrease in strength; decreased bone density and progressive sclerosis of arteries and connective tissue.

This causes greater body fragility, which can lead to immobility, the onset of diseases and an increase in general vulnerability.

2. How does the endocrine system change with age?

With aging the endocrine glands and their hormonal production suffer important variations. The pituitary gland, for example, becomes smaller and slightly decreases the release of growth hormone and prolactin.

As for the thyroid, over the years the metabolism decreases, while in the hypothalamus the anti-diuretic hormone tends to rise, which predisposes to hyponatremia.

With respect to the pancreas, there is a decrease in sensitivity to the action of insulin. On the other hand, the adrenal glands lower the production of aldosterone, cortisol and glucocorticoids, resulting in dizziness and loss of the ability to tolerate stress.

Meanwhile, parathyroid hormone levels tend to rise, contributing to the loss of bone mass and increasing the risks of osteoporosis.

Finally, the sex glands reduce estrogen and testosterone levels, generating the definitive cessation of menstruation, infertility and decreased erectile capacity in men.

3. What are the most frequent endocrine disorders during old age?

The most common are those related to the pancreas and thyroid.
It is estimated that more than 50 percent of people over 80 have glucose intolerance. In addition to the progressive decrease in insulin secretion, the increase in peripheral resistance due to physical inactivity, the increase in abdominal fat and the decrease in lean mass contribute to the deterioration of your metabolism.

On the other hand, thyroid dysfunction is common as you get older. In addition, many elderly people do not ingest enough calcium and have a vitamin D deficiency, which results in secondary hyperparathyroidism associated with muscle weakness, which increases the risk of falls.

4. What endocrine diseases deserve special attention in older adults?

Some conditions to be aware of are Diabetes, Hypothyroidism, Hyperthyroidism, Hypogonadism, Thyroid Cancer, Obesity, Hyperparathyroidism, Sarcopenia and Osteoporosis, among others.

5. What other aspects interfere with the occurrence of chronic ailments in older adults?

In addition to the genetic and age factors, there are also other important external aspects to consider, such as nutrition, lack of physical activity, alcohol consumption and smoking, which favor the appearance of pathologies.

Chapter 174. Nutrition in older adults

Eating well and exercising regularly is important at all stages of life, but it becomes even more essential during old age to stay healthy and active. Eating a healthy and balanced diet is essential for the body to get the nutrients it needs to function.

In addition, this also help control weight and prevent diseases, such as osteoporosis, high blood pressure, heart problems, diabetes and some types of cancer. However, the nutritional requirements are not the same for all ages.

To learn what older people need to consume, we interview Dr. Mario Vega Carbó, a specialist in clinical endocrinology.

Doctor Mario,
1. How do dietary needs change with age?

Older adults need fewer calories than in previous years, but they need many nutrients. Therefore, the foods they consume should be rich in vitamins, minerals, proteins and fiber, with special emphasis on the variety. For example, at this stage it is very important to consume calcium and vitamin D to care for bones, and fiber to prevent stomach and intestinal problems.

Also of iron, since its deficiency is very common in the elderly and causes anemia and other disorders.

2. What types of foods are recommended for older adults?

Within the diet they are advised to include fruits and vegetables; whole grains such as oats, bread and rice; skim milk and dairy; low calorie cheese; fish, shellfish, lean meats, poultry and eggs; and nuts, beans and seeds.

On the other hand, it is important that they consume foods low in saturated fat, trans fat, cholesterol, salt (sodium) and added sugar; and drink enough liquid.

3. How many average calories does an older adult need to eat per day?

The amount of calories will depend on the age, sex and activity level of the person. For a woman over 50, it is estimated that she should consume an average of between 1,600 and 2,000 calories per day, while in a man it varies between 2,000 to 2,800. The more active you are, the more calories you need.

4. What can be done with the elderly who have trouble eating?

If the patient has problems chewing, it is important that he be examined by a dentist. If you have dentures, it may not fit well or you may have injured gums.

If you have trouble swallowing, you can try to drink a lot of liquid with food. They can also be offered purees, juices, creams, minced meat and soft foods in general.

If you lost your taste and smell, you can look to add color and texture to the dishes and use extra spices, herbs or lemon juice to give more flavor. If you are not hungry, you can try to exercise to whet your appetite.

5. What drinks are recommended for older adults?

Older people are more vulnerable to dehydration. Therefore it is important that they drink a lot of water and fruit juices, preferably outside meals and in small quantities. Also, drink milk and yogurt. It is advised to avoid the consumption of tea and coffee, because they alter sleep and are diuretic.

In case of drinking alcohol, only one glass of red wine per day is recommended if medications are not being taken.

6. How does poor diet affect the elderly?

Poor diet weakens the immune system, increasing the risk of infections; causes delayed wound healing; and generates the loss of muscle and bone mass, increasing the chances of falls and fractures, among other problems.

7. What other recommendations are important at this stage?

Older adults are advised to eat slowly and chew food well. Also, if possible, eat at least 5 times a day.

In addition, it is important that they remain active and perform at least 150 minutes of exercise during the week. The activity can be divided into 10-minute sessions, several times a day.

Chapter 175. Sarcopenia and muscle weakness

Sarcopenia is a progressive and widespread loss of muscle mass and power that occurs during aging. Although the weakness and depletion of physical strength is a normal consequence of the passing of the years, when it occurs in an accelerated manner it may be due to other factors.

This ailment mainly affects physically inactive people, although it can also occur in those elderly people who exercise regularly.

Among other disorders, Sarcopenia can hinder the performance of daily tasks, reduce the speed of movements and increase the chances of falls and injuries.

To learn more about this topic, we interview Mario Vega Carbó, an endocrinologist and master in satisfactory longevity with more than 20 years of experience.

Doctor Mario,
1. How is muscle mass affected over the years?

Muscle mass gradually decreases between 3 and 8 percent every decade after age 30, and the process accelerates after 60. This results in a progressive loss of strength that is natural. This process is usually accompanied by other physical changes, such as the increase in fatty tissue, which increase the risks of suffering from hypertension, diabetes, obesity and cardiovascular problems.

2. What causes sarcopenia and who does it affect?

The reasons that cause it are varied. In addition to aging itself, other possible causes are limited or unbalanced food intake, sedentary lifestyle, lack of physical exercise and excessive rest. It can also be a consequence of genetic factors, hormonal problems, weight loss, other diseases or the consumption of certain medications.

It is estimated that Sarcopenia affects 30 percent of those over 60, and 50 percent of those over 80.

3. How is this disorder detected?

Faced with its symptoms, muscle mass is usually measured with assessments of weight, height and perimeters, and a bioimpedanciometry is performed, which evaluates the amount of water, fat and muscle contained in a person. In addition, tests of strength and physical performance are carried out.

4. What is your treatment?

Usually the therapy points to changes in the patient's lifestyle. This includes proper nutrition and programmed resistance exercise.

The recommended diet for a person with Sarcopenia should be balanced but also contain a good amount of protein, including dairy, meat, eggs and fish. As for the exercise, it must be progressive and personalized, aiming to strengthen mainly the lower extremities.

On the other hand, therapies with testosterone, dehydroepiandrosterone and growth hormone are being studied, although their results are still not entirely clear in cornflowers and can cause certain unwanted side effects.

5. What other complications can this disease bring?

People with Sarcopenia often have difficulty moving, getting up from a chair, climbing stairs or walking at a light pace, which increases the risk of falls and fractures.

Complications resulting from a fall constitute the sixth leading cause of death in people over 65 years of age, so appropriate care should be taken.

On the other hand, this medical condition usually increases the risks of suffering from other chronic diseases, such as Osteoporosis and Diabetes.

In addition, Sarcopenia can cause disability, functional independence and profoundly affect the quality of life of a person, so it is important to prevent and detect it early.

6. What other aspects should these patients take into account?

Adequate diet and regular physical activity, including exercises to strengthen the muscles, are essential to prevent sarcopenia, maintain good shape and remain active. This gives the elderly more independence and allows them to cope better with chronic diseases, if they suffer from them.

On the contrary, the lack of physical activity causes the muscle mass to continue decreasing, aggravating the symptoms.

Chapter 176. Osteoporosis in the elderly

Osteoporosis is a disease that thins and weakens the bones, causing them to become brittle and break easily. In older adults, this disease can reduce the quality of life, by hindering the performance of daily tasks, decreasing the speed of movement and increasing the chances of falls and injuries.

It can also cause abnormal curvature of the spine, loss of size and prominent abdomen, in addition to generating acute and chronic pain, respiratory distress, depression and decreased self-esteem. Osteoporosis especially affects the bones of the hip, spine and wrist.

To learn more about this topic, we consulted Dr. Mario Vega Carbó, a specialist in endocrinology and family medicine, in charge of the Vega & Vado Office.

Doctor Mario,
1. Who has more risks of getting Osteoporosis?

This condition is more common in older women who do little physical activity, consume few dairy products, are smokers and have a family history related to this condition. Also in those people who consume certain medications, such as corticosteroids, heparin, lithium or diuretics, and those who suffer from kidney failure and inflammatory, rheumatic, liver and endocrine diseases.

2. How is muscle mass evaluated in older adults?

It is analyzed by clinical and physical exams, and with tests of gait speed, balance, chair lift and stepping up, among others.

3. What aspects increase the risk of fractures?

The chances increase if not enough calcium and vitamin D are consumed or if they are not properly absorbed by the body. The risks also grow as the years go by and with alcohol consumption, smoking, lack of exercise and body weight, malnutrition, certain medications such as prednisone and cortisone and eating disorders.

4. What are the consequences of osteoporosis fractures?

These fractures have a high prevalence in the elderly and increase the risk of death due to illness, cause the loss of independence, deterioration in the quality of life and a high cost in resources.

In addition, a fracture due to Osteoporosis increases the risks of suffering another within the next year, especially of the hip.

5. What is the importance of vitamin D in preventing osteoporosis?

Vitamin D improves muscle function and prevents the risk of further falls and fractures.

6. What causes your deficit in older adults?

In the elderly this can be caused by pigmentation and aging of the skin, since after 60 years 70 percent of vitamin D production decreases. It may also be due to its low intake, malabsorption syndrome, celiac disease, chronic pancreatitis, gastrectomy, anticonvulsants and glucocorticoids.

7. What is the treatment of Osteoporosis in old age?

As a first step it is recommended to maintain healthy lifestyle habits, such as a balanced diet rich in calcium and daily exercise, with control to avoid bumps and falls. In addition, it is advised to avoid tobacco and excessive alcohol consumption.

On the other hand, older adults may need calcium and vitamin D supplements, and bone strengthening medications. Among the latter are bisphosphonates, estrogen and estrogen receptor modulators, which prevent bone loss. On the other hand, teriparatide stimulates the formation of new tissue.

If there is an endocrine, liver or other problem that causes osteoporosis, it should also be treated.

8. What is the importance of preventing falls in the elderly?

Prevention is vital. It is estimated that 35% of older adults fall per year, causing joint numbness, fragility, loss of independence and greater chances of ending up in an asylum.

9. What factors increase the risk of falling?

Some factors that increase the risks are muscle weakness, a history of falls, gait disorders, instability, visual or cognitive problems, depression, the use of certain medications and the age over 80 years.

10. What preventive measures can be taken to prevent falls?

In cases of risk, it is important to make security modifications at home, eliminating possible obstacles and improving the lighting of the environments; and wear appropriate footwear. Also exercise safely, eat healthy, avoid tobacco and alcohol, sleep well and consume adequate amounts of vitamin D.

On the other hand, polypharmacy and the use of psychotropic drugs should be reduced, and hip protectors should be used.

Chapter 177. Obesity in older adults

Obesity is a growing disorder that is present in all ages, causing serious health problems. In older adults, excess body fat decreases physical function and can make them weaker and more fragile, as well as increasing the risk of illness and premature death.

It is estimated that in people with this disorder the life expectancy falls between 8 and 13 years, compared to those who have a normal weight. In most cases, obesity in old age is due more to a decrease in physical activity than to an increase in the amount of calories consumed.

To learn more about this topic, we interview Dr. Mario Vega Carbó, a specialist in endocrinology, and family medicine with more than 20 years of experience.

Doctor Mario,
1. How does obesity occur in old age?

Among the obese elderly are those who were also young and survived, and on the other those who developed this disorder as adults. In old age there are some changes in metabolism and body composition that favor weight gain. For example, the elderly have less ability to oxidize fats and perform less physical activity, which facilitates the accumulation of adiposity.

Sedentary lifestyle makes older adults more vulnerable to this pathology.

2. What problems does this disorder cause in older adults?

Obesity causes an increase in cardiovascular diseases, especially heart disease and stroke, and a deterioration in cognitive function. It also increases the risks of respiratory problems; arterial hypertension; Diabetes; musculoskeletal disorders, especially osteoarthritis; and some types of cancer, such as breast and colon cancer.

On the other hand, it can cause osteoporosis and a progressive loss of muscle mass and power, venous, lymphatic and skin edema problems. The consequences of obesity become more serious as age increases.

3. How does it affect them on a day-to-day basis?

Obesity can cause them to have trouble moving and doing everyday tasks. In addition, the elderly tend to tire faster and may feel short of breath.

On the other hand, this disorder can generate social isolation, low self-esteem and depression.

4. What is the treatment of obesity in the elderly?

The therapy consists mainly of proper diet and physical exercise. The diet should be rich in vitamins, minerals, proteins and fiber, with special emphasis on variety. On the contrary, saturated fats, trans fats, cholesterol, salt and refined sugars should be avoided.

As for exercise, it must be progressive and performed safely. It is important that they reach at least 150 minutes of activity during the week, being able to divide it into 10-minute sessions, several times a day.

On the other hand, it is not proven that drugs to treat obesity, such as orlistat and sibutramine are safe in older adults. About bariatric surgery, it is not recommended in people over 65 years.

5. What other aspects must be taken into account in the case of older adults?

In the elderly, excessive weight loss can be dangerous and cause a deterioration of health, when the body does not get the nutrients it needs to function. Poor diet weakens the immune system, increasing the risk of infections; and generates the loss of muscle and bone mass, increasing the chances of falls and fractures. Therefore, the decrease in the amount of calories consumed should be done following a balanced diet.

Chapter 178. Diabetes in older adults

It is estimated that between 20 and 25 percent of people over 65 have Diabetes and the percentage is expected to increase in the coming decades. This chronic condition reduces the possibility of a quiet aging, by decreasing the functional capacity of the person and increasing the risks of hypertension, coronary heart disease and stroke.

On the other hand, these patients are also more likely to suffer from polypharmacy, cognitive impairment, depression, urinary incontinence and falls.

To learn more about this topic, we interview Mario Vega Carbó, an endocrinologist and a master in satisfactory longevity with more than 20 years of experience.

Doctor Mario,
1. How does the Diabetes approach change in older adults?

In these cases the treatment is much more complex, since it requires the evaluation of physical, mental, functional, family, social and welfare aspects. It is very important to be attentive to complications that can alter the person's ability to move, such as visual and lower limb disorders, and accelerate cognitive impairment.

2. Why do the elderly have more risks of suffering from this disease?

This is due to a combined effect of increased insulin resistance and reduced endocrine pancreatic function. The decrease in sensitivity to insulin action is probably a consequence of the increase in adipose tissue and the decrease in muscle mass, which are associated with poor diet and low physical activity of age.

3. How is diabetes detected in older adults?

Patients may show an increase in hunger, thirst and the need to urinate; infections; sickness; inadequate healing and headache.

In the elderly, the disease can also occur atypically, such as urinary incontinence due to hyperglycemia and polyuria; and falls associated with neuropathy, cognitive or behavioral alterations.

Therefore, for its diagnosis it is necessary to make a comprehensive evaluation that measures and analyzes the functionality, fragility and sarcopenia, depression, cognitive impairment, comorbities, socioeconomic support, nutritional status, vascular complications, history of hypoglycemia and neurosensory alterations.

4. How does diabetes affect the typical problems of old age?

Complications associated with diabetes can accelerate the deterioration of mobility, generating instability, gait disturbance, falls and fractures. In addition, older adults with this disease may present more risks of polypharmacy, muscle weakness, stroke, motor and sensory neuropathy, poor glycemic control, hypoglycemia, orthostatic hypotension and visual disturbances.

On the other hand, Diabetes is linked to changes in the cerebral cortex of the elderly, being able to generate greater mental and motor slowness and increasing cognitive impairment.

It also accelerates the process of general aging, resulting in the appearance of urinary incontinence, sarcopenia and greater fragility, which at the same time stimulate the manifestation of Diabetes, thus causing a vicious cycle.

5. What is the treatment of Diabetes in older adults?

When evaluating a therapy for an elderly person, certain factors must be taken into account, such as their cognitive and self-care capacity, the presence of other diseases, their vulnerability to hypoglycemia and their life expectancy.

In those cases in which the older adult keeps his cognitive and functional capacity intact, with a significant expected survival, he must be treated in a similar way as a young person.

Otherwise, therapy should be more relaxed and aim at family care, with special emphasis on safety and avoiding episodes of symptomatic hyperglycemia.

Finally, in people who are at the end of their lives, treatment should aim to calm the pain, avoid dehydration and hypoglycemia.

Regarding the use of medications, caution is recommended with those that generate hypoglycemia, digestive intolerance and weight loss, and it is advised to opt for simple administration regimens, avoiding polypharmacy and evaluating interactions.

6. What other aspects should be taken into account during the illness?

As excessive food intake and sedentary lifestyle increase your risks, you should also work on a special diet and in adapting a healthier lifestyle.

In that sense, the diet should be rich in vitamins, minerals, proteins and fiber, with special emphasis on the variety. On the contrary, saturated fats, trans fats, cholesterol, salt and refined sugars should be avoided.

As for exercise, it must be progressive and performed safely. Physical activity is essential to preserve muscle mass and maintain strength and balance. In addition, it contributes to glycemic control, improves mobility and prevents falls.

Finally, the consumption of adequate amounts of liquids should be encouraged to avoid dehydration.

Chapter 179. Peripheral Neuropathy and Numbness of Hands and Feet

Peripheral Neuropathy is a condition in which the peripheral nerves, responsible for joining the brain and spinal cord with the rest of the body, do not work properly.

This may be due to damage to one or several nerves, either for hereditary reasons, stretching, pressure or as a consequence of other diseases. Neuropathy is quite common and can be mild or severe, depending on the extent of the injury.

It usually causes numbness, tingling, burning or pain, mainly in the hands and feet, although it can occur anywhere in the body.

In order to learn more about this topic, we interview Mario Vega Carbó, a specialist in endocrinology and family medicine with more than 20 years of experience.

Doctor Mario,
1. What diseases can cause Peripheral Neuropathy?

Peripheral nerves are fragile and easily injured. The most common cause is Diabetes, due to the high levels of blood sugar that cause them damage. Other diseases that can cause it are autoimmune such as Sjögren and Guillain-Barré syndromes; infections such as HIV, herpes or hepatitis C; deficiencies of certain vitamins; an intoxication; tumors; metabolic, kidney or liver problems; and spinal cord disorders.

2. How else can neurological injuries occur?

Nerves can be damaged in an accident or playing sports. Also due to excessive alcohol consumption, the use of certain medications or exposure to cold temperatures or certain toxins.

Other common causes are excessive pressure, as is the case with Carpal Tunnel Syndrome, and hereditary neuropathies.

3. What are the main symptoms of this condition?

The signs will depend on the damaged nerve and the severity of the injury. The most common are tingling and numbness, increased pain or numbness, loss of the ability to detect changes in temperature, lack of coordination and balance, weakness, spasms and muscle cramps, infection and ulcers in feet and legs.

On the other hand, Peripheral Neuropathy can cause excessive sweating, problems swallowing and digesting food, heartburn, dizziness, lightheadedness, fainting and changes in blood pressure.

In addition, as with any state of chronic pain, depression, anxiety and associated sleep problems are frequent.

4. How is it diagnosed?

In view of their symptoms, the patient's history will be analyzed and a series of neurological tests will be performed to see the degree of nerve damage. This may include blood and spinal fluid tests, electromyographs to check muscle activity and nerve conduction studies to see how signals travel through the body. It is also possible for a nerve and skin biopsy.

5. What is the treatment?

The first thing to do is to address the underlying cause of the neurological damage and relieve its symptoms. For example, if neuropathy is a consequence of diabetes, the level of blood sugar must be controlled. If it is due to alcohol intake or the use of a certain medication, they should be avoided. If the cause is an infection, an autoimmune disease or a hormonal deficiency, they must be treated.

If there is pressure on a certain nerve, surgery may be necessary to remove it. Meanwhile, for muscle weakness, it is possible to improve movements with physiotherapy.

On the other hand, a transcutaneous electrical nerve stimulation or a plasma exchange and intravenous immunoglobulin can also be performed to improve certain infections. As for pain, if it is mild it can be treated with pain relievers, such as non-steroidal anti-inflammatory drugs, and with anticonvulsant medications. In addition, some antidepressants are also effective in reducing discomfort.

If the pain is severe, a specialist should be consulted. Splints for hands or feet, a cane or a wheelchair may be necessary. However, timely therapy can prevent permanent damage. Generally controlling the cause, the injuries improve.

6. What else can be done to improve the forecast?

Leading a healthy life, exercising, drinking plenty of fluids and eating well can help reduce the effects of neuropathy. It is also recommended to correct vitamin deficiencies, avoid alcohol and quit smoking, since cigarettes can make symptoms worse.

On the other hand, some patients also feel relief with the practice of alternative medicines, such as acupuncture and the use of certain herbs.

Chapter 180. Reversible Dementias

Dementia is a syndrome characterized by cognitive impairment that affects memory, ability to think, language, social development and behavior. Occasionally, your symptoms can be resolved with proper treatment, recovering the previous intellectual level. In others, partial improvement can be obtained or its progress stopped.

Some potentially reversible conditions are depression, adverse effects of drugs or alcohol, normal pressure hydrocephalus, brain lesions or tumors, hypothyroidism and vitamin B12 deficiency.

Also those cases in which the medical condition is caused by certain medications and the one that has a metabolic origin related to blood sugar, calcium and sodium levels.

Dementia usually occurs in people over 60, so the risks increase as you get older.

To talk about this topic, we interview Mario Vega Carbó, an endocrinologist and master in satisfactory longevity with more than 20 years of experience.

Doctor Mario,
1. In which cases is dementia reversible and in which cases not?

When the changes that occur in the brain are degenerative and progressive, they generally cannot be reversed. This is the case of conditions such as Alzheimer's, vascular dementia and Lewy bodies, Huntington's disease and Parkinson's disease, among others.

On the contrary, when it is a consequence of infections and immune disorders, metabolic problems and endocrine abnormalities, nutritional deficiencies, reactions to medications, subdural hematomas, intoxication, hypoxia, brain tumors, normal pressure hydrocephalus or psychiatric diseases, it can be treated and cured

2. How is dementia detected?

In general, to perform a diagnosis, a complete physical examination and cognitive and neuropsychological tests are performed to assess memory, reasoning, language, movements, senses and attention, among other factors.

A CT scan or MRI of the brain, blood and urine tests that detect physical problems, and a psychiatric exam may also be necessary.

3. How can this ailment be prevented?

There are some factors that are not manageable, such as aging and family history. However, it is possible to help prevent dementia by avoiding abusive alcohol and drug use, controlling cardiovascular and endocrine diseases, not smoking and treating depression and sleep apnea.

Also eating properly, taking enough vitamin D, keeping the mind active and exercising regularly.

4. What type of drugs and drugs can cause dementia?

Some medications related to this disorder are benzodiazepines, anticholinergics, tricyclic antidepressants, neuroleptics, antiepileptics, antirrhythmics, antihistamines, steroids and antiparkinsonians. Polypharmacy can increase the risks of cognitive impairment.

5. In what cases can dementia be due to metabolic and endocrine disorders?

Diseases such as hypothyroidism, diabetes, hyponatremia, hypoglycemia, hypopituitarism and hyperparathyroidism can produce neurological manifestations related to dementia.

Some possible symptoms associated with these disorders are disorientation, apathy, depression, slow thinking, difficulties in resolving situations, memory problems, hallucinations, catatonic states and seizures.

6. How is dementia treated?

The therapy will depend on what is the cause of it. Treatment with antidepressants can improve your symptoms. In cases where dementia results from another disease or disorder, when its signs are controlled they may disappear or stop.

Chapter 181. Hypothyroidism in older adults

Hypothyroidism is a condition in which the thyroid does not produce enough thyroid hormone. It is estimated that between 5 and 7 percent of people over 65 suffer from it, being a little more frequent in women.

Its most common cause in old age is Hashimoto's disease or autoimmune thyroiditis. It can also be the result of previous gland surgery, radiotherapy and radioactive iodine treatments.

Its clinical manifestations in the elderly are usually very varied and in some cases different from those of the young, which sometimes makes diagnosis difficult. In general, hypothyroidism in older adults is accompanied by depression, the reason why this occurs is not entirely clear.

To talk about this topic, we interviewed Dr. Mario Vega Carbó, a specialist in endocrinology and family medicine, who works as an endocrinologist at the Santa Fe Medical Center and the Vega & Vado Office.

Doctor Mario,
1. What are the most frequent symptoms of Hypothyroidism in old age?

The most common signs in the elderly are fatigue and weakness, although a wide range of manifestations may appear. Some of them are intolerance to heat, pain, nausea, constipation, difficulty swallowing, reduced libido, gait disturbances, sexual dysfunction, hair loss, joint stiffness and severe voice.

Also personality changes, memory loss, irritability, psychosis and depression.

2. How are they different from those presented by young people?

In comparison, the elderly gain less weight, have less muscle cramps, cold intolerance and paraesthesia.

3. How is this disease detected in the elderly?

Because the variety of symptoms is so wide, the diagnosis of hypothyroidism in older adults is often complicated. Weakness, fatigue, constipation, gait disturbances, depression and memory loss are often confused with other diseases.

4. What consequences can hypothyroidism bring in older adults?

This medical condition can bring heart problems, peripheral neuropathy, depression and infertility. Also in the elderly is Comme Mixedematous, a serious complication of Hypothyroidism that puts the patient's life at risk.

It can be triggered by a stressful situation, such as sepsis, intoxications, medications or extreme temperatures, and its symptoms are severe intolerance to cold and drowsiness, followed by deep lethargy and loss of consciousness.

5. How is the treatment of hypothyroidism in old age?

The use of Levothyroxine is also recommended for older adults. The doses used are usually lower than in young patients, due to less degradation.

It is important to regulated and control the dose of Levothyroxine, because higher doses can lead to heart diseases, anxiety and osteoporoses.

Chapter 182. Hyperthyroidism in older adults

Hyperthyroidism is a condition in which the thyroid produces too much thyroid hormone. This disorder is rare in the elderly, being more common in women than in men.

The causes that cause it in old age are similar to those of young people, although in older adults the toxic multinodular goiter is more common than Graves' disease. In addition, in that age group it is also usual to be motivated by the intake of large amounts of synthetic thyroid hormone, which may be the result of an error in the supply, inadequate indication or confusion of the patient.

Other possible causes of hyperthyroidism in the elderly are inflammation of the gland due to viral infections, an overactive adenoma and exaggerated iodine consumption.

To talk about this topic, we interviewed Dr. Mario Vega Carbó, a specialist in endocrinology and family medicine, who is in charge of the Vega & Vado Office.

Doctor Mario,
1. What are the most common symptoms of hyperthyroidism in older adults?

In a good part of the elderly the signs of this disease are usually vague and less precise than in the young. They have lower rates of fatigue, weakness, nervousness, sweating, heat intolerance, increased appetite and diarrhea.

On the contrary, mental confusion and cardiac manifestations such as arrhythmias, congestive heart failure and angina pectoris are more common in older adults.

2. What problems does your diagnosis present in the elderly?

Being its most diffuse symptoms, many times its diagnosis is often confused with other medical conditions, such as heart disease, dementia or gastrointestinal problems, or with the changes of old age.

3. What consequences can hyperthyroidism have on older adults?

In the elderly, this disease can cause heart problems and osteoporosis. Excess thyroid hormone generates a low level of thyroid stimulating hormone, which increases the risks of atrial defibrillation, hip fractures and neuropsychiatric problems.

On the other hand, it can also cause a Thyroid Storm, an acute increase in the symptoms of hyperthyroidism that endangers the functioning of the organs and the patient's life. It can be triggered by a situation of stress, systemic infections, surgery, induction of anesthesia and sepsis, and can cause high fever, delirium, hypotension, diarrhea, tachycardia, shock and death.

4. How is this ailment treated in the elderly?

The therapy will depend on the cause of hyperthyroidism, the severity of its symptoms and the general state of health of the patient. In older adults, Graves' disease and toxic multinodular goiter are advised to treat them with radioactive iodine instead of antithyroid drugs.

On the other hand, if the goiter produces compression, surgery is recommended. In the rest of the cases, methimazole can be used in combination with beta-blockers, which help to improve heart rhythm disorders, tremors and anxiety.

Chapter 183. Thyroid Cancer in Older Adults

Thyroid Cancer is a condition whose incidence has increased in recent years in the elderly. It is estimated that 90% of women over 60 and 60% of men over 80 have thyroid nodules. Despite being more frequent in women, the probability of cancer is higher in men.

Within this group its evolution is usually slow and its symptoms are uncommon, often confused with age-specific changes.

To learn more about this topic, we interview Mario Vega Carbó, an endocrinology specialist with more than 20 years of experience.

Doctor Mario,
1. What are the symptoms of Thyroid Cancer?

Your signs may vary depending on the type of cancer. Among the most common are lump or swelling in the neck, cough, difficulty swallowing, enlargement of the thyroid gland, changes in the voice with increased hoarseness, sore throat, breathing problems and swollen lymph nodes.

2. What are the most common types of thyroid cancer in the elderly?

The most common is papillary carcinoma. While it is usually benign, it is usually more aggressive in older adults. On the other hand, the follicular is more frequent in the elderly and increases the chances of metastasis. Anaplastic, meanwhile, is a rare type of cancer, but its frequency increases after 60 years. It is invasive and grows very fast.

Finally, spinal cancer and thyroid lymphoma are less frequent, but most appear during old age.

3. What is your treatment?

Therapy depends on the type of Thyroid Cancer. Before a papillary carcinoma, surgery is usually performed in which all or almost the entire gland is removed. Then, radioactive iodine treatment is continued to reduce the risk of recurrence and, after the operation, synthetic thyroid hormone should be taken for life.

Against follicular carcinoma, radioactive iodine is the therapy chosen for distant metastases. If the tumor does not concentrate properly, external radiation should be evaluated.

In case of anaplastic carcinoma, in addition to radical neck surgery, radiotherapy and chemotherapy should be included. Surgery is recommended for medullary carcinoma, while external radiation and chemotherapy are advised for thyroid lymphoma.

4. What other complications can this disease bring?

This condition can cause injury to the larynx, damage to the vocal cords and hoarseness after surgery, low calcium levels due to accidental removal of the parathyroid glands and spread of cancer to other parts of the body.

Chapter 184. Multiple Myeloma and its disorders

Multiple Myeloma is a cancer in the blood that begins in the plasma cells of the bone marrow. These cells are part of the immune system and are responsible for secreting large amounts of antibodies to fight infections and other diseases.

When this condition is generated, cancer cells grow rapidly and form tumors in areas of solid bones, weakening them. They also replace healthy cells and produce abnormal proteins that can cause different types of complications in the body.

To learn more about this topic, we interview Mario Vega Carbó, a specialist in endocrinology and family medicine with more than 20 years of experience.

Doctor Mario,
1. Why does Multiple Myeloma occur and who does it affect?

The cause of this disease is unknown but it is known that treatment with radiation therapy and exposure to industrial or agricultural toxins may increase the risk of suffering from it. In general it affects adults over 60 years and is more common among men. Those who have a family history with this disease also have more predisposition to suffer it.

2. What are its main signs?

Myeloma cancer cells, when multiplied, displace healthy white and red blood cells. This makes the patient feel fatigue and shortness of breath, is more likely to get infections and has abnormal bleeding.

The disease can also cause bone pain, mainly in the spine, hip and chest; sickness; constipation, loss of appetite; slimming and excessive thirst.

On the other hand, when bones are weakened there are more chances of suffering fractures and numbness in the legs.

3. How is Multiple Myeloma detected?

In the face of its symptoms, a physical examination and blood and urine tests are usually performed. Among other aspects, albumin, calcium and total protein levels are analyzed and renal function tests are carried out.

On the other hand, bone x-rays can show if there are bone problems. In case of suspecting Multiple Myeloma, a bone marrow biopsy will be performed and, if confirmed, further tests will be performed to determine whether it has spread.

4. What is your treatment?

The therapy will depend on the degree of disease progression. In some cases it develops slowly and takes years to present symptoms. If so, it is not necessary to initiate any procedure, but simply to carry out permanent controls.

If there are already signs, the treatment will seek to relieve pain, control the complications of the condition and slow its progress. Certain targeted drugs fight myeloma cells and their actions, and improve the immune system. On the other hand, to mitigate bone discomfort or reduce the tumor, radiotherapy and chemotherapy combined with steroids can be used.

In relatively young patients with an adequate state of health, a bone marrow transplant can be performed, either with own or third-party stem cells. Treatment usually involves a combination of all these procedures.

5. What is the prognosis of this treatment?

Their results will depend on the age of the patient and the stage of the disease. In some cases it progresses very quickly and in others it takes years to appear.

6. What other complications can this ailment bring?

This disease interferes with the normal functioning of the bone marrow, the immune system and the bone renewal mechanisms. That is why it can cause anemia, increased risk of infections, bone problems and kidney failure.

Other complications derived from Multiple Myeloma are high doses of calcium in the blood and loss of movement due to the pressure of the tumor on the spinal cord. His treatment also contemplates the care of these symptoms.

7. What other aspects should be taken into account to face the Multiple Myeloma?

Due to the stress and concern that this disease can cause, psychological support and participation in therapeutic groups with people suffering from the same disease is recommended.

Chapter 185. The practice of exercise in older adults

Adequate food and regular physical activity are essential for older adults to prevent disease and stay in good shape.

Elderly who perform exercises to strengthen the muscles, strength and balance, have more independence and better chronic diseases, if they suffer. Training in the elderly must be progressive and carried out safely, with control to avoid blows and falls.

To learn more about this topic, we interview Mario Vega Carbó, a specialist in endocrinology with more than 20 years of professional experience.

Doctor Mario,
1. What are the main benefits of physical exercise for older adults?

The practice of physical activity helps improve overall health, quality of life and sleep. In addition, it allows to maintain an adequate weight, collaborates in the management of stress and reduces the chances of contracting certain diseases, such as type 2 diabetes, cardiovascular problems, obesity, osteoporosis, joint pain and breast and colon cancer.

Exercise contributes to glycemic control, improves mobility; prevents falls, mental disorders and depression; and stimulates functional capacity and social life. It also helps to whet the appetite in the elderly who have trouble eating.

2. At what age does the natural decline of the body begin?

The decline in muscle mass and bone density generally begins around 50 years of age. However, the practice of physical activity helps to delay this natural decline.

In that sense, it is recommended that older adults perform muscle strengthening tasks at least twice a week, as well as aerobic exercises that allow them to stay active for longer.

3. What benefits does each type of activity offer?

Aerobic or resistance activities, such as walking, running, dancing, swimming or cycling, increase the heart and respiratory rate and strengthen the heart, lungs and blood vessels. They also delay or prevent many diseases that are common in older adults.

On the other hand, strength exercises, such as lifting weights, help strengthen muscles, while balance exercises, such as going down and up stairs and Tai Chi, allow you to prevent falls.

Finally, flexibility, such as yoga, makes it possible to stretch, stay agile and keep the body relaxed.

4. How much physical activity is recommended for older adults?

It is important that those over 60 years of age perform at least 150 minutes of exercises during the week, which can be divided into 10-minute sessions, several times a day. The goal is to achieve at least 30 minutes of moderate intensity resistance activities, every day.

5. What happens to people who reach old age without having exercised?

It is never too late to start exercising and, however minimal, any physical activity is better than doing nothing. These patients who have been inactive for many years are advised to start with a low level of effort and gradually increase the intensity. For starters, for example, walking and swimming are recommended at a comfortable pace.

6. Can people with heart problems, arthritis or other diseases exercise safely?

The vast majority of people can perform controlled physical activity without risk. Contrary to what is thought, its practice can help in the treatment of these and other diseases.

For example, people who suffered a heart attack have fewer risks of having another if they exercise regularly.

7. In which cases is the practice of physical activity contraindicated in older adults?

Contraindications for this group are similar to those of young people. For example, in patients with acute ailments, such as febrile symptoms, chest pains, uncontrolled diabetes, hypertension, asthma or heart failure, it is first necessary to resolve these situations before beginning a training plan.

Similarly, in cases of surgery, hernias, cataracts or muscle or joint injuries, some practices should be avoided until the problem is corrected. If you experience pain or dizziness during exercise it is important to stop with the routine until you consult the doctor.

However, it is usually always possible to perform some type of low intensity physical activity that helps improve the quality of life of patients.

8. What steps can be taken to prevent injuries?

As we mentioned earlier, when starting an exercise plan it is important to start slowly, with a low level of effort, and gradually increase the intensity over time.

It is advisable to wait at least two hours to start the activities after eating, wear appropriate shoes and clothes, make a warm entry before starting the training session and another stretching and cooling at the end, and drink water before, during and after of each practice. In addition, abrupt and abnormal movements should always be avoided.

Finally, the variety of exercises helps reduce monotony and the risk of injury.

Epilogue

In *"I answer 1,500 questions about Hormones, Metabolism and Nutrition,"* Dr. Mario Vega Carbó, an endocrinology specialist, with more than 20 years of experience in the field, addresses the main questions that the public has regarding various diseases and conditions that They affect the complex hormonal mechanisms that control metabolism and are influenced by nutrition.

In this book, 185 chapters are presented in a question and answer design, which provide the reader with the possibility of finding that explanation he seeks in relation to a disease, its causes, its symptoms and treatment options.

It is presented in a structure of questions related to specific topics, which were grouped into chapters. In turn, the chapters on a specific topic (diabetes, pituitary gland, pediatric endocrinology, for example), gathered in parts that represent areas of knowledge in endocrinology. Related parties, were organized into sections on specific topics, metabolism, endocrinology, reproduction and life cycle

In the first section of *metabolism*, we clarify the main doubts about dietetics, knowing the different types of menus available and the myths and realities around them; Nutrition issues were also presented, where the most important issues regarding body weight and its deviations are discussed. Closing this section, we talked about diabetes, explaining through simple questions, what this condition is about, its symptoms, its types, the causes, and especially the treatment and control.

The second section, *endocrinology,* dealt with more specific questions related to complex endocrine diseases. We investigate the thyroid gland, its diseases, the causes, the diagnostic methods and the treatments. Very related to this gland, calcium metabolism, its importance in the body and the processes that regulate it were exposed.

In this section, questions were found that help to understand ailments that affect the adrenal glands and their syndromes (Addison's disease, Cushing's syndrome); and also, it deepens the questions about the pituitary gland, which can be considered as the hormonal center of the body.

The third section explains metabolism issues and hormones related to reproduction and life cycle. Diseases such as polycystic ovary syndrome, female sexual identity disorders, infertility, will be addressed in a chapter on the ovaries. For men, questions about hypogonadism, morphological alterations of the sexual organs, hormonal therapies, will also be developed.

In this last section topics of endocrinology are included in special stages of life, the corresponding questions are clarified in the parts of endocrinology in obstetrics, pediatrics and geriatrics.

The entire book is a synthesis of the most frequent questions that the population has about hormones, metabolism, and endocrinology.

We hope you liked the content on these pages, and that your doubts have been clarified. The purpose is to offer quality content so that the public can better understand endocrinological diseases.

Thank you for purchasing and reading the book *"I answer 1,500 questions about Hormones, Metabolism and Nutrition"!*

The interview

Mario Vega Carbó

Cuban doctor, with more than 20 years of professional experience, specialist in Endocrinology and Family Medicine.

He was received in 1994 at the Institute of Medical Sciences of Havana (ISCMH), then continued his training by completing a Master's Degree in Satisfactory Longevity and Diagnostic Ultrasound, as well as different specializations in Higher Medical Education, finally graduated from the Endocrinology Institute .

His career began at the Municipal Health Department of La Lisa and continued at the Latin American School of Medicine and the National Institute of Endocrinology.

Since 2014 he has been an endocrinologist at the Vega & Vado Office, in Managua, Nicaragua.

He is also a professor of Medical Pathophysiology and a lover of doing good, of family and nature.

Author of several academic and educational books related to his specialty, available in 10 languages.

Social Media:

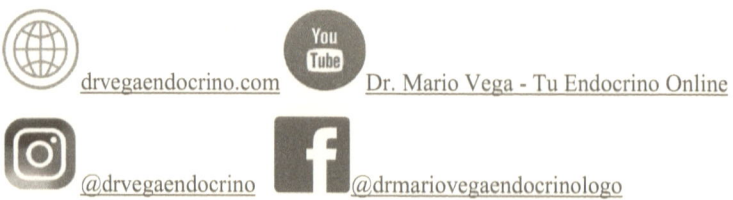

drvegaendocrino.com   Dr. Mario Vega - Tu Endocrino Online

@drvegaendocrino   @drmariovegaendocrinologo

Other books of the author

1. An approach to Natural Endocrinology
2. Endocrine Alerts: Saving Lives
3. ABC of the Endocrinologist, for the non-specialist
4. Recipes of your Endocrine
5. Where hormone queen ... short stories
6. Food myths, vision of the Endocrinologist
7. S.O.S Hormonal toxins, naked truths
8. Vitamin D: An omnipresent hormone?
9. Hormones, exercises and fitness body
10. Obesity, Diabetes, Thyroid and S.O.P

Available in 10 languages!

Interview conducted by:

Mario Enrique Vega Beltran
Estudent ofjournalism
University of La Habana

Synopsis

Nutrition, obesity, diabetes, osteoporosis, short stature in children, early sexual development, menstruation disorders, infertility, erectile dysfunction, abnormal cholesterol and triglyceride levels, hypothyroidism, high blood pressure, glandular tumors, special diets ... and much more!

In *"I answer 1,500 questions about Hormones, Metabolism and Nutrition"*, Dr. Mario Vega Carbó explains, in a simple and simple language, for all audiences, the causes of the main endocrine diseases, their most common symptoms, their risks and the options of treatment.

In addition, the book has special sections on the most significant hormonal disorders in children, pregnant women and the elderly, and a special chapter on diets and feeding advice to prevent and control different conditions.

We invite you to read these pages and enter the world of the endocrine system and its glands, responsible for the natural production of hormones that regulate our body.

www.ingramcontent.com/pod-product-compliance
Lightning Source LLC
Chambersburg PA
CBHW030604220526
45463CB00004B/1161